STUDENT WORKBOOK

Comprehensive Health Insurance
Billing, Coding, and Reimbursement

Second Edition

DEBORAH VINES

ANN BRACELAND

KELLY WILLIAMS

TIFFANY ROSTA

PEARSON

Boston   Columbus   Indianapolis   New York   San Francisco   Upper Saddle River
Amsterdam   Cape Town   Dubai   London   Madrid   Milan   Munich   Paris   Montreal   Toronto
Delhi   Mexico City   São Paulo   Sydney   Hong Kong   Seoul   Singapore   Taipei   Tokyo

Notice: The authors and the publisher of this volume have taken care that the information and technical recommendations contained herein are based on research and expert consultation, and are accurate and compatible with the standards generally accepted at the time of publication. Nevertheless, as new information becomes available, changes in clinical and technical practices become necessary. The reader is advised to carefully consult manufacturers' instructions and information material for all supplies and equipment before use, and to consult with a healthcare professional as necessary. This advice is especially important when using new supplies or equipment for clinical purposes. The authors and publisher disclaim all responsibility for any liability, loss, injury, or damage incurred as a consequence, directly or indirectly, of the use and application of any of the contents of this volume.

10

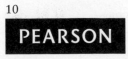

ISBN-13 978-0-13-297302-1
ISBN-10   0-13-297302-2

Contents

How to Use the Workbook

STUDENT WORKBOOK LEARNING OBJECTIVES

After reading the core student textbook and completing the workbook, the student should be able to do the following:

- Define and spell the key terms and abbreviations from each chapter.

- Understand and utilize all chapter objectives.

- Use critical thinking skills and the knowledge presented in the core student textbook to read case-based scenarios and answer critical thinking questions. The student should be able to do the following:

  - Recognize the importance of obtaining certification and membership status.

  - Understand laws, regulations, and penalties associated with coding compliance.

  - Understand the ethics of a medical coder.

  - Prepare for an internal and an external audit.

  - Understand Medicare insurance.

  - Understand Medicaid insurance.

  - Recognize the difference between primary and secondary insurance.

  - Understand workers' compensation insurance and disability insurance.

  - Understand TRICARE and CHAMPVA insurance.

  - Recognize the different types of insurance reimbursement fraud and abuse.

  - Submit a completed insurance claim.

  - Understand the different reasons that an insurance claim may be denied.

  - Know when and how to rebill an insurance claim.

  - Know when and how to appeal a denied insurance claim.

  - Enter necessary data to a patient's account, using medical practice management software.

  - Enter necessary data to prepare an insurance claim, using medical practice management software.

  - Balance the batch at the end of each day.

- Accurately complete practice exercises on coding and creating claim forms using source documents (patient information forms, encounter forms, SOAP notes) and fee schedules. The student should be able to do the following:

  - Select the correct diagnostic codes, using the ICD-9-CM manual, Volumes 1 and 2, and/or the ICD-10-CM Manual.

  - Select the correct hospital procedure codes, using the ICD-9-CM manual, Volume 3, and/or the ICD-10-PCS manual.

  - Select the correct E/M codes for place of service coding, using the CPT manual.

  - Select the correct procedure codes and HCPCS codes, using the CPT manual.

  - Apply CPT modifiers to procedure codes when applicable.

- o Review and analyze medical records and medical documentation for completeness and accuracy.
- o Correctly complete CMS-1500 claim forms for commercial insurance carriers.
- o Correctly complete UB-04 claim forms for hospital billing.
- o Accurately calculate the Medicare fee.
- o Accurately calculate participating and nonparticipating Medicare providers that accept assignment.
- o Accurately calculate nonparticipating Medicare providers that do not accept assignment.
- o Correctly complete a Medicare claim form.
- o Correctly complete a Medicaid claim form.
- o Correctly complete a TRICARE and CHAMPVA claim form.
- o Correctly complete a secondary claim form.
- o Correctly complete a workers' compensation claim form.
- o Write an appeal letter for a denied claim.
- o Accurately calculate and issue a refund.
- o Correctly read and calculate an explanation of benefits form.
- Accurately complete chapter review questions in true–false, short answer, multiple choice, and matching formats to measure understanding of the material presented in the core student text.
- Accurately complete the tests presented at the end of the workbook. These tests can be used by instructors as an outcomes assessment to measure student understanding and mastery of skills. The following tests are offered:
  - o TEST 1: Identify the Correct Diagnostic Code
  - o TEST 2: Coding Hospital Procedures
  - o TEST 3: Coding Outpatient Procedures and Diagnoses
  - o TEST 4: Coding Outpatient Radiology and/or Pathology Procedures and Diagnoses
  - o TEST 5: Coding Procedures and Diagnoses, Using E/M Codes
  - o TEST 6: Explanation of Benefits
  - o TEST 7: Explanation of Benefits
  - o TEST 8: Complete a Medicare Claim
  - o TEST 9: Complete a Medicaid Claim
  - o TEST 10: Complete a Medi-Medi Claim
  - o TEST 11: Complete a TRICARE Claim
  - o TEST 12: Complete a Workers' Compensation Claim
  - o TEST 13: Complete a CMS-1500 Claim Form for Commercial Insurance
  - o TEST 14: Complete a UB-04 Claim Form for Hospital Billing

INSTRUCTIONS TO THE STUDENT

This workbook is designed to be used with your student text, *Comprehensive Health Insurance: Billing, Coding, and Reimbursement, Second Edition*. The workbook will prepare you to complete medical billing and coding procedures, and it will provide opportunities to practice on and further develop your knowledge of the different types of health insurances, medical fees and calculations, proper medical documentation, coding compliance, audits, appeals, and CMS-1500 and UB-04 claim forms. Following are the main features of this workbook:

- Chapter Objectives—a bulleted list taken from the beginning of each chapter in your core textbook appears at the beginning of each workbook chapter.

- Chapter Outlines of your student text are available for your review at the beginning of each workbook chapter. If any content area is unclear, the student is urged to review that area before beginning the workbook exercises.

- Key Terms—medical terminology that correlates with each chapter in the textbook reinforces student spelling and mastery of key vocabulary. Students are directed to use the glossary in their core text to provide definitions of key terminology.

- Critical Thinking Questions—individual, group, and scenario-based questions develop and enhance critical thinking skills and problem-solving skills.

- Practice Exercises—reinforcement practice exercises similar to those found in the core textbook provide additional opportunities for coding, creating claim forms, reading and calculating an explanation of benefits form, and writing a letter of appeal for a denied claim. Practice exercises are designed to measure student mastery of these key skills. Patient information forms, SOAP notes, encounter forms, fee schedules, and blank CMS-1500 and UB-04 claim forms are provided within the workbook to complete all insurance claim practice exercises.

- Chapter Review Questions—each chapter of the workbook contains a variety of questions in matching, multiple choice, true–false, and short answer format, designed to reinforce student learning and mastery of key concepts presented in the core textbook.

- Test Your Knowledge tests, found at the end of the student workbook, can be used at the discretion of the instructor to evaluate student learning and understanding of coding, creating claim forms, and calculating explanation of benefits forms.

CHAPTER 1
Introduction to Professional Billing and Coding Careers

CHAPTER OBJECTIVES

Upon completion of this chapter in your student text, you should be able to do the following:

1. Recognize different types of facilities that would employ allied health personnel.
2. Define job descriptions pertaining to a position.
3. Discuss options available for certification.

CHAPTER OUTLINE

Employment Demand

Facilities
  Physician's Practice
  Multispecialty Clinic
  Hospital
  Centralized Billing Office

Job Titles and Responsibilities
  Medical Office Assistant (MOA)
  Medical Biller
  Medical Coder
  Registered Health Information Technicians (RHIT)
  Payment Poster
  Medical Collector
  Refund Specialist
  Insurance Verification Representative
  Admitting Clerk or Front Desk Representative
  Patient Information Officer

Professional Memberships

Certification
  Medical Office Assistant Certification
  Medical Billing Certifications
  Medical Coding Certifications
  Medical Records Certification

KEY TERMS

Using the highlighted terms and glossary in the textbook, define the following terms.

1. admitting clerk _____

_____

2. centralized billing office (CBO) _____

3. certifications _____

4. insurance verification representative _____

5. medical biller _____

6. medical coder _____

7. patient account services (PAS) _____

8. registered health information technician (RHIT) _____
_____

CRITICAL THINKING QUESTIONS

Using the knowledge you have gained from reading the textbook, apply critical thinking skills to answer the following questions.

1. In your own words, explain the benefits of belonging to a professional organization.

   _____

   _____

   _____

   _____

2. Relate the following questions to your last doctor's appointment:
   a. What type of specialty was/were practiced by the physician(s)? _____
   b. How many physicians worked in this practice? _____
   c. Which one of the following three would this practice qualify as: a solo/private practice, a small-group practice, or a large-group practice? _____

3. Of all the types of medical careers listed in your text, which one would you most like to pursue and why? _____

   _____

   _____

   _____

4. Using an online job search engine, locate all the positions that you will qualify for after completing your schooling. Referring to these open positions, answer the following questions:

a. How many jobs will you qualify for? _____

b. Which of these jobs would you be most interested in doing, and why? _____
_____
_____
_____
_____

c. Describe the position that most interested you, and discuss why this is.
_____
_____
_____
_____
_____
_____
_____
_____
_____
_____
_____
_____
_____
_____
_____
_____
_____

5. Write down the educational, career, and personal goals that you would like to accomplish within the periods defined here (discuss your answers in class):

a. One year _____
_____
_____
_____
_____

b. Five years _____
_____
_____
_____
_____

6. Discuss why it is important to have both career and educational goals. _____

_____

_____

_____

_____

PRACTICE EXERCISES

1. Provide a brief description of the following types of health care organizations that a medical office specialist may work for

    a. Solo/private practice _____

    _____

    _____

    _____

    b. Small-group practice _____

    _____

    _____

    _____

    c. Large-group practice _____

    _____

    _____

    _____

    d. Hospital _____

    _____

    _____

    _____

    e. Patient account services facility (PAS) _____

    _____

    _____

    _____

    f. Centralized billing office (CBO) _____

    _____

    _____

    _____

2. Write the job descriptions for the following different types of medical careers:

    a. Medical office assistant_____

    _____

    _____

    _____

b. Medical biller _____

_____

_____

c. Medical coder _____

_____

_____

d. Registered health information technician (RHIT) _____

_____

_____

e. Payment poster _____

_____

_____

_____

f. Medical collector _____

_____

_____

_____

g. Refund specialist _____

_____

_____

_____

h. Insurance verification representative _____

_____

_____

_____

i. Admitting clerk/front desk representative _____

_____

_____

_____

j. Patient information clerk _____

_____

_____

_____

k. Privacy compliance officer _____

_____

_____

_____

3. Provide a brief description of each different type of medical certification listed next. Access any related websites provided in the Resources section of this chapter, if necessary.

   a. National certified medical office assistant (NCMOA) _____

   _____

   _____

   _____

   b. Certified medical administrative assistant (CMAA) _____

   _____

   _____

   _____

   c. Certified medical billing specialist (CMBS) _____

   _____

   _____

   _____

   d. Certified medical reimbursement specialist (CMRS)_____

   _____

   _____

   _____

   e. Certified coding associate (CCA)_____

   _____

   _____

   _____

   f. Certified professional coder (CPC) _____

   _____

   _____

   _____

   g. Certified professional coder-hospital (CPC-H) _____

   _____

   _____

   _____

   h. Certified coding specialist (CCS) _____

   _____

   _____

   _____

   i. Certified coding specialist-physician (CCS-P) _____

   _____

   _____

   _____

   j. Registered health information technician (RHIT)_____

   _____

   _____

   _____

REVIEW QUESTIONS

MATCHING

Choose the correct answer and write its corresponding letter in the space provided.

a. Certification
b. Allied health employees
c. American Health Information Management Association (AHIMA)
d. National Healthcareer Association (NHA)
e. National Center for Competency Testing (NCCT)

1. _____ Awards the CCA, CCS, and RHIT.
2. _____ Voluntary (optional) credentialing in a professional organization that shows a person's qualifications, involvement, and dedication in a particular field.
3. _____ Awards the CMAA.
4. _____ Awards the NCMOA.
5. _____ Members of the clinical health care profession who work together in a health care team to make the health care system function.

MULTIPLE CHOICE

Circle the letter of the choice that best completes the statement or answers the question.

1. Which of the following has affected physician offices due to managed care?
   a. Additional staff had to be added for daily financial operations to be carried out.
   b. Payments for services were not received up front from the patient.
   c. Money was not readily available for operation costs.
   d. All of the above

2. Which of the following is a benefit of holding a professional membership in your field?
   a. Professional membership provides professional development opportunities.
   b. Professional membership makes available up-to-date information on important issues.
   c. Professional membership provides employment opportunities.
   d. All of the above

3. Which of the following associations is the professional association for coders?
   a. AAPC
   b. AHIMA
   c. AAMT
   d. None of the above

4. A small physician group practice consists of _____.
   a. 10-plus physicians
   b. three through nine physicians
   c. physicians usually practicing the same specialty
   d. Both b and c

5. A large physician group practice consists of _____.
   a. 10-plus physicians
   b. three through nine physicians
   c. physicians who usually practice in different specialties
   d. Both a and c

SHORT ANSWER

Provide the correct response to each question that follows.

1. What did physicians have to do to improve reimbursement once managed care was implemented? ____

   _____

2. Before managed care, when did most patients pay for physician services? _____

   _____

3. What are two other titles for a medical office assistant?

   1. _____

   2. _____

4. What are six other titles for a medical biller?

   1. _____

   2. _____

   3. _____

   4. _____

   5. _____

   6. _____

5. What are four other titles for a medical coder?

   1. _____

   2. _____

   3. _____

   4. _____

TRUE/FALSE

Identify each statement as true (T) or false (F).

1. _____ Physicians and nurses make up 60 percent of all health care providers, wherease the other 40 percent are allied health employees.

2. _____ Medical office specialists work only in outpatient settings.

3. _____ After graduating, the medical office specialist must obtain certification.

4. _____ With managed care it is the responsibility of the physician to file the claim and wait for payment.

5. _____ Certification is an important addition to your resume.

CHAPTER 2
Understanding Managed Care: Insurance Plans

CHAPTER OBJECTIVES

Upon completion of this chapter in your student text, you should be able to do the following:

1. Understand the history and impact of managed care.
2. Be able to discuss the organization of managed care and how it affects the provider, employee, and policyholder.
3. Calculate the financial responsibility of the patient.
4. Identify the type of managed care plan in which the patient is enrolled.
5. Recognize various types of insurance coverage.

CHAPTER OUTLINE

The History of Health Care in America

Medical Reform

Managing and Controlling Health Care Costs
    Discounted Fees for Services
    Medically Necessary Patient Care
    Care Rendered by Appropriate Provider
    Appropriate Medical Care in Least Restrictive Setting
    Withholding Providers' Funds

Types of Managed Care Organizations
    Health Maintenance Organization (HMO)
    Preferred Provider Organization (PPO)
    Point-of-Service (POS) Options
    Criticism of MCOs

Alternative Health Care Plans
    Exclusive Provider Organization
    Independent Physician Association
    Physician–Hospital Organization
    Self-Insured Plan

Insurance Plans
    Commercial Health Insurance

Types of Insurance Coverage
    Indemnity Plan/Fee for Service
    Hospital Insurance
    Hospital Indemnity Insurance
    Medical Insurance
    Surgical Insurance
    Outpatient Insurance
    Major Medical Insurance

KEY TERMS

Using the highlighted terms and glossary in the textbook, define the following terms.

1. assignment of benefits _____
   _____

2. carriers _____
   _____

3. coinsurance _____
   _____

4. commercial health insurance_____
   _____

5. copayment _____
   _____

6. deductible _____
   _____

7. enrollee_____
   _____

8. group insurance _____
   _____

9. health maintenance organization (HMO) _____
   _____

10. inpatient_____
    _____

11. insured _____
    _____

12. managed care _____
    _____

13. managed care organization (MCO) _____
    _____

14. outpatient _____

_____

15. point-of-service (POS) _____

_____

16. policyholder_____

_____

17. preauthorizations _____

_____

18. preexisting condition _____

_____

19. preferred provider organization (PPO) _____

_____

20. premiums_____

_____

21. primary care physician (PCP) _____

_____

22. providers _____

_____

23. referral _____

_____

24. special risk insurance _____

_____

25. subscribers_____

_____

26. utilization_____

_____

CRITICAL THINKING QUESTIONS

Using the knowledge you have gained from reading the textbook, apply critical thinking skills to answer the following questions.

1. A new patient, Lucy Vrabel, has just given you her insurance information. Answer the following questions related to Lucy's insurance plan:

   a. Why is it important to gather insurance information during the first visit and verify it on subsequent visits?

   _____

   _____

   _____

   _____

b. How is insurance verified each time a patient comes in?

_____

_____

c. After establishing Lucy's type of insurance plan, what eight questions should be asked of the insurance company about her plan?

1. _____

2. _____

3. _____

4. _____

5. _____

6. _____

7. _____

8. _____

d. What should be documented after receiving Lucy's insurance information in case of a claim denial or collection problems after services have been rendered?

_____

_____

_____

_____

2. Samuel Ridge just learned that he will be laid off from his job at the end of the week. He works for a corporation of 100-plus employees. Answer the following questions related to Samuel's situation:

a. What is the name of the federal law that will allow Sam, after his termination from the company, to continue the group coverage that he had through his workplace?

_____

b. How long a period is Sam allowed to keep this coverage?

_____

c. What are the two other reasons, besides termination of employment, that a person may qualify for this coverage?

1. _____

2. _____

3. The physician for whom you work does not contract with and accept assignment for the type of insurance Linda has, which is TRICARE.

a. What process is followed when a physician does not accept assignment?

_____

b. Will Linda have to pay up front for these services? Why or why not?

_____

4. Patient Julia Watson needs a surgical procedure that is not covered by her insurance plan. Answer the following questions related to the medical necessity of this procedure:

   a. What must be obtained from Julia's insurance company to allow this procedure?

      _____

   b. If Julia's insurance company's utilization protocol is different from that of the physician and the procedure is denied, what could be the action brought against the provider if this surgical procedure was, in fact, medically necessary?

      _____

      _____

      _____

5. In your own words, explain how health care has changed in America.

_____

_____

_____

_____

_____

_____

_____

_____

PRACTICE EXERCISES

1. In each case scenario that follows, calculate the financial responsibility of the patient and/or carrier and the discounted amount that the physician must write off, and put your answers in the spaces provided.

   a. Felix Grossman was seen today for an upper respiratory infection. Total charges for today's services are $140. The allowed amount is $90.

     _____   _____

     Discount amount   Carrier pays provider

   b. Emma Mastrangelo had a CT scan of the brain today because of recurrent migraines. Total charges are $720.50. Her benefits pay 90 percent of this procedure. The allowed amount is $462.60.

     _____   _____   _____

     Patient responsibility   Discount amount   Carrier pays provider

   c. Mabel Smith was seen in the office today for a checkup on her rheumatoid arthritis. Total charges are $85. The allowed amount is $52. She has a copay of $10.

     _____   _____

     Discount amount   Carrier pays provider

   d. Rufus Durst had a cholecystectomy performed today. Total charges are $2995.70. His benefits pay 60 percent of this procedure. The allowed amount is $1745.32.

     _____   _____   _____

     Patient responsibility   Discount amount   Carrier pays provider

     What amount will the physician write off?_____

2. Answer the following questions in detail:
   a. Phyllis Gould is being seen today for her annual gynecological examination by a physician who is not in her HMO network. Who will be financially responsible for her medical bill?

      _____

      1. Why?

         _____

         _____

   b. Rodger McMurray has an HMO insurance plan. He did not obtain permission from his PCP for today's visit to the orthopedic specialist. Who will be financially responsible for his medical bill?

      _____

      1. Why?

         _____

         _____

3. Discuss usual, reasonable, and customary fees, and describe all three terms in detail.

   _____

   _____

   _____

   _____

4. How do MCOs provide high-quality care while managing and controlling costs?

   _____

   _____

   _____

   _____

5. Provide answers to the following questions:
   a. What are the six advantages of managed care as presented in the textbook?
      1. _____
      2. _____
      3. _____
      4. _____
      5. _____
      6. _____
   b. What are the six disadvantages of managed care as listed in the textbook?
      1. _____
      2. _____
      3. _____
      4. _____
      5. _____
      6. _____

c. List the different characteristics of each type of MCO:

HMO

1. _____
2. _____
3. _____
4. _____
5. _____
6. _____

PPO

1. _____
2. _____
3. _____
4. _____

EPO

1. _____
2. _____
3. _____
4. _____

POS

1. _____
2. _____
3. _____
4. _____
5. _____
6. _____

IPA Model HMO

1. _____
2. _____

Staff Model HMO

1. _____
2. _____
3. _____

Group Model HMO

1. _____
2. _____

Network Model HMO

1. _____
2. _____

d. In what way does an MCO withholding program encourage or discourage physician incentives?

_____

_____

_____

_____

_____

_____

e. Describe the following different types of insurance coverage:
1. Hospital _____

_____

_____

2. Hospital indemnity _____

_____

_____

3. Medical _____

_____

_____

4. Surgical _____

_____

_____

5. Outpatient _____

_____

_____

6. Major medical _____

_____

_____

7. Special risk _____

_____

_____

8. Catastrophic _____

_____

_____

9. Short-term _____

_____

_____

10. Full-service _____

_____

_____

11. Long-term _____

_____

_____

12. Supplemental _____

_____

_____

 f. List three ways in which MCOs can create administrative burdens on physicians.

  1. _____

  2. _____

  3. _____

REVIEW QUESTIONS

MATCHING

Choose each correct answer and write its corresponding letter in the space provided.

a. utilization
b. capitation
c. PCP
d. outpatient
e. copay

1. ____ Fixed amount that is paid for each office visit or hospital encounter.
2. ____ Fixed fees paid monthly by health insurance plans, calculated on the basis of the number of enrollees seen by the physician
3. ____ Gatekeeper
4. ____ Person who receives medical care at a medical facility, but does not require admittance for more than 24 hours
5. ____ The process of a health insurance company reviewing patient data to establish medically necessary health care

MULTIPLE CHOICE

Circle the letter of the choice that best completes the statement or answers the question.

1. A fee agreed on by a physician and that is reimbursed by an insurance carrier for services rendered is the _____

 a. contracted fee
 b. controlled fee
 c. discounted fee
 d. Both a and c

2. Which of the following helps an MCO determine whether a medical service is medically necessary?
 a. Premium
 b. Utilization
 c. Special risk insurance
 d. All of the above

3. A person who is covered under an insurance policy is known as the _____
 a. subscriber
 b. insured
 c. policyholder
 d. All of the above

4. What is a written authorization obtained by the provider before a hospital admission or certain procedures?
   a. Special risk insurance
   b. Preauthorization
   c. Referral
   d. Premium

5. What law establishes guidelines to ensure patient privacy compliance and health plan portability provisions?
   a. OSHA
   b. HMO
   c. HIPAA
   d. POS

SHORT ANSWER

Provide the correct response to each question that follows.

1. Discuss the terms *coinsurance* and *copayments*. What is the difference between the two?

   _____
   _____
   _____
   _____
   _____

2. What are three terms (other than *subscriber*) that can be used interchangeably to refer to a subscriber of an insurance plan?
   1. _____
   2. _____
   3. _____

3. Provide three examples of preventative medical procedures covered by HMOs.
   1. _____
   2. _____
   3. _____

4. List three types of health care providers with which a PPO or an HMO may enter into a contract.
   1. _____
   2. _____
   3. _____

5. In the spaces that follow, describe a group insurance plan, an individual insurance plan, and a self-insured employers plan, highlighting the differences between the three plans.
   1. Group insurance _____
   _____
   _____

2. Individual insurance _____

_____

_____

3. Self-insured employers plan _____

_____

_____

TRUE/FALSE

Identify each statement as true (T) or false (F).

1. _____ Subscribers to HMOs and PPOs will not have out-of-pocket expenses when they see physicians who are out of the network.

2. _____ It is the physician's responsibility to make sure that he or she is compensated for services rendered to patients.

3. _____ Defensive medicine is aiding in curbing the rising costs of health care delivery.

4. _____ The medical office specialist should collect insurance information up front and verify on each subsequent visit.

5. _____ Many physicians are joining larger groups of physicians to aid in financial burdens and create a greater patient load opportunity.

CHAPTER 3
Understanding Managed Care: Medical Contracts and Ethics

CHAPTER OBJECTIVES

Upon completion of this chapter in your student text, you should be able to do the following:

1. Understand the key elements of a managed care contract that dictates the provider's compensation for services.

2. Identify covered services for patients, which can include preventive medical services and types of office visits.

3. Recognize the obligation of a medical office specialist to uphold a standard of ethics.

4. Know the definitions that are used in a managed care contract in order to understand the contract and discuss claims issues with the patient and carrier.

5. Conduct discussions with the patient regarding accounts, following the Patient's Bill of Rights.

CHAPTER OUTLINE

Purpose of a Contract

A Legal Agreement

Compensation and Billing Guidelines
   Covered Medical Expenses
   Payment

Ethics in Managed Care
   Changes in Healthcare Delivery
   MCO and Provider Credentialing
   Ethics of the Medical Office Specialist

Contract Definitions

Compensation for Services

Patient's Bill of Rights

KEY TERMS

Using the highlighted terms and glossary in the textbook, define the following terms.

1. National Committee for Quality Assurance (NCQA) _____

_____

2. network _____

_____

3. nonparticipating provider (non-PAR) _____

_____

4. participating provider (PAR)_____

_____

5. schedule of benefits _____

_____

CRITICAL THINKING QUESTIONS

Using the knowledge you have gained from reading the textbook, apply critical thinking skills to answer the following questions.

1. As the medical office specialist (MOS), you are asked by the physician to review a managed care contract. List the compensation and billing guidelines information that should be reviewed for each of the following processes:

   a. Submitting claims _____

   _____

   _____

   b. Coordination of benefits_____

   _____

   _____

   c. Capitated plan payment _____

   _____

   _____

   d. Fee schedule _____

   _____

   _____

2. In your own words, explain how managed care organizations (MCOs) are reducing costs in relationship to the patient and the provider.

   _____

   _____

   _____

   _____

3. What are some of the corporate business values that are making their way into the healthcare sector now that managed care has been implemented? Are these positive or negative changes?

_____

_____

_____

_____

_____

4. Read the following scenario, and determine whether the medical billing specialist is acting ethically concerning the physician's office billing procedures:

   a. Randi Collins, the medical billing specialist, is coding an office wart removal procedure. She bills this procedure as complicated, but the patient's chart does not specify that it was a complicated wart removal. She knows that part of her job is to code all procedures to the highest level of specificity for proper reimbursement. Is this an ethical billing practice? _____

   If she is unsure of the clarity of the diagnosis, what should she do before billing this procedure as complicated? _____

5. The physician you work for demands that you code a patient's diagnosis falsely. You explain to him that you are not comfortable doing this, and you refuse. He threatens your job. What should you do? _____

_____

   a. What could happen to you and the physician for falsifying this document?

_____

PRACTICE EXERCISES

1. In layperson's terms, define the following managed care organization (MCO) contract terms for patient Fredrick Call:

   a. Benefit plan

   _____

   _____

   b. Contracted services

   _____

   _____

   c. Coordination of Benefits (COB)

   _____

   _____

   d. Copayment

   _____

   _____

   e. Covered person

   _____

   _____

f. Covered services

_____

_____

g. Emergency services

_____

_____

h. Fee maximum

_____

_____

i. Medical director

_____

_____

j. Medically necessary

_____

_____

k. Participating hospital

_____

_____

l. Participating provider

_____

_____

m. Nonparticipating provider

_____

_____

2. Using the sample contents of a managed care contact in your text (Figure 3.1), define in your own words the following MCO contract terms for compensation for services rendered by the provider.

a. Billing

_____

_____

b. Coordination of benefits (COB) recoveries

_____

_____

c. Third-party liability recoveries and subrogation

_____

_____

d. Payment

_____

_____

e. No balance bill

_____

_____

f. Limitations regarding payment

_____

_____

g. Hold harmless provision for utilization review decision

_____

_____

3. What is the Patient's Bill of Rights, and how is it used by MCOs and providers?

_____

_____

_____

_____

_____

_____

_____

_____

_____

_____

_____

_____

4. Explain what a managed care organization's (MCO's) credentialing process for a provider consists of.

_____

_____

_____

_____

5. Why does credentialing need to be done for providers within the MCO?

_____

_____

_____

_____

_____

REVIEW QUESTIONS

MATCHING

Choose each correct answer and write its corresponding letter in the space provided.

a. coordination of benefits
b. fee-for-service
c. rebundle
d. per case
e. capitation

1. ____ Type of managed care contract payment where the payer compensates the provider on a predetermined rate for each episode of care provided

2. ____ Type of managed care contract payment where covered services are compensated at a discount of the provider's usual and customary charges

3. ____ Determining which payer should be billed first when a patient has two payers

4. ____ When an MCO adds to the covered services included to a single fee or amends any terms of the compensation arrangement without prior review by the provider

5. ____ Type of managed care contract payment where a provider is compensated for covered services at a fixed monthly payment (per-member-per-month amount)

MULTIPLE CHOICE

Circle the letter of the choice that best completes the statement or answers the question.

1. Which of the following are standards for licensed personnel and other employees of medical practices?
   a. Courtesy
   b. Ethics
   c. Respect
   d. All the above are standards for providers

2. Which of the following is *not* another name for a policyholder?
   a. Owner
   b. Enrollee
   c. Member
   d. All the above are names for a policyholder.

3. Which of the following is *not* a type of preventative medicine service?
   a. Physical examination
   b. Pap smear
   c. Both a and b
   d. None of the above

4. The usual time limit for submitting claims to an MCO is _____.
   a. 6 to 12 months
   b. 4 to 12 months
   c. 3 to 6 months
   d. 4 to 6 months

5. On which day(s) of the month do most capitation plans pay a provider?
   a. 1st
   b. 15th
   c. 30th
   d. Both b and c

SHORT ANSWER

Provide the correct response to each question that follows.

1. What is the medical office specialist's role when it comes to managed care contracts? _____
   _____

2. List the four most common types of managed care contract payment arrangements.
   1. _____
   2. _____
   3. _____
   4. _____

3. When should an MCO contract agreement be modified or amended regarding the best interest of the provider? _____
   _____
   _____

4. What are laws called that set forth principles of protection for all patients concerning health care delivery?
   _____
   _____

5. What organization requires that an MCO plan being reviewed for accreditation demonstrate that it conducts a thorough credentialing process of providers? _____
   _____

TRUE/FALSE

Identify the statement as true (T) or false (F).

1. _____ An MCO should not contract with a physician who has a questionable background.
2. _____ A participating provider is a provider that is under contract with the MCO.
3. _____ A provider does not have to sign a contract with an MCO to be in its network.
4. _____ MCO contracts do not network with laboratories.
5. _____ A medical office specialist must document, sign, and date all conversations regarding a patient's account, whether the conversation is with the provider, insurance carrier, or even the patient.

CHAPTER 4
Introduction to the Health Insurance Portability and Accountability Act (HIPAA)

CHAPTER OBJECTIVES

Upon completion of this chapter in your student text, you should be able to do the following:

1. Describe the responsibility of the medical office specialist to protect all protected health information (PHI).
2. Discuss what is required to disclose patient information to family members, friends, and when ordered by courts or government entities.
3. Understand the patient's right to request access or correction to his or her medical records.
4. Explain HIPAA security standards that require a healthcare provider to have security policies and procedures.
5. Discuss the penalties and fines involved for not being in compliance with HIPAA regulations.
6. Understand HITECH's mandatory requirements for healthcare providers to implement "meaningful use" by managing patient information and treatment through electronic health records (EHR).

CHAPTER OUTLINE

HIPAA Privacy Rule
  Legal Request
  Pharmacies and Durable Medical Equipment
  Language Barrier
  Patient Access and Corrections

Transactions and Code Set Rule

Uniform Code Sets

Security Rule
  Electronic Medical Record
  Electronic Health Record

Unique Identifiers Rule
  National Provider Identifier

HIPAA Enforcement Rule
  Civil Penalties
  Federal Criminal Penalties

HITECH Act
  Meaningful Use

Privacy and Security Protection

Healthcare Reform

KEY TERMS

Using the highlighted terms and glossary in the textbook, define the following terms.

1. civil money penalty (CMP) _____

2. computerized patient order entry (CPOE) _____

3. covered entities (CE) _____

4. durable medical equipment (DME) _____

5. electronic data interchange (EDI) _____

6. electronic health record (EHR) _____

7. electronic medical record (EMR) _____

8. electronic protected health information (EPHI) _____

9. encrypted _____

10. Food and Drug Administration (FDA) _____

11. Health and Human Services (HHS) _____

12. Health Information Technology for Economic and Clinical Health (HITECH) Act _____

13. meaningful use _____

14. National Provider Identifier (NPI) _____

15. Office of Civil Rights (OCR) _____

16. Office of the National Coordinator (ONC) for Health Information _____

17. Privacy Compliance Officer _____

18. protected health information (PHI) _____

CRITICAL THINKING QUESTIONS

Using the knowledge you have gained from reading the textbook, apply critical thinking skills to answer the following questions.

1. If a patient comes into the office and wants to access their medical records, what should be done before they are given access, and why? _____

   _____

   _____

2. Discuss the differences between an EHR and EMR. _____

   _____

   _____

3. You are working as an office manager and are asked to outline the purpose of the HIPAA Security Rules to share with new employees. Discuss the following areas of the HIPAA Security Rule:

   a. Administrative safeguards _____

   _____

   b. Physical safeguards _____

   _____

   c. Technical safeguards _____

   _____

4. Discuss the three unique identifiers and what they are used for. _____

   _____

   _____

5. What is the HITECH Act, and how does it relate to meaningful use? _____

   _____

   _____

PRACTICE EXERCISES

1. Discuss the three rules that are a part of the Health Insurance Portability and Accountability Act.

   a. Privacy Rule _____

   _____

   _____

   b. Security Rule _____

   _____

   _____

   c. Transactions and Code Set Rule _____

   _____

   _____

2. Write a job description for the following position: privacy compliance officer. _____

   _____

   _____

   _____

3. Give the five reasons for most of the HIPAA privacy complaints.

1. _____

   _____

   _____

2. _____

   _____

   _____

3. _____

   _____

   _____

4. _____

   _____

   _____

5. _____

   _____

   _____

4. Refer to Figure 4.1 in your book. What information is required on the legal request for information?

_____

_____

_____

5. What are the four examples of when patient information may be released without a patient consent?

_____

_____

_____

_____

REVIEW QUESTIONS

MATCHING

Choose the correct answer and write its corresponding letter in the space provided.

a. Privacy Compliance Officer
b. Office of Civil Rights
c. encryption
d. Uniform Code Sets
e. computerized provider order entry (CPOE)

1. ____ Method for the provider to enter orders via the electronic record
2. ____ Person who is responsible for receiving and responding to records requests
3. ____ When the information is scrambled during transmission
4. ____ Agency responsible for overseeing HIPAA regulations
5. ____ Uniform set of medical codes to simplify the process of submitting claims

MULTIPLE CHOICE

Circle the letter of the choice that best completes the statement or answers the question.

1. What are the civil penalties that will be imposed for violating the HIPAA regulations?
   a. $100 per person up to $50,000 person
   b. $100 per person up to $25,000 person
   c. $100 per person up to $75,000 person
   d. $100 per person up to $150,000 person

2. What are the criminal penalties that will be imposed for violating the HIPAA regulations?
   a. $25,000 to $250,000 and 1–10 years in prison
   b. $50,000 to $250,000 and 5–10 years in prison
   c. $50,000 to $250,000 and 1–10 years in prison
   d. $50,000 to $250,000 and 1–20 years in prison

3. What organization would you contact to file a HIPAA complaint?
   a. ONC
   b. OIG
   c. HHS
   d. All of the above

4. Who is responsible for training all employees on HIPAA?
   a. Security officer
   b. Privacy compliance officer
   c. Compliance officer
   d. All of the above

5. Which of the following safeguards includes encryption?
   a. Physical safeguards
   b. Administrative safeguards
   c. Technical safeguards
   d. All of the above

SHORT ANSWER

Provide the correct response to each question that follows.

1. What are the criminal penalties for violating HIPAA?
   a. _____
   b. _____
   c. _____

2. What must a CPOE allow a provider to be able to do?
   a. _____
   b. _____
   c. _____
   d. _____
   e. _____
   f. _____
   g. _____

3. What types of criteria will be included in Stage II of meaningful use? _____
_____

4. What types of healthcare professionals are eligible for Medicare incentives under meaningful use? __
_____

5. Who has the authority to grant authorization for uses and disclosures of PHI? _____
_____

TRUE/FALSE

Identify each statement as true (T) or false (F).

1. _____ Incentives for meaningful use will begin in 2015.
2. _____ EMRs and EHRs are basically the same.
3. _____ The privacy rule protects each patient's PHI.
4. _____ The National Provider Identifier is considered a unique patient identifier.
5. _____ Several covered entities have developed their own proprietary EDI systems.

CHAPTER 5

ICD-9-CM Medical Coding

CHAPTER OBJECTIVES

Upon completion of this chapter in your student text, you should be able to do the following:

1. Understand the history of coding.
2. State the purpose of the ICD-9-CM.
3. Define abbreviations, symbols, typefaces, punctuation, and formatting conventions.
4. Utilize the correct volume of ICD-9-CM to find the appropriate code.
5. Code to the highest level of certainty and specificity.
6. Assign the correct code in the proper order.
7. List the nine steps of accurate ICD-9-CM coding.

CHAPTER OUTLINE

Definition of Diagnosis Coding

History of Diagnosis Coding

Purpose of ICD-9-CM Coding

Addenda

The Three Volumes of the ICD-9-CM
    Volume 1: Tabular List of Diseases and Injuries
    Volume 2: Alphabetic Index of Diseases and Injuries
    Volume 3: Tabular and Alphabetic Index of Procedures

ICD-9-CM Conventions

Use of the Two Main Volumes
    Use the Alphabetic Index (Volume 2) First
    Use the Tabular List (Volume 1) Next

How to Code

Key Coding Guidelines
    Primary Diagnosis First, Followed by Current Coexisting Conditions
    Code to the Highest Level of Certainty
    Code to the Highest Level of Specificity
    Surgical Coding
    Coding Late Effects
    Acute and Chronic Conditions
    Combination Codes: Multiple Coding

KEY TERMS

Using the highlighted terms and glossary in the textbook, define the following terms:

1. addenda _____
   _____

2. adverse effect _____
   _____

3. combination code _____
   _____

4. complication code _____
   _____

5. conventions _____
   _____

6. diagnosis _____
   _____

7. diagnostic statement _____
   _____

8. eponym _____
   _____

9. etiology _____
   _____

10. ICD-9-CM _____
    _____

11. late effect _____
    _____

12. main term _____
    _____

13. manifestation _____

_____

14. morphology _____

_____

15. NEC (not elsewhere classified) _____

_____

16. NOS (not otherwise specified) _____

_____

17. primary diagnosis _____

_____

18. principal diagnosis _____

_____

19. residual effect _____

_____

20. rule out _____

_____

21. secondary _____

_____

22. sign _____

_____

23. subterms _____

_____

24. supplementary terms _____

_____

25. symbols _____

_____

26. symptom _____

_____

CRITICAL THINKING QUESTIONS

Using the knowledge you have gained from reading the textbook, apply critical thinking skills to answer the following questions:

1. Discuss the various ways that ICD-9-CM coding is used throughout the United States. Why is accuracy in coding so important?

_____

_____

_____

_____

_____

2. In your own words, answer the following questions related to the ICD-9-CM:

   a. What impact does the ICM-9-CM manual have on health care and medicine in today's world?

   _____

   _____

   _____

   _____

   b. Your office just received the new annual edition of the ICM-9-CM. What updates will be included?

   _____

   _____

   _____

3. Answer the following questions related to the three volumes of the ICD-9-CM, and if applicable, supply an example, using the manual:

   a. Give an example of a chapter heading in the Classification of Diseases and Injuries.

   _____

   b. Give an example of a category and supply the code.

   _____

   c. Give an example of a subcategory and supply the code.

   _____

   d. Give an example of a subheading in the Classification of Diseases and Injuries.

   _____

   e. Find a fifth-digit subcategory code. What additional information does the fifth digit supply to the code?

   _____

   _____

   _____

   f. In your own words, what is the difference between a V code and an E code?

   _____

   _____

   _____

   g. When would a coder need to use a code from the Table of Drugs and Chemicals?

   _____

   _____

   _____

   h. Using the ICD-9-CM, where would you find a code for thyroid cancer, primary?

   _____

   _____

   _____

4. a. What volume does Crawford Hospital need to use to code procedures?

   _____

   b. Can Crawford Outpatient Radiology use this volume to code procedures?

   _____

5. Define the following conventions and symbols found in the ICD-9-CM, and if applicable, provide an example, using the manual:

a. main term _____
_____

b. sub term _____
_____

c. supplementary terms _____
_____

d. carryover lines/turnover lines _____
_____

e. see _____
_____

f. see also _____
_____

g. see category _____
_____

h. see also category _____
_____

i. eponym _____
_____

j. NEC _____
_____

k. : _____
_____

l. NOS _____
_____

m. [ ] _____
_____

n. ( ) _____
_____

o. instructional notes _____
_____

p. use additional code _____
_____

q. code first underlying disease _____
_____

r. includes _____
_____

s. excludes _____
_____

t. ▲ _____

u. ● _____

v. What symbols alert the coder to add a fourth and fifth digit?

_____

_____

w. Uncertain behavior of a neoplasm _____

_____

x. Unspecified behavior of a neoplasm _____

_____

PRACTICE EXERCISES

1. Place a double underline below the main terms and a single underline below any subterms in each of the following medical conditions:

a. rheumatoid arthritis

b. first-degree burn

c. myocardial infarction

d. dog bite

e. Parkinson's dementia

f. paroxysmal atrial fibrillation

g. acute pharyngitis

h. hand pain

i. heart palpitations

j. squamous cell melanoma

k. kidney stones

l. chronic alcoholism

m. malignant hypertension

n. chronic kidney failure

o. polycystic ovarian disease

p. atopic dermatitis

q. cerebrovascular accident

2. Using the ICD-9-CM manual, code the following medical conditions:
   a. Signs and symptoms
      1. headache _____
      2. facial pain _____
      3. weight loss _____
      4. epistaxis _____
      5. abnormal liver function test _____
      6. vocal cord abscess _____
      7. absent bowel sounds _____
   b. Illnesses/Diseases/Disorders
      1. hypothyroidism _____
      2. Bell's palsy _____
      3. diaper rash _____
      4. spousal abuse _____
      5. cystic acne _____
      6. gastroesophageal reflux disease_____
      7. ectopic pregnancy _____
      8. premature birth _____
      9. moderate retardation _____
      10. congestive heart failure _____
      11. DM I, uncontrolled _____
      12. gestational diabetes _____
      13. acute MI, anterolateral wall, initial _____
      14. erectile dysfunction _____
      15. strep infection, group A _____
      16. Kaposi's sarcoma of skin M code _____
      17. hip fracture, depressed _____
   c. Combination codes (Note: Some conditions will have one code; others will have two.)
      1. acute and chronic bronchitis _____
      2. acute and chronic pancreatitis _____

3. hypertension with chronic kidney disease _____

4. hypertension with heart failure _____

5. DM II with cataract _____

6. DM I with coma _____

7. comminuted finger and thumb fracture _____

8. brain concussion, loss of consciousness 40 min _____

9. urinary infection due to *E-coli* _____

10. compound fracture of fibula with simple fracture of tibia _____

d. HTN/Neoplasm/Drug and Chemical Tables

   1. benign hypertension _____

   2. HTN, unspecified _____

   3. cancer of bladder _____

   4. bone cancer, coccyx, secondary _____

   5. uterine cancer, behavior unknown _____

   6. Carcinoma of brain metastasized from lungs _____

   7. M codes _____

   8. ingested Clorox, accidental _____

   9. OD barbituate, suicide attempt _____

   10. anaphylaxis due to prescription cephalosporin _____

e. Late effects

   1. Speech deficit due to CVA

      Cause _____ Residual _____

      Code(s) _____

   2. Arthritis due to past ankle fracture

      Cause _____ Residual _____

      Code(s) _____

   3. Dysphasia due to CVA

      Cause _____ Residual _____

      Code(s) _____

f. Burns

   1. First-degree burns of nose, second-degree burns of cheek and chin, and third-degree burns of forehead _____

g. V codes

   1. HIV positive _____

   2. Hearing exam _____

   3. Sickle-cell trait screen _____

   4. Denture fitting _____

   5. Physical, child for school _____

   6. Contact with rabies _____

   7. Blood alcohol testing _____

   8. Admission for peritoneal cath dialysis _____

9. Chemotherapy visit for pancreatic cancer _____

10. Encounter for oral birth control _____

11. Removal of surgical dressing of wound _____

12. Hospice care _____

13. DTP vaccination _____

14. Allergy desensitization _____

15. History of pulmonary embolism _____

16. Family history of ovarian cancer _____

17. History of colon polyps _____

   h. E codes

     1. Heel injury (wound) due to broken glass _____

     2. Concussion due to MVA that hit a tree _____

3. Read the following diagnostic statements, determine the primary and secondary diagnoses, and write the appropriate codes:

   a. Patient presents with an elevated white blood cell count. Patient has staph infection due to infection of surgical wound.

     Primary diagnosis _____ Code(s) _____

     Secondary diagnosis _____ Code(s) _____

   b. Patient's mammogram shows evidence of left breast mass. There is a family history of breast cancer.

     Primary diagnosis _____ Code(s) _____

     Secondary diagnosis _____ Code(s) _____

   c. Patient experiencing syncope and epistaxis. Patient has essential HTN, malignant.

     Primary diagnosis _____ Code(s) _____

     Secondary diagnosis _____ Code(s) _____

   d. Patient is seen today for acute and chronic sinusitis and swollen glands.

     Primary diagnosis _____ Code(s) _____

     Secondary diagnosis _____ Code(s) _____

   e. Patient has unstable angina. He has an old MI from 5 years ago.

     Primary diagnosis _____ Code(s) _____

     Secondary diagnosis _____ Code(s) _____

   f. Patient with DM II presents with ulceration on right thigh.

     Primary diagnosis _____ Code(s) _____

     Secondary diagnosis _____ Code(s) _____

4. What are the nine steps for accurate ICD-9-CM coding?

   1. _____

   2. _____

   3. _____

   4. _____

   5. _____

   6. _____

   7. _____

8. _____

9. _____

5. What are the three coding guidelines that will help medical office specialists as they code claims?

   1. _____

   2. _____

   3. _____

6. Using volume 3 of the ICD-9-CM, code the following hospital procedures:

   1. Hemorrhoidectomy _____

   2. Cholecystectomy _____

   3. Dilation and curettage _____

   4. Knee arthroscopy _____

   5. Blood transfusion _____

   6. Chemotherapy infusion _____

   7. Biopsy, needle aspiration of right breast _____

   8. Coronary artery bypass graft, one vessel _____

   9. Cast application _____

   10. Atrial cardioversion _____

   11. Gastric lavage _____

   12. Bilateral tubal ligation _____

   13. Bladder catheter replacement _____

   14. Spinal tap _____

   15. Chest x-ray _____

   16. Abdominal ultrasound _____

   17. CT scan, thyroid _____

REVIEW QUESTIONS

MATCHING

Choose each correct answer, and place its corresponding letter in the space provided.

a. primary diagnosis
b. principal diagnosis
c. benign
d. malignant
e. carcinoma in situ

1. ____ Slow progression; not cancerous
2. ____ Represents the patient's most serious condition, regardless of the reason for encounter
3. ____ Tumor cells that have cancerous changes, but do not extend beyond the point of origin or invade surrounding normal tissue
4. ____ The final diagnosis after tests and examination has been performed.
5. ____ Rapid progression; cancerous

MULTIPLE CHOICE

Circle the letter of the choice that best completes the statement or answers the question.

1. Which of the following determines the percentage of body surface area that has been burned?
   a. Burn Mass index
   b. Rule of Nines
   c. Neither a nor b
   d. Both a and b

2. What law mandated the use of ICD-9-CM for Medicare claims?
   a. Health Insurance Portability and Accountability Act of 1996
   b. World Health Organization Act of 1982
   c. Medicare Catastrophic Act of 1988
   d. None of the above

3. Which of the following terms alerts a coder to a combination code?
   a. Due to
   b. Without
   c. Following
   d. All of the above

4. Which of the following terms alerts a coder that a code may be an E-code?
   a. Illness
   b. Injury
   c. Caused by
   d. Both b and c

5. Which is *not* a reason for agencies or organizations to use the ICD-9-CM?
   a. To forecast healthcare needs and evaluate facilities and services
   b. To conduct studies of trends in diseases over the years
   c. To review costs
   d. All of the above are reasons that the ICD-9-CM is used by agencies and organizations.

SHORT ANSWER

Provide the correct response to each question that follows:

1. When are volumes 1, 2, and 3 of the ICD-9-CM updated?

   _____

   _____

2. What are the three main steps to coding accurately?

   1. _____
   2. _____
   3. _____

3. What is a subclassification in the ICD-9-CM?

   _____

   _____

4. What is an adverse reaction?

   _____

   _____

   _____

5. Discuss V codes and how they are used for coding encounters.

   _____

   _____

   _____

TRUE/FALSE

Identify the statement as true (T) or false (F).

1. _____ A diagnosis does not need to match a procedure to prove medical necessity.

2. _____ Only E codes can be used as the primary diagnosis.

3. _____ Volume 1 of the ICD-9-CM is needed only to find an accurate code.

4. _____ Medicaid and most private insurance carriers adopt rules and regulations for health care reimbursement that are based on Medicare.

5. _____ Conventions can vary per the ICD-9-CM publishing company.

CHAPTER 6

ICD-10-CM Medical Coding

CHAPTER OBJECTIVES

Upon completion of this chapter in your student text, you should be able to do the following:

1. Understand the similarities and variances between ICD-9 and ICD-10 codes.
2. Recognize the difference between a crosswalk and mapping.
3. Compare ICD-9 and ICD-10 general coding guidelines.
4. Discuss new features found in ICD-10-PCS.

CHAPTER OUTLINE

The Future of Diagnosis Coding: ICD-10
    Transition to ICD-10

Conversion Tools

Similarities and Variances between the Two Coding Systems

New Features Found in ICD-10-CM

General Coding Guidelines for ICD-10-CM

New Features Found in ICD-10-PCS
    Completeness
    Expandability
    Multiaxial
    Standardized Terminology

KEY TERMS

Using the highlighted terms and glossary in the textbook, define the following terms.

1. Coordination and Maintenance (C & M) Committee_____

_____

2. crosswalk _____

_____

3. General Equivalence Mappings (GEM) files _____

_____

4. health information management (HIM) _____

_____

5. ICD-10 Procedure Coding System (ICD-10-PCS) _____

_____

6. *International Classification of Diseases*, Tenth Revision (ICD-10-CM) _____

_____

7. mapping _____

_____

8. National Center for Health Statistics (NCHS) _____

_____

9. World Health Organization (WHO) _____

_____

CRITICAL THINKING QUESTIONS

Using the knowledge you have gained from reading the textbook, apply critical thinking skills to answer the following questions:

1. After reviewing the differences between ICD-9-CM and ICD-10-CM coding, how do you think the use of ICD-10-CM coding will change the way coders and billers do their jobs?

_____

_____

_____

_____

_____

_____

_____

_____

_____

_____

2. In your own words, answer the following questions regarding annual updates:
   a. What are reasons for providing annual updates for the ICD-9 and ICD-10 codes?

   _____

   _____

   _____

   b. Why is there a freeze on annual updates for ICD-9 and ICD-10 codes until ICD-10 is implemented?

   _____

   _____

   _____

3. Answer the following questions related to the volumes of the ICD-10-CM, and if applicable, supply an example, using the manual:
   a. Give an example of a chapter from the Tabular List of Diseases and Injuries.

   _____

b. Give an example of a category and supply the code.

_____

c. Give an example of a subcategory and supply the code.

_____

d. Give an example of a chapter heading in the *Classification of Diseases and Injuries*.

_____

e. Find a sixth-digit subcategory code. What additional information does the fifth digit supply to the code?

_____

_____

_____

f. In your own words, what are Z codes, and how do they compare to the V codes from the ICD-9-CM?

_____

_____

_____

g. How are codes for External Causes to Injury and Illness looked up in the ICD-10-CM?

_____

_____

_____

h. Using the ICD-10-CM, where would you find a code for lung cancer, primary?

_____

_____

_____

4. a. What would be used to look up procedure codes for the hospital?

_____

b. Can outpatient procedures be coded using this system? Why or why not?

_____

5. What are GEMs, and how will they be used for conversion from ICD-9 to ICD-10?

_____

_____

PRACTICE EXERCISES

1. Use the following GEM Web site to convert the ICD-9-CM codes to ICD-10-CM: http://www.aapc.com/icd-10/codes/

   a. 784.0 _____

   b. 346.90 _____

   c. 410.91 _____

   d. 710.0 _____

   e. 959.9 _____

f. 731.0 _____

g. 714.0 _____

h. 825.00 _____

2. Using the ICD-10-CM manual code the following medical conditions:

a. Signs and Symptoms

1. leg pain _____

2. malaise and fatigue _____

3. hematochezia _____

4. abdominal pain _____

5. painful urination _____

6. sore throat _____

7. tarry stools _____

b. Illnesses/Diseases/Disorders

1. hyperemesis gravidarum _____

2. cerebral palsy _____

3. thrush, oral _____

4. suicide attempt _____

5. supraventricular tachycardia _____

6. gastroesophageal reflux disease with esophagitis _____

7. fibromyalgia _____

8. newborn jaundice, unspecified _____

9. trimalleolar fracture _____

10. knee osteoarthritis _____

c. HTN/Neoplasm/Drug and Chemical Tables

1. malignant hypertension _____

2. hypertension due to renal failure _____

3. malignant melanoma, lip _____

4. malignant neoplasm, bone, limb _____

5. opioid abuse _____

d. Burns

1. First-degree burn of face _____

e. Z codes

1. Family history diabetes _____

2. Newborn hearing screen after failed exam _____

3. Prep care for renal dialysis _____

4. Administration chemotherapy for lung cancer _____

5. Encounter for emergency contraception _____

3. Read the following diagnostic statements, determine the primary and secondary diagnoses, and write the appropriate codes:

a. Patient presents with wrist pain and after examination is found to have carpal tunnel syndrome and trigger finger, thumb.

Primary diagnosis _____ Code(s) _____

Secondary diagnosis _____ Code(s) _____

b. Patient's colonoscopy shows the patient has a polyp. The patient has a history of polyps.

Primary diagnosis _____ Code(s) _____

Secondary diagnosis _____ Code(s) _____

c. Patient experiencing syncope during pregnancy reveals a normal pregnancy.

Primary diagnosis _____ Code(s) _____

Secondary diagnosis _____ Code(s) _____

4. What are three differences between the coding guidelines for ICD-10-CM and ICD-9-CM?

1. _____

2. _____

3. _____

5. List the six new features of the ICD-10-CM.

1. _____

2. _____

3. _____

4. _____

5. _____

6. _____

REVIEW QUESTIONS

MATCHING

Choose each correct answer and place its corresponding letter in the space provided.

a. GEMs
b. mapping
c. crosswalks
d. WHO
e. laterality

1. ____ Right, left, bilateral

2. ____ World Health Organization, responsible for developing ICD-10-CM and ICD-10-PCS

3. ____ Mapping between ICD-9 to ICD-10 and vice versa

4. ____ Reflects the complexity of the codes rather than oversimplifying

5. ____ Direct match, one-to-one relationship

MULTIPLE CHOICE

Circle the letter of the choice that best completes the statement or answers the question.

1. Use of ICD-10 codes will provide the following once implemented?
   a. Better tracking and statistics
   b. Use of data for quality and safety
   c. More efficiency
   d. All of the above

2. How many characters is ICD-10-PCS?
   a. 7 alphanumeric characters
   b. 5 numerical characters
   c. 3–7 alphanumeric characters
   d. None of the above

3. When was the last regular update of both the ICD-9 and ICD-10?
   a. October 1, 2011
   b. October 1, 2010
   c. October 1, 2012
   d. None of the above

4. Which of the following terms alerts a coder that a code may be a Z code?
   a. Illness
   b. Injury
   c. Administration
   d. Both a and c

5. Which is *not* a major modification to the ICD-10-CM?
   a Added trimesters for obstetric codes
   b Less codes than ICD-9-CM
   c Revisions to diabetic codes
   d All of the above are reasons that the ICD-9-CM is used by agencies and organizations.

SHORT ANSWER

Provide the correct response to each question that follows.

1. Which volume(s) will ICD-10-CM replace?
   _____
   _____

2. What are some of the chapters that the seventh digit is used for in the ICD-10-CM?
   _____
   _____

3. What are some of the areas that ICD-9 lacks when compared to ICD-10?
   _____
   _____

4. What are the four major attributes that the ICD-10-PCS is working toward incorporating?
   1. _____
   2. _____
   3. _____
   4. _____

5. List the features of the ICD-10-PCS.

_____

_____

_____

TRUE/FALSE

Identify the statement as true (T) or false (F).

1. _____ With ICD-10-PCS, each character has 34 different possible values.
2. _____ With ICD-10-CM, Z codes cannot be used as the principal diagnosis.
3. _____ A three-digit code can be used routinely with ICD-10-CM.
4. _____ ICD-10-CM is a system of classification used for procedure codes.
5. _____ The letters O and I are not used with ICD-10-PCS to avoid confusion.

CHAPTER 7
Introduction to CPT® and Place of Service Coding

CHAPTER OBJECTIVES

Upon completion of this chapter in your student text, you should be able to do the following:

1. Understand the history of CPT.
2. Understand evaluation and management (E/M) services.
3. Explain the three types of CPT categories.
4. Distinguish the need for modifiers.
5. Distinguish between a new and established patient.
6. Know the three key elements in choosing an E/M code.
7. Determine the correct E/M code.

CHAPTER OUTLINE

Current Procedural terminology (CPT)

CPT Categories
    CPT Category I
    CPT Category II
    CPT Category III

CPT Nomenclature
    Symbols
    Guidelines

CPT Modifiers
    Evaluation and Management Modifiers

Coding to the Place of Service
    Other Services Provided in the E/M Section

Office versus Hospital Services
    Emergency Department Services
    Preventive Medicine Services

Type of Patient
    New Patient
    Established Patient
    Referral
    Consultation

CPT is a registered trademark of the American Medical Association.

Level of E/M Service
    Extent of Patient's History
    Extent of Examination
    Complexity of Medical Decision Making
    Additional Components
    Assigning the Code

KEY TERMS

Using the highlighted terms and glossary in the textbook, define the following terms.

1. American Medical Association (AMA) _____

    _____

2. Centers for Medicare and Medicaid Services (CMS) _____

    _____

3. chief complaint (CC) _____

    _____

4. consultation _____

    _____

5. counseling _____

    _____

6. Current Procedural Terminology (CPT) _____

    _____

7. E/M codes _____

    _____

8. established patient _____

    _____

9. examination _____

    _____

10. history _____

    _____

11. history of present illness (HPI) _____

    _____

12. medical decision making (MDM) _____

    _____

13. modifiers _____

    _____

14. nature of the presenting problem _____

    _____

15. new patient _____

    _____

16. nomenclature _____

    _____

17. past, family, and social history (PFSH) _____

_____

18. review of systems (ROS) _____

_____

CRITICAL THINKING QUESTIONS

Using the knowledge you have gained from reading the textbook, apply critical thinking skills to answer the following questions:

1. What is the history of CPT coding? Write a summary describing how it has changed throughout the years.

_____

_____

_____

_____

_____

_____

2. Samuel Lewis, MD, is coding an E/M service for patient Marge Mahoney. What are three important components for Dr. Lewis to use when selecting the appropriate code for Mrs. Mahoney's visit?

   1. _____

   2. _____

   3. _____

3. Read the following scenarios, and determine what part of the medical history it identifies:

   a. The patient's mother had diabetes.

   _____

   b. The patient smokes cigarettes, 1 pack per day.

   _____

   c. The patient has a history of herpes simplex virus.

   _____

   d. The patient currently takes Prednisone t.i.d.

   _____

   e. The patient had a cholecystectomy in 1998.

   _____

4. Determine whether the following is/are considered a body area or an organ system, as recognized by the CPT manual:

   a. The patient's neurologic exam reveals orientation X3.

   _____

   b. The abdomen is soft, nontender.

   _____

   c. The head presents as normocephalic, atraumatic.

   _____

d. Skin shows no lesions, bruises, or rashes.

_____

e. Eyes: Pupils are equal, round, and reactive to light. Sclera is white.

_____

f. Ears, nose, mouth, and throat are unremarkable.

_____

g. Psychiatric: Patient's mood is pleasant and upbeat.

_____

h. Chest: No wheezes, rubs, or rhonci.

_____

5. A patient's E/M code is 99214. The physician spent over 25 minutes of counseling and coordination of care time with this patient. What code(s), if any, should be reported to ensure the maximum reimbursement level for this service?

_____

PRACTICE EXERCISES

1. Using the CPT manual, choose the correct E/M code for each scenario that follows:

a. A new patient is seen today for an infection on the right index finger. The nail is examined and has evidence of a fungal infection. Patient is started on antibiotics.

E/M code _____

b. A patient is seen for a checkup on arthritis of the knees and for hypertension. The patient has no new complaints. His blood pressure is stable with medication therapy, and his arthritis has presented only mild symptoms since the last visit.

E/M code _____

c. A patient being seen for an initial hospital visit, presents with unstable angina and elevated cardiac enzymes. The patient has a history of hypertension, DM II, and smoking two packs of cigarettes per day for 12 years.

E/M code _____

d. A patient is being seen for the second day of admission for an emergency appendectomy. Patient is healthy otherwise and presents stable.

E/M code _____

e. A patient is being discharged after an episode of shingles. The physician completes the discharge within 20 minutes.

E/M code _____

f. A patient is seeing the endocrinologist for his rheumatoid arthritis follow-up. The progression has slowly advanced since the last visit. Labs are unremarkable.

E/M code _____

g. A patient's internal medicine doctor orders a neurologist consult for the patient regarding seizure disorder. The patient was admitted for cellulitis and has begun to seizure.

E/M code _____

h. A patient presents to the ER with complaints of an asthma attack. The patient also has COPD. After administration of medications, CXR, and lab, the patient is stable and is discharged.

E/M code _____

i. The physician spends 1 hour and 40 minutes providing critical care to a CCU patient.

E/M code _____

j. The physician visits a newborn for day three in the neonatal ICU. The child should be able to be released in a couple more days.

E/M code _____

k. A newborn weighing 1600 g is admitted to the neonatal ICU.

E/M code _____

l. A patient is being examined for the first time in a long-term care facility. The patient's health consists of glaucoma due to DM I, old MI, and recent CVA. The patient has hemipeligia of her dominant side. A full ROS is completed.

E/M code _____

m. A patient who was admitted yesterday to skilled nursing is being seen today for postop surgery of left hip replacement. The patient shows no signs of infection and is eating and eliminating well.

E/M code _____

n. A physician spends 40 minutes redeveloping a care plan for a patient in a nursing home.

E/M code _____

o. A physician spends an extra 35 minutes with a new patient discussing fertility options.

E/M code _____

p. A physician reassesses the anticoagulant management of a patient.

E/M code _____

q. A new patient, age 15, is seen for a physical examination. Exam is unremarkable.

Patient was given the first series of hepatitis B vaccination.

E/M code _____

r. An established patient, age 25, is seen for an annual gynecological exam.

E/M code _____

s. A 2-year-old is seen today for a well-child exam. Patient is developing normally.

E/M code _____

t. The physician spends 30 minutes counseling a patient on a weight-loss program.

E/M code _____

u. A patient is seen today for a disability evaluation. The patient has congestive heart failure and renal failure.

E/M code _____

v. A patient is seen in the hospital on the first hospital day. Patient is an inpatient. Patient has been admitted for chest pain. The physician sees the patient for 30 minutes.

E/M code _____

2. Using the CPT manual, code the following scenarios and apply the appropriate E/M modifier:

a. A patient is seen by his family doctor for chronic bronchitis. A chest x-ray was performed. The patient also complains of numbness and tingling in his right hand and wrist. An x-ray of the right hand and wrist was also performed.

E/M code and modifier _____

b. The Social Security Administration required a 40-year-old disabled patient to be seen today for an annual physical exam.

E/M code and modifier _____

c. The orthorhinolaryngologist sees a referred patient for chronic sinusitis. The physician explains to the patient that the sinusitis is not getting better and determines that surgery is the best option.

E/M code and modifier _____

d. A patient presents for postop care due to a hysterectomy. The patient has a new complaint of four lesions that have appeared on her perineal area. She has a history of herpes simplex virus.

Modifier _____

e. A patient is prepped and going in to have a colonoscopy. The procedure is discontinued due to problems with the patient's heart.

Modifier _____

3. Think of your last doctor's visit. Without identifying any personal information, select the appropriate E/M code that would have been used for the visit. Use the CPT manual to complete this exercise.

E/M code _____

REVIEW QUESTIONS

MATCHING

Choose the correct answer and write its corresponding letter in the space provided.

a. inpatient
b. outpatient
c. new patient
d. established patient
e. observation status

1. ____ Person who has *not* been seen by a physician or practice for 3 years
2. ____ Medical care provided at a doctor's office or outside health facility
3. ____ Patients who are being observed to see if they should be admitted to the hospital
4. ____ Admittance to the hospital, a skilled nursing facility, or a nursing home for 24+ hours
5. ____ Person who *has* been seen by a physician or practice within 3 years

MULTIPLE CHOICE

Circle the letter of the choice that best completes the statement or answers the question.

1. Which of the following CPT symbols alerts the coder to new or revised text enclosed?

   a. ▲
   b. ●
   c. ▶◀
   d. +

2. Which of the following CPT symbols alerts the coder to a revised code that has been changed?

   a. ▲

   b. ●

   c. ►◄

   d. +

3. Which of the following CPT symbols alerts the coder that the code is new to the edition?

   a. ▲

   b. ●

   c. ►◄

   d. +

4. Which of the following describes the purpose of CPT modifiers?

   a. Describe the procedure

   b. Describe issues with the procedure

   c. Describe an alteration to the procedure

   d. None of the above

5. Which association/organization publishes the CPT manual?

   a. HIPAA

   b. AMA

   c. WHO

   d. CMS

SHORT ANSWER

Provide the correct response to each question that follows.

1. What are the eight sections of the CPT manual and their respective code ranges?

   1. _____

   2. _____

   3. _____

   4. _____

   5. _____

   6. _____

   7. _____

   8. _____

2. Out of the eight sections just listed, in which sections are Category I codes found? _____

   _____

3. Where are the CPT guidelines found in the manual, and what is their purpose? _____

   _____

   _____

4. Why is the use of modifiers that are added to a code so important? _____

   _____

   _____

   _____

   _____

5. The E/M section is divided into broad services. What are some examples of these services?

_____

_____

_____

TRUE/FALSE

Identify each statement as true (T) or false (F).

1. _____ Category II codes contain performance management tracking codes.

2. _____ The CPT may have some procedures that appear in certain sections other than those sections where these procedures may seem to ordinarily be classified.

3. _____ You must first determine the place of service when coding from the E/M section.

4. _____ Most services for established patients and subsequent care require all three key components when the appropriate E/M code is being chosen.

5. _____ A referred patient and a consultation mean the same thing.

CHAPTER 8
Coding Procedures and Services

CHAPTER OBJECTIVES

Upon completion of this chapter in your student text, you should be able to do the following:

1. Correctly use the CPT® index.
2. Understand the four primary classes of main entries in the CPT index.
3. Understand code ranges and conventions.
4. Discuss the purpose of each section and the guidelines.
5. Know how to use modifiers correctly.
6. Use add-on codes properly.
7. Review codes for accuracy.
8. Given procedural statements, apply coding guidelines to determine the correct CPT codes.

CHAPTER OUTLINE

Organization of the CPT Index
    Instructions for Using the CPT
    Code Range

Formatting and Cross-References
    Formattting
    Cross-references

Section Guidelines

Modifiers

Add-on Codes (+)

Coding Steps
    Coding for Anesthesia

Surgical Coding

Separate Procedure

Surgical Package or Global Surgery Concept

Supplies and Services

Radiology Codes

Pathology and Laboratory Codes

Medicine Codes

CPT is a registered trademark of the American Medical Association.

KEY TERMS

◾

Using the highlighted terms and glossary in the textbook, define the following terms:

1. add-on codes _____

   _____

2. bundled code _____

   _____

3. Clinical Laboratory Improvement Amendment (CLIA) _____

   _____

4. cross-references _____

   _____

5. descriptor _____

   _____

6. fragmented billing _____

   _____

7. global period _____

   _____

8. global surgical concept _____

9. panel _____

10. physical status modifier _____

    _____

11. primary procedure _____

    _____

12. professional component _____

    _____

13. secondary procedure _____

    _____

14. separate procedure _____

    _____

15. special report _____

    _____

16. surgical package _____

    _____

17. technical component _____

    _____

18. unbundling _____

_____

CRITICAL THINKING QUESTIONS

Using the knowledge you have gained from reading the textbook, apply critical thinking skills to answer the following questions:

1. Answer each of the following as it relates to the CPT index:

    a. What are the four primary classes of entries in the main index? Give an example for each.

    1. _____

    2. _____

    3. _____

    4. _____

    b. When codes are sequential, what are they separated by? When codes are not sequential, what are they separated by? _____

    _____

2. Answer each of the following as it relates to the CPT format:

    a. Using the CPT, locate the following descriptors for code 15780, and answer the given three questions related to this code:

    1. What is the full descriptor for this parent code?

    _____

    2. What is the full descriptor for the indented code 15781?

    _____

    3. What is the full descriptor for the indented code 15782?

    _____

    b. Code 15786 is for abrasion of a single lesion. What code(s) would be used to bill for abrasion of five lesions?

    _____

    c. Where in the CPT manual would you find vital supplemental information that is used to correctly code from each section?

    _____

3. Answer the following questions related to anesthesia coding:

    a. To bill anesthesia services correctly, what guide would you use?

    _____

    _____

    b. Maryann Grull is having a partial hysterectomy. What services are included in the anesthesia code?

    _____

    _____

c. When does Maryann's anesthesia period begin and end during her surgery?

_____

_____

4. Answer the following questions related to CPT coding:
   a. When a patient has a major procedure, what services and/or care would be part of the surgical package?

   _____

   _____

   _____

   b. What services and/or care would not be part of the patient's surgical package?

   _____

   _____

   _____

   c. Read each procedure that follows. Identify whether each procedure is normally bundled in a surgical package by writing **YES** in the space provided. If the procedure is *not* normally bundled in a surgical package, write **NO** is the space provided.
      1. _____ Administration of sedative, local or regional anesthesia by the performing physician
      2. _____ Complicated debridement of traumatized tissue and lysis of adhesions
      3. _____ Application of a cast, sling, or splint
      4. _____ Removal of polyps or other benign lesions during a colonoscopy
      5. _____ Surgical supplies
      6. _____ Administration of general anesthesia by the anesthesiologist
   d. In your own words, what would be some examples of situations where a modifier would be used?

   _____

   _____

   _____

5. What are the three steps to perform procedural coding? Give a brief explanation for each.
   1. _____

   _____

   _____

   2. _____

   _____

   _____

   3. _____

   _____

   _____

PRACTICE EXERCISES

1. Using the CPT manual, choose the correct codes for each procedure that follows:

   Anesthesia

   Liver transplantation on a patient who will not live unless the surgery is performed:

   Code(s) _____

   Surgical wrist arthroscopy on a healthy patient:

   Code(s) _____

   Burr hole on a 72-year-old patient in severe distress:

   Code(s) _____

   Skin

   Destruction of seven lesions by laser:

   Code(s) _____

   I&D of cyst, simple:

   Code(s) _____

   Simple repair of wounds of the scalp 0.5 cm, neck 1.2 cm, and shoulder 3.6 cm:

   Code(s) _____

   Biopsy of right breast by needle core with image guidance, percutaneous:

   Code(s) _____

   Local treatment of first-degree burn, initial:

   Code(s) _____

   Moh's surgery of arm, first stage, four tissue blocks:

   Code(s) _____

   Musculoskeletal

   Closed treatment of acetabular fracture, skeletal traction:

   Code(s) _____

   Application of short cast:

   Code(s) _____

   Bone biopsy of greater trochanter:

   Code(s) _____

   Amputation of ankle:

   Code(s) _____

   Local arthrodesis of elbow joint:

   Code(s) _____

   Fracture, two ribs, open treatment:

   Code(s) _____

   Closed treatment, acetabulum with manipulation:

   Code(s) _____

   Reinsertion of spinal fixation device:

   Code(s) _____

Respiratory

Direct laryngoscopy with biopsy:

Code(s) _____

Removal of a rock lodged in the nose:

Code(s) _____

Thoracotomy; with exploration

Code(s) _____

Lobectomy, two:

Code(s) _____

Sinusotomy of the frontal sinuses:

Code(s) _____

Bronchoscopy with bronchial alveolar lavage:

Code(s) _____

Cardiovascular

Pulmendartectomy with embolectomy:

Code(s) _____

CABG, three coronary vessels:

Code(s) _____

Insertion of ventricular pacemaker:

Code(s) _____

Ruptured aneurysm repair of the abdominal aorta, hypogastric, direct:

Code(s) _____

Closure of atrial septal and ventricular septal defect, direct:

Code(s) _____

Coronary endarterectomy; open:

Code(s) _____

Hemic and Lymphatic

Partial splenectomy:

Code(s) _____

Resection of the diaphragm, complex:

Code(s) _____

Lymph biopsy of left axillea, deep:

Code(s) _____

Digestive

Upper GI endoscopy with biopsy:

Code(s) _____

Destruction of herpetic lesion of the anus by cryosurgery:

Code(s) _____

Repair of strangulated umbilical hernia:

Code(s) _____

Hemorrhoidopexy:

Code(s) _____

Cleft palate repair, hard and soft:

Code(s) _____

Esophagogastroduodenoscopy; with biopsy:

Code(s) _____

Urinary

Closure of pyelocutaneous fistula:

Code(s) _____

Urodynamic uroflowmetry, complex:

Code(s) _____

Ureterectomy, abdominal approach:

Code(s) _____

Cystourethroscopy with internal urethrotomy, female patient:

Code(s) _____

Nephrotomy for renal calculi:

Code(s) _____

Male

Circumcision with clamp on newborn:

Code(s) _____

Urethroplasty of 2.7 cm hypospadias:

Code(s) _____

Circumcision, adult:

Code(s) _____

Destruction of penis lesion, laser technique:

Code(s) _____

Punch biopsy of the prostate:

Code(s) _____

Female

Hysteroscopy of the endometrium with biopsy and D&C:

Code(s) _____

Total hysterectomy:

Code(s) _____

Colpopexy, vaginal; extraperitoneal approach:

Code(s) _____

Perineal biopsy of one lesion:

Code(s) _____

Partial oophorectomy, one ovary:

Code(s) _____

Tubal ligation, vaginal approach:

Code(s) _____

Maternity Care and Delivery

Induced abortion by evacuation with D&C:

Code(s) _____

Fetal contraction stress test:

Code(s) _____

Antepartum, delivery, and postpartum care after previous C-section:

Code(s) _____

Surgical treatment of ectopic pregnancy, with salpingectomy, vaginal:

Code(s) _____

Cesarean delivery only:

Code(s) _____

Endocrine

Removal of carotid bay tumor:

Code(s) _____

Thyroidectomy, subtotal for malignancy with radical neck dissection:

Code(s) _____

Nervous

Stereotactic stimulation of spinal cord, percutaneous:

Code(s) _____

Subdural hematoma drainage by burr hole technique:

Code(s) _____

Implant of intrathecal catheter with laminectomy:

Code(s) _____

5.1 cm meningocele repair:

Code(s) _____

Cervical laminoplasty with decompression, two vertebral segments:

Code(s) _____

Sciatic neuroplasty:

Code(s) _____

Eye and Ocular Adnexa

Nonperforated cornea laceration repair:

Code(s) _____

Removal of embedded glass from right eyelid with simple skin repair, 1.0 cm:

Code(s) _____

Removal of cataract of right eye, secondary:

Code(s) _____

Auditory

Removal foreign body from external auditory canal, without anesthesia:

Code(s) _____

Radiology

Cholangiography

Code(s) _____

Saline infused sonohysterography with Doppler color flow:

Code(s) _____

CT, soft tissue of neck without contrast, followed by contrast:

Code(s) _____

DXA scan, axial skeleton:

Code(s) _____

Retrograde intravenous urography with KUB:

Code(s) _____

CXR, complete, 4 views:

Code(s) _____

Bilateral mammogram, diagnostic:

Code(s) _____

Swallowing function test with cineradiography:

Code(s) _____

Percutaneous transhepatic biliary drainage with contract monitoring:

Code(s) _____

Radiation treatment delivery, single area with simple blocking, 8 MeV:

Code(s) _____

Radiation treatment, five treatments:

Code(s) _____

Single thyroid uptake study:

Code(s) _____

Pathology

Total creatine kinase:

Code(s) _____

ANA titer:

Code(s) _____

Hepatitis panel:

Code(s) _____

Aerobic stool culture for salmonella:

Code(s) _____

Quantitative HCG:

Code(s) _____

Semen analysis:

Code(s) _____

Western Blot with interpretation and report:

Code(s) _____

ABO blood typing:

Code(s) _____

Surgical pathology, needle biopsy of the prostate:

Code(s) _____

Bone marrow smear with interpretation:

Code(s) _____

CBC with differential:

Code(s) _____

ESR, automated:

Code(s) _____

Quantitative Quinidine assay:

Code(s) _____

Pap smear screen, thin layer, automated:

Code(s) _____

Cocaine screen and confirmation:

Code(s) _____

Surgical pathology, uterus and tubes after prolapse:

Code(s) _____

Medicine

Family psychotherapy:

Code(s) _____

MMR vaccination for 2-year-old boy:

Code(s) _____

ESRD, full month for 69-year-old female:

Code(s) _____

Intranasal influenza immunization:

Code(s) _____

IV hydration infusion, four hours:

Code(s) _____

Psychiatric diagnostic interview examination:

Code(s) _____

Hepatitis A vaccination, adult:

Code(s) _____

Ophthalmology examination, new patient, intermediate:

Code(s) _____

Fitting for spectacles, monofocal:

Code(s) _____

Visual field exam:

Code(s) _____

Hearing aid check, left ear:

Code(s) _____

Pure tone audiometry:

Code(s) _____

Echocardiography with realtime 2-D imaging, M-mode with Doppler:

Code(s) _____

Elective cardioversion:

Code(s) _____

Telephonic pace analysis for dual chamber pacemaker:

Code(s) _____

Arterial and venous duplex, bilateral:

Code(s) _____

Pulse oximetry on exercise:

Code(s) _____

Laser treatment for psoriasis, 190 sq. cm:

Code(s) _____

Allergy injection, two:

Code(s) _____

Physical therapy evaluation:

Code(s) _____

EMG of the arm, bilateral:

Code(s) _____

Central nervous system chemotherapy administration with spinal puncture:

Code(s) _____

Chiropractic spinal manipulation treatment:

Code(s) _____

Home health visit for stoma care:

Code(s) _____

2. Using the CPT manual, apply the appropriate modifier for the following procedures:

Liver transplantation with surgical team:

Code(s) _____

Radical mastectomy, bilateral:

Code(s) _____

TURP, second stage:

Code(s) _____

Arthroscopy, knee, infected from surgery, with medial meniscus repair performed by two surgeons:

Code(s) _____

Stopped, treadmill exercise stress test, myocardial perfusion imaging, multiple studies:

Code(s) _____

Repeat bleeding time:

Code(s) _____

Lead testing performed by outside lab:

Code(s) _____

Avulsion, vagus nerve, abdominal, surgical care only:

Code(s) _____

Laparoscopic hysterectomy of uterus weighing 24 lbs; was to be total, but was determined to be partial removal at the time of surgery:

Code(s) _____

Emergency endotracheal intubation on infant weighing 3.5 kg:

Code(s) _____

Discontinued outpatient breast biopsy by fine needle due to patient reaction to regional anesthetic:

Code(s) _____

3. Using the CPT and the ICD-9-CM manuals, code the following scenarios:

   a. A patient is seen for a follow-up after cholecystomy 2 weeks ago. Patient is not having diarrhea. Review of the abdomen is unremarkable.

   Code(s) _____

   b. A patient is seen for the first time by the allergist for asthma and allergic rhinitis. A prick allergy test is administered for 15 allergens. Reaction is present for grass pollen, dust mites, and dog dander. The patient was started on Allegra-D and Singulair, and Claritin was administered after the testing. The patient is to return in 1 month to assess the advisability of allergy injections.

   Code(s) _____

   c. A new patient sees a family physician for missed menses × 2 weeks. A urine pregnancy test is performed in the office, which is negative. The patient is referred to her gynecologist for further evaluation.

   Code(s) _____

REVIEW QUESTIONS

MATCHING

Choose the correct answer and place its corresponding letter in the space provided.

a. modifier TC
b. professional component (S&I)
c. See, or Use
d. See Also
e. Ø

1. ____ Direction in the CPT to look under another main term to reference a code
2. ____ Denotes that a code cannot be used with a particular modifier, such as −51
3. ____ Technical component; used when a test is performed, but the physician does not interpret
4. ____ Points to another code and also denotes synonyms, eponyms, and abbreviations
5. ____ A cardiologist interprets and reports a Holter monitor report for a family physician

MULTIPLE CHOICE

Circle the letter of the choice that best completes the statement or answers the question.

1. Procedures and services for laboratory are listed in the index under which of the following terms?
   a. Panels
   b. Name of the test
   c. Panel, blood test, or hormone assay
   d. All of the above

2. Which of the following procedures and services are found in the medicine section?
   a. Audiology
   b. Otorhinolaryngology
   c. Physical therapy, speech therapy, and rehabilitation
   d. All of the above

3. How many codes are needed to code an immunization?
   a. 1
   b. 2
   c. 3
   d. None of the above

4. What do anesthesia codes usually cover?
   a. Postoperative follow-up visits
   b. Preop and postop care
   c. Administration of fluids
   d. All of the above
   e Both b and c are correct

5. Which of the following is true regarding bundled codes?
   a. Related procedures are covered by a single code.
   b. Separate procedures cannot be coded under bundled codes.
   c. Bundled codes include usual procedures that are performed together.
   d. Both a and c are correct.

SHORT ANSWER

Provide the correct response to each question that follows:

1. What code do physicians use to keep track of the number of post-op visits?
   _____

2. What code is used to report supplies not covered under a procedure?
   _____

3. What symbol is used when the codes given in the index are a range of codes? What if the codes are two codes either sequential or not? _____

   _____

   _____

4. What are the two routes of contrast administration that should be coded as "without contrast"?
   1. _____
   2. _____

5. To code tests from the pathology 8000 series, you will need a code for the _____
   and another code to report the _____ of the specimen.

TRUE/FALSE

Identify each statement as true (T) or false (F):

1. _____ The medical office specialist should always check the main text to verify accuracy of the code given.

2. _____ A panel blood test can be coded if most of the tests in it are performed.

3. _____ A patient's diagnosis may determine the need for modifiers.

4. _____ Besides physicians, other health care professionals can code from the medicine section of the CPT.

5. _____ An unlisted or a new procedure does not usually require a special report from the reporting physician.

CHAPTER 9

HCPCS and Coding Compliance

CHAPTER OBJECTIVES

Upon completion of this chapter in your student text, you should be able to do the following:

1. Understand the two levels of HCPCS.
2. Recognize the need for HCPCS coding and when to report HCPCS codes.
3. Learn how to use HCPCS modifiers.
4. Interpret and identify correct code linkages.
5. Review the coding for accuracy.
6. Understand federal laws, regulations, and penalties that pertain to coding compliance.
7. Understand the responsibilities of coding and coding compliance.
8. Explain the National Correct Coding Initiative.
9. Understand medical ethics for the medical coder.

CHAPTER OUTLINE

History of HCPCS

HCPCS Level of Codes
    Level I: CPT® Codes
    Level II: HCPCS National Codes

HCPCS Modifiers
    Use of the GA Modifier

HCPCS Index

Coding Compliance

Code Linkage

Billing CPT Codes
    Fraudulent Claims
    Physician Self-Referral
    Government Investigations and Advice
    Errors Relating to Code Linkage and Medical Necessity
    Errors Relating to the Coding Process
    Errors Relating to the Billing Process

National Correct Coding Initiative

Fraudulent Actions

Federal Compliance
How to Be Compliant
Benefits of a Compliance Program
Ethics for the Medical Coder

KEY TERMS

Using the highlighted terms and glossary in the textbook, define the following terms:

1. abuse _____

   _____

2. advanced beneficiary notice (ABN) _____

   _____

3. advisory opinion _____

   _____

4. assumption coding _____

   _____

5. code linkage _____

   _____

6. durable medical equipment (DME) _____

   _____

7. fraud _____

   _____

8. HCPCS _____

   _____

9. Level I HCPCS _____

   _____

10. Level II HCPCS _____

    _____

11. National Correct Coding Initiative (NCCI) _____

    _____

12. OIG fraud alerts _____

    _____

13. OIG Work Plan _____

    _____

CRITICAL THINKING QUESTIONS

Using the knowledge you have gained from reading the textbook, apply critical thinking skills to answer the following questions.

1. What are the five reasons that the CMS has maintained HCPCS?

    1. _____

    2. _____

    3. _____

    4. _____

    5. _____

2. Answer the following questions related to the two levels of HCPCS:

    a. In your own words, briefly describe Level I codes.

    _____

    _____

    _____

    _____

    b. In your own words, briefly describe Level II codes.

    _____

    _____

    _____

    _____

    _____

    _____

    c. How do you look up the HCPCS codes, and how does this compare to locating CPT codes?

    _____

    _____

    _____

    _____

    _____

3. Answer the following questions related to HCPCS modifiers:

a. Discuss HCPCS modifiers and how they are used.

_____

_____

_____

_____

_____

b. Identify the correct HCPCS modifier for each scenario that follows:

1. A patient has trigger finger release on right 2nd finger.

_____

2. A patient is seen by a locum tenens physician in the clinic.

_____

3. A patient has a blepharoplasty on the right upper eyelid.

_____

4. A patient had a surgical procedure for her left, fourth-digit hammer toe.

_____

c. A patient has a tummy tuck following a gastric bypass. The tummy tuck may not be covered under his insurance policy. What form needs to be signed by this patient and filed in his chart?

_____

_____

d. Why would this form need to be signed and filed?

_____

_____

e. How would you notify the insurance carrier that this form was obtained?

_____

_____

4. Answer the following questions related to compliance:

a. In your own words, what is the Federal Register and what is its purpose?

_____

_____

_____

_____

_____

b. You are assigned the duty of creating a compliance plan for your office. What important information can be obtained from the Compliance Program Guidance that will help you to implement a compliance plan?

_____

_____

_____

_____

_____

PRACTICE EXERCISES

1. Referring to Chapter 9 in your text, read each of the given scenarios and identify what type of billing and/or coding error has occurred. Write **CL** for an error in code linkage, **CP** for an error in the coding process, and **BP** for an error in the billing process.

    a. _____ The medical office specialist submits a claim before the physician documents the visit.

    b. _____ The physician asks the coder to code for a procedure that is not performed, and the coder does this for him.

    c. _____ The coder changes a diagnosis for a procedure that does not meet medical necessity.

    d. _____ The physician orders a head CT for a patient with COPD.

2. Using HCPCS codes, code the following:

    1. Ambulance emergency service with BLS
    Code _____

    2. Replacement of tubing for breast pump
    Code _____

    3. Blood glucose reagent strips for home monitoring, 50 strips
    Code _____

    4. Above-the-knee surgical stockings (2)
    Code _____

    5. Dome and mouthpiece for small-volume ultrasonic nebulizer
    Code _____

    6. Enteral nutrition infusion pump with alarm
    Code _____

    7. Pair of wooden underarm crutches
    Code _____

    8. Raised toilet seat
    Code _____

    9. Hospital bed with mattress, semi-electric
    Code _____

    10. Standard adult manual wheelchair
    Code _____

    11. 40 mg of methylprednisolone acetate, injection
    Code _____

    12. Chemotherapy administration by push
    Code _____

    13. Surgical boot, left foot
    Code _____

3. In your own words, how can you help to code medical services and procedures ethically?

    _____

    _____

    _____

    _____

    _____

REVIEW QUESTIONS

MATCHING

Choose the correct answer and place its corresponding letter in the space provided.

a. progress note
b. clean claim
c. fraud
d. Federal Civil False Claims Act
e. abuse

1. _____ Intentional deception when submitting or coding claims
2. _____ Updates the patient's clinical course of treatment and summarizes the assessment and plan of care
3. _____ An action that misuses the money that the government has allocated, such as Medicare funds
4. _____ A claim without errors that displays proper code linkage
5. _____ Prohibits making fraudulent statements or representation in connection with a claim and outlines liability of these fraudulent acts

MULTIPLE CHOICE

Circle the letter of each choice that best completes the statement or answers the question.

1. Which of the following is a type of law that can prohibit a physician from practicing as a provider to government health programs?
   a. Civil
   b. Criminal
   c. Administrative
   d. None of the above

2. Which of the following is a type of law that requires that an individual who is found guilty can be subject to serving a jail sentence?
   a. Civil
   b. Criminal
   c. Administrative
   d. None of the above

3. Which of the following is a type of law that requires that if an individual is found guilty, awards monies and can order fines?
   a. Civil
   b. Criminal
   c. Administrative
   d. None of the above

4. Which of the following does the Stark law govern?
   a. Compliance plans
   b. Fraud and abuse
   c. Physician self-referral
   d. All of the above

5. Which of the following is *not* a benefit of having a voluntary compliance program?

    a. Reducing the chances of an external audit

    b. Avoiding conflicts with the self-referral and antikickbacks statutes

    c. Speeding and optimizing proper payment of claims

    d. All of the above are benefits of having a voluntary compliance program.

SHORT ANSWER

Provide the correct response to each question that follows.

1. What are seven consequences of inaccurate coding and incorrect billing?

    1. _____

    2. _____

    3. _____

    4. _____

    5. _____

    6. _____

    7. _____

2. What five questions can you ask yourself to ensure that a claim is "clean" for submittal?

    1. _____

    2. _____

    3. _____

    4. _____

    5. _____

3. What are HCPCS codes that begin with J usually used for?

    _____

    _____

4. What program was created by HIPAA to uncover fraud and abuse in Medicare and Medicaid programs?

    _____

    _____

5. What are the four parts of government that investigate and prosecute suspected medical fraud and abuse under the HIPAA program described in question #4?

    1. _____

    2. _____

    3. _____

    4. _____

TRUE/FALSE

Identify each statement as true (T) or false (F).

1. _____ If a physician has poor documentation, this opens up the clinic to issues with fraud and abuse.

2. _____ It doesn't matter in what order procedure codes are listed on the CMS-1500 claim form, as long as the claim includes every procedure rendered.

3. _____ To encourage whistleblowing of suspected fraud and abuse against the government, the reporting persons involved can be offered protection and rewards.

4. _____ Occasional billing and coding errors can be interpreted as possible fraud.

5. _____ If a physician claims that he/she didn't know about billing and coding guidelines, then he/she will not be held liable for errors.

CHAPTER 10

Auditing

CHAPTER OBJECTIVES

Upon completion of this chapter in your student text, you should be able to do the following:

1. Understand and know how to implement a coding audit.
2. Be able to review and analyze medical records.
3. Know how to use an audit tool.
4. Recognize the content and documentation requirements.
5. Demonstrate the ability to review for coding accuracy.

CHAPTER OUTLINE

Purpose of an Audit

Types of Audits
    External Audit
    Internal Audit
    Accreditation Audits

Private Payer Regulations

Medical Necessity for E/M Services

Audit Tool

Key Elements of Service
    History
    Examination
    Medical Decision Making

Tips for Preventing Coding Errors with Specific E/M Codes

KEY TERMS

Using the highlighted terms and glossary in the textbook, define the following terms:

1. audit _____

    _____

2. code edits _____

    _____

3. downcode _____

    _____

4. external audit _____

_____

5. internal audit _____

_____

6. Patient Protection and Affordable Care Act (PPACA) _____

_____

7. prospective audit _____

_____

8. retrospective audit _____

_____

9. upcode _____

_____

CRITICAL THINKING QUESTIONS

Using the knowledge you have gained from reading the textbook, apply critical thinking skills to answer the following questions:

1. Answer the following questions related to medical audits:

   a. In your own words, what is the main purpose of an audit?

   _____

   _____

   _____

   _____

   _____

   b. Why should a medical office perform an internal audit?

   _____

   _____

   _____

   _____

   c. Medicare has scheduled an audit with your medical practice. What will the auditor check during the audit?

   _____

   _____

   _____

   _____

   _____

2. What is medical necessity for the E/M codes based on?

   _____

   _____

   _____

3. a. Read the following scenarios, and determine which type of HPI is being conducted in each one:

1. A patient is seen for asthma, chronic bronchitis, and chronic sinusitis. The patient complains of facial pain for three days now. He has been coughing up greenish-brown mucus. He denies any chest tightness or wheezing.

2. A patient presents in the office with complaints of watering, redness, and pain in her left eye that started this morning.

b. Read the following scenarios and determine which type of ROS is being conducted in each one:

1. A patient is seen for asthma, chronic bronchitis, and chronic sinusitis. The patient complains of facial pain for three days now. He has been coughing up greenish-brown mucus. He denies any chest tightness or wheezing. The Physician examines the ears, nose, and throat. TMs are clear. The nose is red and swollen. The throat shows postnasal drip. On A&P, the chest presents with congestion. No wheezing or rub is heard. Bowels sounds are normal. Skin shows no clubbing, cyanosis, or breaks.

2. A patient is seen for a follow-up on congestive heart failure (CHF), hypertension (HTN), and hypothyroidism. She has no complaints at this time. Vitals are stable. BP: 132/70, P: 82, R: 14. HEENT: Normocephalic, atraumatic. Eyes are clear. Pupils are equal, round, and reactive to light. TMs are clear. Oropharynx is clear. Back exam is negative. Chest is negative for wheezes, rubs, or rhonchi. CARDIOVASCULAR: S1, S2 present with normal rhythm and rate. GI: Bowel sounds normal. No visceromegaly, nausea, vomiting, diarrhea, or constipation. Abdomen is soft, non-tender. GU: No urinary retention is noted. HEMIC/LYMPHATIC: No lymphadenopathy. MS: No pain or injuries. EXTREMITIES: No bruising or clubbing. Pedal pulses normal. No pitting edema present. SKIN: No lesions or rashes. NEUROLOGIC: Patient is oriented ×3. PSYCHIATRIC: Mood and affect is upbeat and pleasant.

c. Read the following scenario and determine which type of PFSH is being conducted:

1. Patient has no known drug allergies (KNDA). He is a nonsmoker. He drinks two to three glasses of wine a month. Patient lives with his wife. He has no children. His mother is alive and well. She has DM II. Father's health is unknown. He has one sibling that also has DM II. He has had no operations. He was hospitalized at age 21 with cellulitis as a result of an infected tattoo on his right calf.

d. Refer back to question #3 in b 2. What type of exam is being performed on this patient?

4. Answer the following questions related to proper documentation for the selection of a correct E/M code under auditing compliance:

a. You are reviewing the physician's documentation for a patient's ROS. The physician has written that the patient's blood count is abnormal. There is no other specific data entered concerning the abnormal blood count. Is this acceptable documentation? Why or why not?

b. A physician does not examine the patient's abdomen, but documents that exam is normal. Is this acceptable documentation? Why or why not?

_____

_____

_____

c. A physician documents EENT as negative, but did not review the eyes. Is this acceptable? Why or why not?

_____

_____

_____

d. A physician has documented that a patient's cardiovascular system is "unremarkable." Is this acceptable documentation? Why or why not?

_____

_____

_____

5. Answer the following questions related to medical decision making (MDM) in selection of a proper E/M code:

a. How can the number and type of diagnosed tests performed help the coder to select the proper MDM?

_____

_____

_____

b. What information must be included for a physician to properly document the number of diagnoses and/or treatment options for a patient?

1. _____

2. _____

3. _____

4. _____

c. What information needs to be included for a physician to properly document the amount and/or complexity of data reviewed?

1. _____

2. _____

3. _____

4. _____

5. _____

6. _____

d. What types of health risks to a patient are taken into consideration by physicians when selecting the correct E/M code?

1. _____

2. _____

3. _____

PRACTICE EXERCISES

1. From Chapter 10 in your text, read the scenarios described next and identify what type of coding error has occurred. Write your answer in the space provided.

a. A physician sees a patient in the ER for an ear infection. The E/M code used is 99285.

_____

b. A physician bills for reviewing x-rays with the patient, but does not document this in the chart.

_____

c. A new patient is seen for abdominal pain; only one key component is documented.

_____

d. An established patient is seen for chest pain and has several issues; all five key components are documented.

_____

e. The attending physician sees a patient for an initial inpatient visit. The RN has already documented the HPI. The physician documents only the diagnoses and treatment plans.

_____

f. A physician codes for critical care for a patient. The chart does not indicate any direct personal management or frequent personal assessment and manipulation.

_____

g. A neurologist submits a code for an inpatient consultation. There is no clear order in this patient's chart. The coding specialist codes for the consultation.

_____

2. What two steps should be taken to prepare for an internal audit?

1. _____

2. _____

3. Using the audit tools and tables provided in Chapter 10 of your text, read the following scenarios and identify the correct E/M code for each:

a. A patient is seen for the first time by her family physician, complaining of a shooting left-leg pain that starts in her lumbar spine and travels down to her toes. This started about a month ago and occurs every couple of days. She says that it lasts for almost the whole day. She has a family history of heart disease. She denies smoking, taking drugs, and alcohol use. She does work as a relay operator for BU&U. Her job requires her to sit for long periods of time. ROS reveals associated pain with palpation on her left lumbar region. The rest of the musculoskeletal system is negative for pain, edema, or ROM limitations. The cardiovascular system shows no signs of bruit, heart murmur, or circulatory problems. Pedal pulses X 3. BP: 118/72, P: 80. She denies headaches. No blurred vision. Skin intact without clubbing, cyanosis, or rash.

GI: No distention, heartburn, or diarrhea. Abdomen is soft to palpation and nontender. Patient is pleasant, alert, and oriented X 3. The severity and location of the pain can lead to impairment if not treated immediately. Diagnosis of sciatica. Patient to start Medrol Dose Pak, have x-ray of lumbar spine and left leg, upper. Patient to return in 1 week to assess the nature of physical therapy versus surgery. If the x-rays are negative, she will be sent for an MRI of the lumbar spine.

1. Is this patient being seen as an inpatient or outpatient?

_____

2. Is this patient new or established?

_____

3. What is the proper E/M code?

_____

b. A patient is seeing his PCP for a cough and scratchy throat that started 3 days ago. He also admits to sneezing more often than usual. The patient is a smoker: Two packs a day X 6 years. He has no past history of allergies. On review, HEENT shows watery, red eyes, inflammation in the nasal mucosa, and a reddened throat. Head and ears are unremarkable to exam. There is noted postnasal drainage. Chest is clear to auscultation and percussion. Diagnosis is acute sinusitis with allergic rhinitis. He is prescribed amoxicillin and Nasonex. Patient is to use Claritin OTC. He is to return to the office if his seasonal allergies persist.

1. Is this patient being seen as an inpatient or outpatient?

_____

2. Is this patient new or established?

_____

3. What is the proper E/M code?

_____

c. A patient is being seen for the second day of her hospital course for CHF. She has a history of malignant hypertension that has affected her kidney function in the past. She has never smoked and doesn't drink. She denies any increased salt intake before this episode. ROS is consistent with HPI and past history. Kidneys show worsened state than yesterday, and the thoracentesis will have to be postponed until the patient's kidney function is stable.

1. Is this patient being seen as an inpatient or outpatient?

_____

2. Is this initial or subsequent care?

_____

3. What is the proper E/M code?

_____

d. A patient is being seen today by the dermatologist, per her PCP. This patient presents with complaints of adult cystic acne that keeps getting worse as he ages. It started when he was 19 years old. He has tried OTC products and prescription medication, without relief. He is here to discuss his options. He denies any family members with cystic acne. On exam, there is cystic acne noted on the face, shoulders, and back. He was here last month and started on oral and topical antibiotics. Since then, there is no improvement. His face appears dry and cracked. The option of using Accutane for the treatment of his acne was discussed. He is given the information and is told to read it thoroughly. He will need to obtain fasting labs before and during treatment to assess any liver, sugar, or circulatory problems. He is to call the office with any questions before his next appointment in a week. He will need to sign all consenting papers and return them at this appointment.

He understands the treatment, side effects, and possible adverse reactions, including suicidal tendencies. If the labs present as normal and he consents to this treatment, we will proceed with the prescription and regimen.

1. Is this patient being seen as an inpatient or outpatient?

_____

2. What type of encounter is this?

_____

3. What is the proper E/M code?

_____

REVIEW QUESTIONS

MATCHING

Choose the correct answer and write its corresponding letter in the space provided.

a. HPI
b. PFSH
c. ROS
d. organ systems
e. chief complaint

1. ____ Elements that include operations, hospitalizations, and personal health
2. ____ Elements that include eyes, ears, nose, throat, skin, and psychiatric
3. ____ An inventory of body systems obtained by a series of questions
4. ____ Elements that include the patient's current health problem in the patient's own words
5. ____ Elements that include timing, duration, location, severity, and context

MULTIPLE CHOICE

Circle the letter of each choice that best completes the statement or answers the question.

1. Who would normally perform an internal audit?
   a. Outside agency
   b. Consultant
   c. Employee
   d. Both b and c

2. Which types of CPT codes are audited the most?
   a. Surgery
   b. Radiology
   c. E/M
   d. Medicine

3. The first step in determining an E/M code is to
   a. count all diagnoses.
   b. determine whether the patient is new or established.
   c. determine whether the encounter involves a complete ROS.
   d. Both a and c

4. Which of the following questions alerts the coder *not* to code as a consultation?

    a. Has the provider provided a written report of opinion/advice to the referring physician?

    b. Was a request for an opinion from another physician received?

    c. Will the provider's opinion be used by and affect the requesting physician's own management of the patient?

    d. All of the above.

5. Which of the following qualifies for coding critical care services?

    a. There is a lack of documented work.

    b. The physician consulted the surrogate decision-making family member.

    c. The specific time spent is not recorded.

    d. Time spent performing procedures is included.

SHORT ANSWER

Provide the correct response to each question that follows.

1. What are two ways an audit can be performed? _____

    1. _____

    2. _____

2. What are the two main ways that medical necessity of E/M services is generally expressed?

    1. _____

    2. _____

3. If the OIG finds an auditing problem in a certain area, what will be the result?

_____

4. When is time considered the key factor to assigning a proper E/M code?

_____

5. What are the 15 top coding and documentation errors?

    1. _____

    2. _____

    3. _____

    4. _____

    5. _____

    6. _____

    7. _____

    8. _____

    9. _____

    10. _____

    11. _____

    12. _____

    13. _____

    14. _____

    15. _____

TRUE/FALSE

Identify each statement as true (T) or false (F).

1. _____ The auditor should check to see that the physician properly documents and compare with code assignment.

2. _____ Even though most third-party payers may have their own rules for submitting a clean claim, most states do not require third-party payers to give a reason for a denied claim.

3. _____ A physician can perform both a multisystem and single-organ exam during one encounter.

4. _____ An audit tool can be used for internal audits, as well as external audits.

5. _____ Auditing software will always match all third-party payers' policies for a clean claim.

CHAPTER 11
Physician Medical Billing

CHAPTER OBJECTIVES

Upon completion of this chapter in your student text, you should be able to do the following:

1. Differentiate and complete medical claim forms accurately, both manually and electronically.
2. Define claim form parts, sections, and required information.
3. Exhibit the ability to complete claim forms without omitting information.
4. Understand the common reasons why claim forms are delayed or rejected, and submit a claim without payer rejection.
5. File a secondary claim.

CHAPTER OUTLINE

Patient Information

Superbills

Types of Insurance Claims: Paper vs. Electronic

Optical Character Recognition

CMS-1500 Provider Billing Claim Form

Completing the CMS-1500 Claim Form
Form Locators for the CMS-1500 Form

Physicians' Identification Numbers
Practice Exercises

Common Reasons for Delayed or Rejected CMS-1500 Claim Forms

HIPAA Compliance Alert

Filing Secondary Claims
Determining Primary Coverage
Practice Exercises

KEY TERMS

Using the highlighted terms and glossary in the textbook, define the following terms:

1. assignment of benefits form _____

_____

2. audit/edit report _____

_____

3. billing services _____

_____

4. birthday rule _____

_____

5. claim attachment _____

_____

6. clean claims _____

_____

7. clearinghouse _____

_____

8. CMS-1500 claim form _____

_____

9. coordination of benefits (COB) _____

_____

10. dirty claim _____

_____

11. electronic claims, electronic media claims (EMCs) _____

_____

12. encryption _____

_____

13. employer identification number (EIN) _____

_____

14. facility provider number (FPN) _____

_____

15. form locators _____

_____

16. group provider number (GPN) _____

_____

17. guarantor _____

_____

18. optical character recognition (OCR) _____

_____

19. patient information form _____

_____

20. provider identification number (PIN) _____

_____

21. release of information form _____

    _____

22. secondary insurance _____

    _____

23. state license number _____

    _____

24. superbills _____

    _____

25. supplemental insurance _____

    _____

26. tax identification number (TIN) _____

    _____

27. UB-04 claim form _____

    _____

28. verification of benefits (VOB) form _____

    _____

CRITICAL THINKING QUESTIONS

Using the knowledge you have gained from reading the textbook, apply critical thinking skills to answer the following questions.

1. Answer the following questions related to verification of a patient's insurance benefits:

    a. By what three steps can verifying insurance benefits for a patient be accomplished?

        1. _____

        2. _____

        3. _____

    b. Charles Bingham, Jr., is a new patient with your office. What nine pertinent pieces of information do you need when verifying his insurance benefits?

        1. _____

        2. _____

        3. _____

        4. _____

        5. _____

        6. _____

        7. _____

        8. _____

        9. _____

c. Now that you have gathered all nine pieces of pertinent information to verify Mr. Bingham's insurance benefits, what are the standard questions that you ask his insurance carrier for this verification?

1. _____

2. _____

3. _____

4. _____

5. _____

6. _____

7. _____

8. _____

2. What is the superbill, and how is it used for billing?

1. _____

2. _____

3. _____

3. Answer the following questions related to medical claim forms:

a. What claim form does the following type of provider use for reimbursement?

1. Physicians _____

2. Hospitals _____

b. List the three advantages of electronic claim forms.

1. _____

2. _____

3. _____

_____

_____

_____

c. What do you do if an insurance carrier requires additional information for an electronic claim?

_____

_____

_____

d. What are the three advantages of an electronic claim?

1. _____

2. _____

3. _____

e. What are the four disadvantages of an electronic claim?

1. _____
2. _____
3. _____
4. _____

f. What are two advantages of OCR devices?

1. _____
2. _____

4. a. What is the purpose of the HIPAA security standard rules?

_____
_____
_____
_____

b. Work together in a small group to list the six ways that your office complies with the HIPAA security standard rules. Discuss your answers with the class.

1. _____
2. _____
3. _____
4. _____
5. _____
6. _____

c. What could be the result of breaching a patient's confidentiality?

_____
_____
_____
_____

5. a. Read the following scenarios and determine which insurance policy is the primary insurance:

1. Sara Lind is has both Medicare and Blue Cross/Blue Shield insurance. She is retired, but is covered under her husband's Blue Cross/Blue Shield plan. Mr. Lind works for the postal service. Which insurance will be her primary insurance?

_____

2. Miranda Lee has two insurance policies under which she is the primary policyholder for both. Which insurance will be her primary insurance?

_____

3. Benjamin Nadzam has two insurance policies. He is the policyholder of his Aetna plan, but he is also covered as a dependent under his father's Health America plan. Which insurance will be his primary insurance?

_____

4. Nolan Espinosa has health insurance coverage through his employer's Blue Cross/Blue Shield plan. He is also covered through Medicare. Which insurance will be his primary insurance?

_____

5. Cheyenne Yanul has insurance through both of her parents. Her parents are still married. Which insurance will be her primary insurance?

_____

6. If Cheyenne's parents are divorced and do not share joint custody of Cheyenne, how can her primary insurance plan be determined?

_____

_____

_____

b. How would you submit a secondary claim?

_____

_____

_____

PRACTICE EXERCISES

1. Using the form locator information supplied in your textbook, write each form locator's directions for the CMS-1500 on an index card. Flag each form locator for easy referencing.

2. Define the following CMS-1500 abbreviations:
    1. CCYY _____
    2. CHAMPUS _____
    3. INFO _____
    4. CMS _____
    5. CPT _____
    6. ICD-9-CM _____
    7. ID _____
    8. MM _____
    9. CLIA _____
   10. M _____
   11. EIN_____
   12. DD _____
   13. EMG _____

3. The case studies that follow are provided for additional practice in completing the CMS-1500 claim form for physician outpatient billing. By applying what you have learned in your student text, you are to accurately code and complete each case study. Patient demographics and a brief case history are provided. Complete the cases on the basis of the following criteria:

- All patients have release of information and assignment of benefit signatures on file.

- All providers are participating and accept assignment by contractual agreement. Item 27 is not marked.

- The group practice is the billing entity.

- The national transition to NPI numbers is complete, and legacy PINs of individual payers are no longer used. If legacy PINs are still being used by selected payers in your region, your instructor may provide legacy PINS in addition to the NPI.

- 2012 ICD-9-CM and CPT codes are used.

- Use eight-digit dates for birthdates. Use six-digit dates for all other dates.

- All street names should be entered with standard postal abbreviations, even if they are spelled out on the source documents.

- Enter ICD-9 codes in the order in which they appear on the encounter form.

- When entering CPT codes, enter the E/M code first. Enter remaining codes in descending price order.

To determine the correct fees, refer to the Capital City Medical Fee Schedule, a copy of which is located after each case's source documents. Use the blank CMS-1500 form provided after each case.

a. Using the given source documents, the Capital City Medical Fee Schedule (Figure 11-1), and the blank CMS-1500 form provided (Figure 11-2), complete the following case study for patient Hayden Montana (case 11-1):

CASE 11-1

Capital City Medical—123 Unknown Boulevard, Capital City, NY 12345-2222 (555) 555-1234 Phil Wells, MD, Mannie Mends, MD, Bette R. Soone, MD	**Patient Information Form** Tax ID: 75-0246810 Group NPI: 1513171216

Patient Information:

Name: (Last, First) <u>Montana, Hayden</u> ❑ Male ☒ Female Birth Date: <u>06/26/2010</u>

Address: <u>60 Grove St. Capital City, NY 12345</u> Phone: (555) <u>555-1253</u>

Social Security Number: <u>346-82-3077</u> Full-Time Student: ❑ Yes ☒ No

Marital Status: ☒ Single ❑ Married ❑ Divorced ❑ Other

Employment:

Employer: <u>N/A</u> Phone: ( ) _____

Address: _____

Condition Related to: ❑ Auto Accident ❑ Employment ❑ Other Accident

Date of Accident: _____ State: _____

Emergency Contact: _____ **Phone: ( )** _____

Primary Insurance: <u>Blue Cross Blue Shield</u> Phone: ( ) _____

Address: <u>379 Blue Plaza, Capital City, NY 12345</u>

Insurance Policyholder's Name: <u>Jordan Montana</u> ☒ M ❑ F DOB: <u>05/12/1979</u>

Address: <u>Same</u>

Phone: ( ) _____ Relationship to Insured: ❑ Self ❑ Spouse ☒ Child ❑ Other

Employer: <u>Capital City Police Department</u> Phone: (555) <u>555-0911</u>

Employer's Address: <u>3055 Samaritan Blvd, Capital City, NY 12345</u>

Policy/ID No: <u>YYZ401333213</u> Group No: <u>064835</u> Percent Covered: ___% Copay Amt: $<u>25.00</u>

Secondary Insurance: <u>Aetna</u> Phone: ( ) _____

Address: <u>1625 Healthcare Bldg, Capital City, NY 12345</u>

Insurance Policyholder's Name: <u>Riley Montana</u> ❑ M ☒ F DOB: <u>08/19/1979</u>

Address: <u>Same</u>

Phone: ( ) _____ Relationship to Insured: ❑ Self ❑ Spouse ☒ Child ❑ Other

Employer: <u>The Daily Globe Co.</u> Phone: (555) <u>555-5757</u>

Employer's Address: <u>19 W. Eastern Rd, Capital City, NY 12345</u>

Policy/ID No: <u>32059138</u> Group No: <u>3132</u> Percent Covered: <u>80</u> % Copay Amt: $_____

Reason for Visit: <u>Rash and fever</u>

Known Allergies: _____

Referred by: _____

CASE 11-1
SOAP

02/11/20XX
Assignment of Benefits: Y
Signature on File: Y
Referring Physician: N

S: Hayden Montana presents in the office with her mother today for complaints of a fever and a rash.

O: The rash appeared two days ago and seems to be getting worse. She does have a temperature of 101.8°F. There is no vomiting at this time.

A: 1. Measles–055.9

P: 1. Liquid diet and plenty of rest.
2. Children's Tylenol.
3. Go to ER if temperature elevates.
4. Home from school until next appointment.
5. Return in 7 days.

_____

Phil Wells, MD
Family Practice
NPI: 1234567890

CASE 11-1

Patient Name Hayden Montana

Capital City Medical
123 Unknown Boulevard, Capital City, NY 12345-2222

Date of Service
02-11-20XX

New Patient			Arthrocentesis/Aspiration/Injection			Laboratory	
Problem Focused	99201		Small Joint		20600	Amylase	82150
Expanded Problem, Focused	99202		Interm Joint		20605	B12	82607
Detailed	99203		Major Joint		20610	CBC & Diff	85025
Comprehensive	99204		**Other Invasive/Noninvasive**			Comp Metabolic Panel	80053
Comprehensive/High Complex	99205		Audiometry		92552	Chlamydia Screen	87110
Well Exam Infant (up to 12 mos.)	99381		Cast Application			Cholesterol	82465
Well Exam 1–4 yrs.	99382		Location Long Short			Digoxin	80162
Well Exam 5–11 yrs.	99383		Catheterization		51701	Electrolytes	80051
Well Exam 12–17 yrs.	99384		Circumcision		54150	Ferritin	82728
Well Exam 18–39 yrs.	99385		Colposcopy		57452	Folate	82746
Well Exam 40–64 yrs.	99386		Colposcopy w/Biopsy		57454	GC Screen	87070
			Cryosurgery Premalignant Lesion			Glucose	82947
			Location (s):			Glucose 1 HR	82950
						Glycosylated HGB A1C	83036
Established Patient			Cryosurgery Warts			HCT	85014
Post-Op Follow Up Visit	99024		Location (s):			HDL	83718
Minimum	99211		Curettement Lesion			Hep BSAG	87340
Problem Focused	99212	X	Single		11055	Hepatitis panel, acute	80074
Expanded Problem Focused	99213		2–4		11056	HGB	85018
Detailed	99214		>4		11057	HIV	86703
Comprehensive/High Complex	99215		Diaphragm Fitting		57170	Iron & TIBC	83550
Well Exam Infant (up to 12 mos.)	99391		Ear Irrigation		69210	Kidney Profile	80069
Well exam 1–4 yrs.	99392		ECG		93000	Lead	83655
Well Exam 5–11 yrs.	99393		Endometrial Biopsy		58100	Liver Profile	80076
Well Exam 12–17 yrs.	99394		Exc. Lesion Malignant			Mono Test	86308
Well Exam 18–39 yrs.	99395		Benign			Pap Smear	88155
Well Exam 40–64 yrs.	99396		Location			Pregnancy Test	84703
Obstetrics			Exc. Skin Tags (1–15)		11200	Obstetric Panel	80055
Total OB Care	59400		Each Additional 10		11201	Pro Time	85610
Injections			Fracture Treatment			PSA	84153
Administration Sub. / IM	90772		Loc			RPR	86592
Drug			w/Reduc	w/o Reduc		Sed. Rate	85651
Dosage			I & D Abscess Single/Simple		10060	Stool Culture	87045
Allergy	95115		Multiple or Comp		10061	Stool O & P	87177
Cocci Skin Test	86490		I & D Pilonidal Cyst Simple		10080	Strep Screen	87880
DPT	90701		Pilonidal Cyst Complex		10081	Theophylline	80198
Hemophilus	90646		IV Therapy—To One Hour		90760	Thyroid Uptake	84479
Influenza	90658		Each Additional Hour		90761	TSH	84443
MMR	90707		Laceration Repair			Urinalysis	81000
OPV	90712		Location Size Simp/Comp			Urine Culture	87088
Pneumovax	90732		Laryngoscopy		31505	Drawing Fee	36415
TB Skin Test	86580		Oximetry		94760	Specimen Collection	99000
TD	90718		Punch Biopsy			**Other:**	
Unlisted Immun	90749		Rhythm Strip		93040		
Tetanus Toxoid	90703		Treadmill		93015		
Vaccine/Toxoid Admin <8 Yr Old w/ Counseling	90465		Trigger Point or Tendon Sheath Inj.		20550		
Vaccine/Toxoid Administration for Adult	90471		Tympanometry		92567		

Diagnosis/ICD-9: **055.9**

I acknowledge receipt of medical services and authorize the release of any medical information necessary to process this claim for healthcare payment only. I do authorize payment to the provider.

Patient Signature _Jordan Montana_

Total Estimated Charges: _____

Payment Amount: _____

Next Appointment: _____

Figure 11-1

Capital City Medical
Fee Schedule

New Patient OV		Punch Biopsy various codes	$80
Problem Focused 99201	$45	Nebulizer various codes	$45
Expanded Problem Focused 99202	$65	Cast Application various codes	$85
Detailed 99203	$85	Laryngoscopy 31505	$255
Comprehensive 99204	$105	Audiometry 92552	$85
Comprehensive/High Complex 99205	$115	Tympanometry 92567	$85
Well Exam infant (less than 1 year) 99381	$45	Ear Irrigation 69210	$25
Well Exam 1–4 yrs. 99382	$50	Diaphragm Fitting 57170	$30
Well Exam 5–11 yrs. 99383	$55	IV Therapy (up to one hour) 90760	$65
Well Exam 12–17 yrs. 99384	$65	Each additional hour 90761	$50
Well Exam 18–39 yrs. 99385	$85	Oximetry 94760	$10
Well Exam 40–64 yrs. 99386	$105	ECG 93000	$75
Established Patient OV		Holter Monitor various codes	$170
Post Op Follow Up Visit 99024	$0	Rhythm Strip 93040	$60
Minimum 99211	$35	Treadmill 93015	$375
Problem Focused 99212	$45	Cocci Skin Test 86490	$20
Expanded Problem Focused 99213	$55	X-ray, spine, chest, bone—any area various codes	$275
Detailed 99214	$65	Avulsion Nail 11730	$200
Comprehensive/High Complex 99215	$75	**Laboratory**	
Well exam infant (less than 1 year) 99391	$35	Amylase 82150	$40
Well Exam 1–4 yrs. 99392	$40	B12 82607	$30
Well Exam 5–11 yrs. 99393	$45	CBC & Diff 85025	$95
Well Exam 12–17 yrs. 99394	$55	Comp Metabolic Panel 80053	$75
Well Exam 18–39 yrs. 99395	$65	Chlamydia Screen 87110	$70
Well Exam 40–64 yrs. 99396	$75	Cholestrerol 82465	$75
Obstetrics		Digoxin 80162	$40
Total OB Care 59400	$1700	Electrolytes 80051	$70
Injections		Estrogen, Total 82672	$50
Administration 90772	$10	Ferritin 82728	$40
Allergy 95115	$35	Folate 82746	$30
DPT 90701	$50	GC Screen 87070	$60
Drug various codes	$35	Glucose 82947	$35
Influenza 90658	$25	Glycosylated HGB A1C 83036	$45
MMR 90707	$50	HCT 85014	$30
OPV 90712	$40	HDL 83718	$35
Pneumovax 90732	$35	HGB 85018	$30
TB Skin Test 86580	$15	Hep BSAG 83740	$40
TD 90718	$40	Hepatitis panel, acute 80074	$95
Tetanus Toxoid 90703	$40	HIV 86703	$100
Vaccine/Toxoid Administration for Younger		Iron & TIBC 83550	$45
Than 8 Years Old w/ counseling 90465	$10	Kidney Profile 80069	$95
Vaccine/Toxoid Administration for Adult 90471	$10	Lead 83665	$55
Arthrocentesis/Aspiration/Injection		Lipase 83690	$40
Small Joint 20600	$50	Lipid Panel 80061	$95
Interm Joint 20605	$60	Liver Profile 80076	$95
Major Joint 20610	$70	Mono Test 86308	$30
Trigger Point/Tendon Sheath Inj. 20550	$90	Pap Smear 88155	$90
Other Invasive/Noninvasive Procedures		Pap Collection/Supervision 88142	$95
Catheterization 51701	$55	Pregnancy Test 84703	$90
Circumcision 54150	$150	Obstetric Panel 80055	$85
Colposcopy 57452	$225	Pro Time 85610	$50
Colposcopy w/Biopsy 57454	$250	PSA 84153	$50
Cryosurgery Premalignant Lesion various codes	$160	RPR 86592	$55
Endometrial Biopsy 58100	$190	Sed. Rate 85651	$50
Excision Lesion Malignant various codes	$145	Stool Culture 87045	$80
Excision Lesion Benign various codes	$125	Stool O & P 87177	$105
Curettement Lesion		Strep Screen 87880	$35
Single 11055	$70	Theophylline 80198	$40
2–4 11056	$80	Thyroid Uptake 84479	$75
>4 11057	$90	TSH 84443	$50
Excision Skin Tags (1–15) 11200	$55	Urinalysis 81000	$35
Each Additional 10 11201	$30	Urine Culture 87088	$80
I & D Abscess Single/Simple 10060	$75	Drawing Fee 36415	$15
Multiple/Complex 10061	$95	Specimen Collection 99000	$10
I & D Pilonidal Cyst Simple 10080	$105		
I & D Pilonidal Cyst Complex 10081	$130		
Laceration Repair various codes	$60		

HEALTH INSURANCE CLAIM FORM

APPROVED BY NATIONAL UNIFORM CLAIM COMMITTEE 08/05

Figure 11-2

b. Using the given source documents, the Capital City Medical Fee Schedule (Figure 11-3), and the blank CMS-1500 form provided (Figure 11-4), complete the following case study for patient Eric Avery (Case 11-2):

CASE 11-2

Capital City Medical—123 Unknown Boulevard, Capital City, NY 12345-2222 (555) 555-1234	Patient Information Form
	Tax ID: 75-0246810
Phil Wells, MD, Mannie Mends, MD, Bette R. Soone, MD	Group NPI: 1513171216

Patient Information:

Name: (Last, First) Avery, Eric   ☒ Male   ☐ Female   Birth Date: 09/21/1997

Address: 803 Highland Ave, Capital, NY 12345   Phone: (555) 555-1759

Social Security Number: 298-22-3647   Full-Time Student: ☐ Yes   ☒ No

Marital Status: ☒ Single   ☐ Married   ☐ Divorced   ☐ Other

Employment:

Employer: N/A   Phone: ( )

Address:

Condition Related to: ☐ Auto Accident   ☐ Employment   ☐ Other Accident

Date of Accident: State:

Emergency Contact: **Phone: ( )**

Primary Insurance: Blue Cross Blue Shield   Phone: ( )

Address: 379 Blue Plaza, Capital City, NY 12345

Insurance Policyholder's Name: Lex Avery   ☒ M   ☐ F   DOB: 07/14/1980

Address: Same

Phone: ( )   Relationship to Insured: ☐ Self   ☐ Spouse   ☒ Child   ☐ Other

Employer: Avery and Associates   Phone: (555) 555-0911

Employer's Address: 4587 Plaza South, Capital City, NY 12345

Policy/ID No: YYZ236548722   Group No: 789654 Percent Covered: ____% Copay Amt: $15.00

Secondary Insurance: Phone: ( )

Address:

Insurance Policyholder's Name: ☐ M   ☐ F   DOB:

Address:

Phone: ( )   Relationship to Insured: ☐ Self   ☐ Spouse   ☐ Child   ☐ Other

Employer: Phone: ( )

Employer's Address:

Policy/ID No: Group No: ____ Percent Covered: ____% Copay Amt: $____

Reason for Visit: Rash and fever

Known Allergies:

Referred by:

CASE 11-2
SOAP

05/18/20XX
Assignment of Benefits: Y
Signature on File: Y
Referring Physician: N

S: Eric Avery is being seen today for a rash on his lower abdomen. He noticed it yesterday. It is itchy and painful.

O: On review, this rash is found to be infected and appears tender. The infection looks localized at this time. The Pt. denies vomiting, diarrhea, and tiredness. Presently, a student at his school does have a case of MRSA.

A: 1. Methicillin-resistant staphylococcus aureus (MRSA)—041.11, V09.0, 686.9

P: 1. Will treat with oral antibiotics and hydrocortisone cream.

2. Home from school until next appointment.

3. Pt. to stay indoors.

4. Keep linens and clothing clean.

5. Mother and father aware of progressive symptoms, and to call if infection and/or symptoms worsen.

6. Return in 5 days.

Phil Wells, MD
Family Practice
NPI: 1234567890

CASE 11-2

Patient Name Eric Avery

Capital City Medical
123 Unknown Boulevard, Capital City, NY 12345-2222

Date of Service
05-18-20XX

New Patient			Other Invasive/Noninvasive			Laboratory	
Problem Focused	99201		Arthrocentesis/Aspiration/Injection			Amylase	82150
Expanded Problem, Focused	99202		Small Joint	20600		B12	82607
Detailed	99203		Interm Joint	20605		CBC & Diff	85025
Comprehensive	99204		Major Joint	20610		Comp Metabolic Panel	80053
Comprehensive/High Complex	99205		**Other Invasive/Noninvasive**			Chlamydia Screen	87110
Well Exam Infant (up to 12 mos.)	99381		Audiometry	92552		Cholesterol	82465
Well Exam 1–4 yrs.	99382		Cast Application			Digoxin	80162
Well Exam 5–11 yrs.	99383		Location Long Short			Electrolytes	80051
Well Exam 12–17 yrs.	99384		Catheterization	51701		Ferritin	82728
Well Exam 18–39 yrs.	99385		Circumcision	54150		Folate	82746
Well Exam 40–64 yrs.	99386		Colposcopy	57452		GC Screen	87070
			Colposcopy w/Biopsy	57454		Glucose	82947
			Cryosurgery Premalignant Lesion			Glucose 1 HR	82950
			Location (s):			Glycosylated HGB A1C	83036
Established Patient			Cryosurgery Warts			HCT	85014
Post-Op Follow Up Visit	99024		Location (s):			HDL	83718
Minimum	99211		Curettement Lesion			Hep BSAG	87340
Problem Focused	99212		Single	11055		Hepatitis panel, acute	80074
Expanded Problem Focused	99213	X	2–4	11056		HGB	85018
Detailed	99214		>4	11057		HIV	86703
Comprehensive/High Complex	99215		Diaphragm Fitting	57170		Iron & TIBC	83550
Well Exam Infant (up to 12 mos.)	99391		Ear Irrigation	69210		Kidney Profile	80069
Well exam 1–4 yrs.	99392		ECG	93000		Lead	83655
Well Exam 5–11 yrs.	99393		Endometrial Biopsy	58100		Liver Profile	80076
Well Exam 12 17 yrs.	99394		Exc. Lesion Malignant			Mono Test	86308
Well Exam 18–39 yrs.	99395		Benign			Pap Smear	88155
Well Exam 40–64 yrs.	99396		Location			Pregnancy Test	84703
Obstetrics			Exc. Skin Tags (1–15)	11200		Obstetric Panel	80055
Total OB Care	59400		Each Additional 10	11201		Pro Time	85610
Injections			Fracture Treatment			PSA	84153
Administration Sub. / IM	90772		Loc			RPR	86592
Drug			w/Reduc w/o Reduc			Sed. Rate	85651
Dosage			I & D Abscess Single/Simple	10060		Stool Culture	87045
Allergy	95115		Multiple or Comp	10061		Stool O & P	87177
Cocci Skin Test	86490		I & D Pilonidal Cyst Simple	10080		Strep Screen	87880
DPT	90701		Pilonidal Cyst Complex	10081		Theophylline	80198
Hemophilus	90646		IV Therapy—To One Hour	90760		Thyroid Uptake	84479
Influenza	90658		Each Additional Hour	90761		TSH	84443
MMR	90707		Laceration Repair			Urinalysis	81000
OPV	90712		Location Size Simp/Comp			Urine Culture	87088
Pneumovax	90732		Laryngoscopy	31505		Drawing Fee	36415
TB Skin Test	86580		Oximetry	94760		Specimen Collection	99000
TD	90718		Punch Biopsy			**Other:**	
Unlisted Immun	90749		Rhythm Strip	93040			
Tetanus Toxoid	90703		Treadmill	93015			
Vaccine/Toxoid Admin <8 Yr Old w/ Counseling	90465		Trigger Point or Tendon Sheath Inj.	20550			
Vaccine/Toxoid Administration for Adult	90471		Tympanometry	92567			

Diagnosis/ICD-9: **041.11, V09.0, 686.9**

I acknowledge receipt of medical services and authorize the release of any medical information necessary to process this claim for healthcare payment only. I do authorize payment to the provider.

Patient Signature Lex Avery

Total Estimated Charges: _____

Payment Amount: _____

Next Appointment: _____

Figure 11-3

Capital City Medical
Fee Schedule

New Patient OV		Punch Biopsy various codes	$80
Problem Focused 99201	$45	Nebulizer various codes	$45
Expanded Problem Focused 99202	$65	Cast Application various codes	$85
Detailed 99203	$85	Laryngoscopy 31505	$255
Comprehensive 99204	$105	Audiometry 92552	$85
Comprehensive/High Complex 99205	$115	Tympanometry 92567	$85
Well Exam infant (less than 1 year) 99381	$45	Ear Irrigation 69210	$25
Well Exam 1–4 yrs. 99382	$50	Diaphragm Fitting 57170	$30
Well Exam 5–11 yrs. 99383	$55	IV Therapy (up to one hour) 90760	$65
Well Exam 12–17 yrs. 99384	$65	Each additional hour 90761	$50
Well Exam 18–39 yrs. 99385	$85	Oximetry 94760	$10
Well Exam 40–64 yrs. 99386	$105	ECG 93000	$75
Established Patient OV		Holter Monitor various codes	$170
Post Op Follow Up Visit 99024	$0	Rhythm Strip 93040	$60
Minimum 99211	$35	Treadmill 93015	$375
Problem Focused 99212	$45	Cocci Skin Test 86490	$20
Expanded Problem Focused 99213	$55	X-ray, spine, chest, bone—any area various codes	$275
Detailed 99214	$65	Avulsion Nail 11730	$200
Comprehensive/High Complex 99215	$75	**Laboratory**	
Well exam infant (less than 1 year) 99391	$35	Amylase 82150	$40
Well Exam 1–4 yrs. 99392	$40	B12 82607	$30
Well Exam 5–11 yrs. 99393	$45	CBC & Diff 85025	$95
Well Exam 12–17 yrs. 99394	$55	Comp Metabolic Panel 80053	$75
Well Exam 18–39 yrs. 99395	$65	Chlamydia Screen 87110	$70
Well Exam 40–64 yrs. 99396	$75	Cholestrerol 82465	$75
Obstetrics		Digoxin 80162	$40
Total OB Care 59400	$1700	Electrolytes 80051	$70
Injections		Estrogen, Total 82672	$50
Administration 90772	$10	Ferritin 82728	$40
Allergy 95115	$35	Folate 82746	$30
DPT 90701	$50	GC Screen 87070	$60
Drug various codes	$35	Glucose 82947	$35
Influenza 90658	$25	Glycosylated HGB A1C 83036	$45
MMR 90707	$50	HCT 85014	$30
OPV 90712	$40	HDL 83718	$35
Pneumovax 90732	$35	HGB 85018	$30
TB Skin Test 86580	$15	Hep BSAG 83740	$40
TD 90718	$40	Hepatitis panel, acute 80074	$95
Tetanus Toxoid 90703	$40	HIV 86703	$100
Vaccine/Toxoid Administration for Younger		Iron & TIBC 83550	$45
Than 8 Years Old w/ counseling 90465	$10	Kidney Profile 80069	$95
Vaccine/Toxoid Administration for Adult 90471	$10	Lead 83665	$55
Arthrocentesis/Aspiration/Injection		Lipase 83690	$40
Small Joint 20600	$50	Lipid Panel 80061	$95
Interm Joint 20605	$60	Liver Profile 80076	$95
Major Joint 20610	$70	Mono Test 86308	$30
Trigger Point/Tendon Sheath Inj. 20550	$90	Pap Smear 88155	$90
Other Invasive/Noninvasive Procedures		Pap Collection/Supervision 88142	$95
Catheterization 51701	$55	Pregnancy Test 84703	$90
Circumcision 54150	$150	Obstetric Panel 80055	$85
Colposcopy 57452	$225	Pro Time 85610	$50
Colposcopy w/Biopsy 57454	$250	PSA 84153	$50
Cryosurgery Premalignant Lesion various codes	$160	RPR 86592	$55
Endometrial Biopsy 58100	$190	Sed. Rate 85651	$50
Excision Lesion Malignant various codes	$145	Stool Culture 87045	$80
Excision Lesion Benign various codes	$125	Stool O & P 87177	$105
Curettement Lesion		Strep Screen 87880	$35
Single 11055	$70	Theophylline 80198	$40
2–4 11056	$80	Thyroid Uptake 84479	$75
>4 11057	$90	TSH 84443	$50
Excision Skin Tags (1–15) 11200	$55	Urinalysis 81000	$35
Each Additional 10 11201	$30	Urine Culture 87088	$80
I & D Abscess Single/Simple 10060	$75	Drawing Fee 36415	$15
Multiple/Complex 10061	$95	Specimen Collection 99000	$10
I & D Pilonidal Cyst Simple 10080	$105		
I & D Pilonidal Cyst Complex 10081	$130		
Laceration Repair various codes	$60		

HEALTH INSURANCE CLAIM FORM
APPROVED BY NATIONAL UNIFORM CLAIM COMMITTEE 08/05

	PICA							PICA	

1. MEDICARE   **MEDICAID**   **TRICARE**   **CHAMPVA**   **GROUP**   **FECA**   **OTHER**
CHAMPUS   HEALTH PLAN   BLK LUNG

☐ *(Medicare #)*   ☐ *(Medicaid #)*   ☐ *(Sponsor's SSN)*   ☐ *(Member ID#)*   ☐ *(SSN or ID)*   ☐ *(SSN)*   ☐ *(ID)*

1a. INSURED'S I.D. NUMBER   (For Program in Item 1)

2. PATIENT'S NAME (Last Name, First Name, Middle Initial)

3. PATIENT'S BIRTH DATE   **SEX**
MM   DD   YY   M☐   F☐

4. INSURED'S NAME (Last Name, First Name, Middle Initial)

5. PATIENT'S ADDRESS (No., Street)

6. PATIENT RELATIONSHIP TO INSURED
Self☐   Spouse☐   Child☐   Other☐

7. INSURED'S ADDRESS (No, Street)

CITY   **STATE**

8. PATIENT STATUS
Single☐   Married☐   Other☐

CITY   **STATE**

ZIP CODE   **TELEPHONE (Include Area Code)**
(   )

Full-Time   Part-Time
Employed☐   Student☐   Student☐

ZIP CODE   **TELEPHONE (Include Area Code)**
(   )

9. OTHER INSURED'S NAME (Last Name, First Name, Middle Initial)

10. IS PATIENT'S CONDITION RELATED TO:

11. INSURED'S POLICY GROUP OR FECA NUMBER

a. OTHER INSURED'S POLICY OR GROUP NUMBER

a. EMPLOYMENT? (Current or Previous)
☐YES   ☐NO

a. INSURED'S DATE OF BIRTH   **SEX**
MM   DD   YY   M☐   F☐

b. OTHER INSURED'S DATE OF BIRTH   **SEX**
MM   DD   YY   M☐   F☐

b. AUTO ACCIDENT?   **PLACE (State)**
☐YES   ☐NO

b. EMPLOYER'S NAME OR SCHOOL NAME

c. EMPLOYER'S NAME OR SCHOOL NAME

c. OTHER ACCIDENT?
☐YES   ☐NO

c. INSURANCE PLAN NAME OR PROGRAM NAME

d. INSURANCE PLAN NAME OR PROGRAM NAME

10d. RESERVED FOR LOCAL USE

d. IS THERE ANOTHER HEALTH BENEFIT PLAN?
☐YES   ☐NO   *If yes*, return to and complete item 9 a-d.

READ BACK OF FORM BEFORE COMPLETING & SIGNING THIS FORM.

12. PATIENT'S OR AUTHORIZED PERSON'S SIGNATURE I authorize the release of any medical or other information necessary to process this claim. I also request payment of government benefits either to myself or to the party who accepts assignment below.

SIGNED _____ DATE _____

13. INSURED'S OR AUTHORIZED PERSON'S SIGNATURE I authorize payment of medical benefits to the undersigned physician or supplier for services described below.

SIGNED _____

14. DATE OF CURRENT: ILLNESS (First symptom) OR
MM   DD   YY   ◄   INJURY (Accident) OR
PREGNANCY (LMP)

15. IF PATIENT HAS HAD SAME OR SIMILAR ILLNESS,
GIVE FIRST DATE   MM   DD   YY

16. DATES PATIENT UNABLE TO WORK IN CURRENT OCCUPATION
MM   DD   YY   MM   DD   YY
FROM   TO

17. NAME OF REFERRING PHYSICIAN OR OTHER SOURCE

17a.
17b.   NPI

18. HOSPITALIZATION DATES RELATED TO CURRENT SERVICES
MM   DD   YY   MM   DD   YY
FROM   TO

19. RESERVED FOR LOCAL USE

20. OUTSIDE LAB?   **$ CHARGES**
☐YES   ☐NO

21. DIAGNOSIS OR NATURE OF ILLNESS OR INJURY (Relate Items 1,2,3 or 4 to Item 24E by Line)

1. |___.___   3. |___.___
2. |___.___   4. |___.___

22. MEDICAID RESUBMISSION
CODE   ORIGINAL REF. NO.

23. PRIOR AUTHORIZATION NUMBER

24. A. DATE(S) OF SERVICE		B. PLACE OF SERVICE	C. EMG	D. PROCEDURES, SERVICES, OR SUPPLIES (Explain Unusual Circumstances)		E. DIAGNOSIS POINTER	F. $ CHARGES	G. DAYS OR UNITS	H. EPSDT Family Plan	I. ID. QUAL.	J. RENDERING PROVIDER ID. #
From MM DD YY	To MM DD YY			CPT/HCPCS	MODIFIER						
1										NPI	
2										NPI	
3										NPI	
4										NPI	
5										NPI	
6										NPI	

25. FEDERAL TAX I.D. NUMBER   SSN EIN ☐☐

26. PATIENT'S ACCOUNT NO.

27. ACCEPT ASSIGNMENT?
(For govt. claims, see back)
☐YES   ☐NO

28. TOTAL CHARGE $

29. AMOUNT PAID $

30. BALANCE DUE $

31. SIGNATURE OF PHYSICIAN OR SUPPLIER INCLUDING DEGREES OR CREDENTIALS
(I certify that the statements on the reverse apply to this bill and are made a part thereof.)

SIGNED _____ DATE _____

32. SERVICE FACILITY LOCATION INFORMATION

a. NPI   b.

33. BILLING PROVIDER INFO & PH. # (   )

a. NPI   b.

NUCC Instruction Manual available at: www.nucc.org
WCMS-1500CS

APPROVED OMB 0938-0999 FORM CMS-1500 (08/05)

Figure 11-4

Vertical text (left margin): SECOND FOLD   FIRST FOLD   WHCF-10-ENV / WHCF-10-ENV-SS

Vertical text (right margin): CARRIER   PATIENT AND INSURED INFORMATION   PHYSICIAN OR SUPPLIER INFORMATION

c. Using the given source documents, the Capital City Medical Fee Schedule (Figure 11-5), and the blank CMS-1500 form provided (Figure 11-6), complete the following case study for patient Darpin Ramin (Case 11-3):

CASE 11-3

| Capital City Medical—123 Unknown Boulevard, Capital City, NY 12345-2222 (555) 555-1234 Phil Wells, MD, Mannie Mends, MD, Bette R. Soone, MD | Patient Information Form Tax ID: 75-0246810 Group NPI: 1513171216 |

Patient Information:

Name: (Last, First) Ramin, Darpin ❑ Male ☒ Female   Birth Date: 03/28/1989

Address: 51 Garfield Ave, Capital City, NY 12345   Phone: (555) 555-8881

Social Security Number: 950-60-8027   Full-Time Student: ❑ Yes ☒ No

Marital Status: ☒ Single ❑ Married ❑ Divorced ❑ Other

Employment:

Employer: Satellite Broadcasting   Phone: (555) 555-2330

Address: 1232 Columbus Highway, Capital City, Ny 12345

Condition Related to: ❑ Auto Accident ❑ Employment ❑ Other Accident

Date of Accident: _____ State _____

Emergency Contact: _____ Phone: ( ) _____

Primary Insurance: Aetna   Phone: ( ) _____

Address: 1625 Healthcare Bldg, Capital City, NY 12345

Insurance Policyholder's Name: Same   ❑ M ❑ F DOB: _____

Address: _____

Phone: ( ) _____ Relationship to Insured: ☒ Self ❑ Spouse ❑ Child ❑ Other

Employer: _____   Phone: ( ) _____

Employer's Address: _____

Policy/ID No: 2565799   Group No: 6235   Percent Covered: ___% Copay Amt: $20.00

Secondary Insurance: _____   Phone: ( ) _____

Address: _____

Insurance Policyholder's Name: _____   ❑ M ❑ F DOB: _____

Address: _____

Phone: ( ) _____ Relationship to Insured: ❑ Self ❑ Spouse ❑ Child ❑ Other

Employer: _____   Phone: ( ) _____

Employer's Address: _____

Policy/ID No: _____   Group No: _____ Percent Covered: ___% Copay Amt: $_____

Reason for Visit: I am here for a check on anemia.

Known Allergies: _____

Referred by: _____

CASE 11-3
SOAP

11/08/20XX
Assignment of Benefits: Y
Signature on File: Y
Referring Physician: N

S: Darpin Ramin is here to have a check on her anemia.

O: Pt. still complains of tiredness. Her blood values have not shown improvement. Vitals are normal.

A: 1. Iron deficiency anemia—280.9

P: 1. Continue iron supplement.
2. Refer to the hospital dietician for diet counseling.
3. Return in 3 months.

_____

Phil Wells, MD
Family Practice
NPI: 1234567890

CASE 11-3

Patient Name Darpin Ramin

Capital City Medical
123 Unknown Boulevard, Capital City, NY 12345-2222

Date of Service _____

New Patient			Other Invasive/Noninvasive			Laboratory		
Problem Focused	99201		Arthrocentesis/Aspiration/Injection			Amylase	82150	
Expanded Problem, Focused	99202		Small Joint	20600		B12	82607	
Detailed	99203		Interm Joint	20605		CBC & Diff	85025	
Comprehensive	99204		Major Joint	20610		Comp Metabolic Panel	80053	
Comprehensive/High Complex	99205		**Other Invasive/Noninvasive**			Chlamydia Screen	87110	
Well Exam Infant (up to 12 mos.)	99381		Audiometry	92552		Cholesterol	82465	
Well Exam 1–4 yrs.	99382		Cast Application			Digoxin	80162	
Well Exam 5–11 yrs.	99383		Location Long Short			Electrolytes	80051	
Well Exam 12–17 yrs.	99384		Catheterization	51701		Ferritin	82728	
Well Exam 18–39 yrs.	99385		Circumcision	54150		Folate	82746	
Well Exam 40–64 yrs.	99386		Colposcopy	57452		GC Screen	87070	
			Colposcopy w/Biopsy	57454		Glucose	82947	
			Cryosurgery Premalignant Lesion			Glucose 1 HR	82950	
			Location (s):			Glycosylated HGB A1C	83036	
Established Patient			Cryosurgery Warts			HCT	85014	X
Post-Op Follow Up Visit	99024		Location (s):			HDL	83718	
Minimum	99211		Curettement Lesion			Hep BSAG	87340	
Problem Focused	99212	X	Single	11055		Hepatitis panel, acute	80074	
Expanded Problem Focused	99213		2–4	11056		HGB	85018	X
Detailed	99214		>4	11057		HIV	86703	
Comprehensive/High Complex	99215		Diaphragm Fitting	57170		Iron & TIBC	83550	
Well Exam Infant (up to 12 mos.)	99391		Ear Irrigation	69210		Kidney Profile	80069	
Well exam 1–4 yrs.	99392		ECG	93000		Lead	83655	
Well Exam 5–11 yrs.	99393		Endometrial Biopsy	58100		Liver Profile	80076	
Well Exam 12–17 yrs.	99394		Exc. Lesion Malignant			Mono Test	86308	
Well Exam 18–39 yrs.	99395		Benign			Pap Smear	88155	
Well Exam 40–64 yrs.	99396		Location			Pregnancy Test	84703	
Obstetrics			Exc. Skin Tags (1–15)	11200		Obstetric Panel	80055	
Total OB Care	59400		Each Additional 10	11201		Pro Time	85610	
Injections			Fracture Treatment			PSA	84153	
Administration Sub. / IM	90772		Loc			RPR	86592	
Drug			w/Reduc w/o Reduc			Sed. Rate	85651	
Dosage			I & D Abscess Single/Simple	10060		Stool Culture	87045	
Allergy	95115		Multiple or Comp	10061		Stool O & P	87177	
Cocci Skin Test	86490		I & D Pilonidal Cyst Simple	10080		Strep Screen	87880	
DPT	90701		Pilonidal Cyst Complex	10081		Theophylline	80198	
Hemophilus	90646		IV Therapy—To One Hour	90760		Thyroid Uptake	84479	
Influenza	90658		Each Additional Hour	90761		TSH	84443	
MMR	90707		Laceration Repair			Urinalysis	81000	
OPV	90712		Location Size Simp/Comp			Urine Culture	87088	
Pneumovax	90732		Laryngoscopy	31505		Drawing Fee	36415	X
TB Skin Test	86580		Oximetry	94760		Specimen Collection	99000	
TD	90718		Punch Biopsy			**Other:**		
Unlisted Immun	90749		Rhythm Strip	93040				
Tetanus Toxoid	90703		Treadmill	93015				
Vaccine/Toxoid Admin <8 Yr Old w/ Counseling	90465		Trigger Point or Tendon Sheath Inj.	20550				
Vaccine/Toxoid Administration for Adult	90471		Tympanometry	92567				

Diagnosis/ICD-9: **280.9**

I acknowledge receipt of medical services and authorize the release of any medical information necessary to process this claim for healthcare payment only. I do authorize payment to the provider.

Patient Signature _Darpin Ramin_

Total Estimated Charges: _____

Payment Amount: _____

Next Appointment: _____

Figure 11-5

Capital City Medical
Fee Schedule

New Patient OV			Punch Biopsy various codes	$80
Problem Focused 99201	$45		Nebulizer various codes	$45
Expanded Problem Focused 99202	$65		Cast Application various codes	$85
Detailed 99203	$85		Laryngoscopy 31505	$255
Comprehensive 99204	$105		Audiometry 92552	$85
Comprehensive/High Complex 99205	$115		Tympanometry 92567	$85
Well Exam infant (less than 1 year) 99381	$45		Ear Irrigation 69210	$25
Well Exam 1–4 yrs. 99382	$50		Diaphragm Fitting 57170	$30
Well Exam 5–11 yrs. 99383	$55		IV Therapy (up to one hour) 90760	$65
Well Exam 12–17 yrs. 99384	$65		Each additional hour 90761	$50
Well Exam 18–39 yrs. 99385	$85		Oximetry 94760	$10
Well Exam 40–64 yrs. 99386	$105		ECG 93000	$75
Established Patient OV			Holter Monitor various codes	$170
Post Op Follow Up Visit 99024	$0		Rhythm Strip 93040	$60
Minimum 99211	$35		Treadmill 93015	$375
Problem Focused 99212	$45		Cocci Skin Test 86490	$20
Expanded Problem Focused 99213	$55		X-ray, spine, chest, bone—any area various codes	$275
Detailed 99214	$65		Avulsion Nail 11730	$200
Comprehensive/High Complex 99215	$75		**Laboratory**	
Well exam infant (less than 1 year) 99391	$35		Amylase 82150	$40
Well Exam 1–4 yrs. 99392	$40		B12 82607	$30
Well Exam 5–11 yrs. 99393	$45		CBC & Diff 85025	$95
Well Exam 12–17 yrs. 99394	$55		Comp Metabolic Panel 80053	$75
Well Exam 18–39 yrs. 99395	$65		Chlamydia Screen 87110	$70
Well Exam 40–64 yrs. 99396	$75		Cholestrerol 82465	$75
Obstetrics			Digoxin 80162	$40
Total OB Care 59400	$1700		Electrolytes 80051	$70
Injections			Estrogen, Total 82672	$50
Administration 90772	$10		Ferritin 82728	$40
Allergy 95115	$35		Folate 82746	$30
DPT 90701	$50		GC Screen 87070	$60
Drug various codes	$35		Glucose 82947	$35
Influenza 90658	$25		Glycosylated HGB A1C 83036	$45
MMR 90707	$50		HCT 85014	$30
OPV 90712	$40		HDL 83718	$35
Pneumovax 90732	$35		HGB 85018	$30
TB Skin Test 86580	$15		Hep BSAG 83740	$40
TD 90718	$40		Hepatitis panel, acute 80074	$95
Tetanus Toxoid 90703	$40		HIV 86703	$100
Vaccine/Toxoid Administration for Younger			Iron & TIBC 83550	$45
Than 8 Years Old w/ counseling 90465	$10		Kidney Profile 80069	$95
Vaccine/Toxoid Administration for Adult 90471 $10			Lead 83665	$55
Arthrocentesis/Aspiration/Injection			Lipase 83690	$40
Small Joint 20600	$50		Lipid Panel 80061	$95
Interm Joint 20605	$60		Liver Profile 80076	$95
Major Joint 20610	$70		Mono Test 86308	$30
Trigger Point/Tendon Sheath Inj. 20550	$90		Pap Smear 88155	$90
Other Invasive/Noninvasive Procedures			Pap Collection/Supervision 88142	$95
Catheterization 51701	$55		Pregnancy Test 84703	$90
Circumcision 54150	$150		Obstetric Panel 80055	$85
Colposcopy 57452	$225		Pro Time 85610	$50
Colposcopy w/Biopsy 57454	$250		PSA 84153	$50
Cryosurgery Premalignant Lesion various codes$160			RPR 86592	$55
Endometrial Biopsy 58100	$190		Sed. Rate 85651	$50
Excision Lesion Malignant various codes	$145		Stool Culture 87045	$80
Excision Lesion Benign various codes	$125		Stool O & P 87177	$105
Curettement Lesion			Strep Screen 87880	$35
Single 11055	$70		Theophylline 80198	$40
2–4 11056	$80		Thyroid Uptake 84479	$75
>4 11057	$90		TSH 84443	$50
Excision Skin Tags (1–15) 11200	$55		Urinalysis 81000	$35
Each Additional 10 11201	$30		Urine Culture 87088	$80
I & D Abscess Single/Simple 10060	$75		Drawing Fee 36415	$15
Multiple/Complex 10061	$95		Specimen Collection 99000	$10
I & D Pilonidal Cyst Simple 10080	$105			
I & D Pilonidal Cyst Complex 10081	$130			
Laceration Repair various codes	$60			

HEALTH INSURANCE CLAIM FORM
APPROVED BY NATIONAL UNIFORM CLAIM COMMITTEE 08/05

CARRIER

☐☐☐ PICA

1. MEDICARE	MEDICAID	TRICARE CHAMPUS	CHAMPVA	GROUP HEALTH PLAN	FECA BLK LUNG	OTHER	1a. INSURED'S I.D. NUMBER	(For Program in Item 1)
☐ (Medicare #)	☐ (Medicaid #)	☐ (Sponsor's SSN)	☐ (Member ID#)	☐ (SSN or ID)	☐ (SSN)	☐ (ID)		

2. PATIENT'S NAME (Last Name, First Name, Middle Initial)	3. PATIENT'S BIRTH DATE SEX	4. INSURED'S NAME (Last Name, First Name, Middle Initial)
	MM ┊ DD ┊ YY M☐ F☐	

5. PATIENT'S ADDRESS (No., Street)	6. PATIENT RELATIONSHIP TO INSURED	7. INSURED'S ADDRESS (No, Street)
	Self☐ Spouse☐ Child☐ Other☐	

CITY	STATE	8. PATIENT STATUS	CITY	STATE
		Single☐ Married☐ Other☐		

ZIP CODE	TELEPHONE (Include Area Code)		ZIP CODE	TELEPHONE (Include Area Code)
	( )	Employed☐ Full-Time Student☐ Part-Time Student☐		( )

9. OTHER INSURED'S NAME (Last Name, First Name, Middle Initial)	10. IS PATIENT'S CONDITION RELATED TO:	11. INSURED'S POLICY GROUP OR FECA NUMBER
a. OTHER INSURED'S POLICY OR GROUP NUMBER	a. EMPLOYMENT? (Current or Previous) ☐YES ☐NO	a. INSURED'S DATE OF BIRTH SEX MM ┊ DD ┊ YY M☐ F☐
b. OTHER INSURED'S DATE OF BIRTH SEX MM ┊ DD ┊ YY M☐ F☐	b. AUTO ACCIDENT? PLACE (State) ☐YES ☐NO	b. EMPLOYER'S NAME OR SCHOOL NAME
c. EMPLOYER'S NAME OR SCHOOL NAME	c. OTHER ACCIDENT? ☐YES ☐NO	c. INSURANCE PLAN NAME OR PROGRAM NAME
d. INSURANCE PLAN NAME OR PROGRAM NAME	10d. RESERVED FOR LOCAL USE	d. IS THERE ANOTHER HEALTH BENEFIT PLAN? ☐YES ☐NO If yes, return to and complete item 9 a-d.

READ BACK OF FORM BEFORE COMPLETING & SIGNING THIS FORM.
12. PATIENT'S OR AUTHORIZED PERSON'S SIGNATURE I authorize the release of any medical or other information necessary to process this claim. I also request payment of government benefits either to myself or to the party who accepts assignment below.

SIGNED _____   DATE _____

13. INSURED'S OR AUTHORIZED PERSON'S SIGNATURE I authorize payment of medical benefits to the undersigned physician or supplier for services described below.

SIGNED _____

14. DATE OF CURRENT: ◀ ILLNESS (First symptom) OR MM ┊ DD ┊ YY INJURY (Accident) OR PREGNANCY (LMP)	15. IF PATIENT HAS HAD SAME OR SIMILAR ILLNESS, GIVE FIRST DATE MM ┊ DD ┊ YY	16. DATES PATIENT UNABLE TO WORK IN CURRENT OCCUPATION MM ┊ DD ┊ YY MM ┊ DD ┊ YY FROM TO
17. NAME OF REFERRING PHYSICIAN OR OTHER SOURCE	17a. 17b. NPI	18. HOSPITALIZATION DATES RELATED TO CURRENT SERVICES MM ┊ DD ┊ YY MM ┊ DD ┊ YY FROM TO
19. RESERVED FOR LOCAL USE		20. OUTSIDE LAB? $ CHARGES ☐YES ☐NO

21. DIAGNOSIS OR NATURE OF ILLNESS OR INJURY (Relate Items 1,2,3 or 4 to Item 24E by Line)		22. MEDICAID RESUBMISSION CODE ORIGINAL REF. NO.
1. └___.___ 3. └___.___ 2. └___.___ 4. └___.___		23. PRIOR AUTHORIZATION NUMBER

24. A. DATE(S) OF SERVICE						B. PLACE OF SERVICE	C. EMG	D. PROCEDURES, SERVICES, OR SUPPLIES (Explain Unusual Circumstances) CPT/HCPCS MODIFIER		E. DIAGNOSIS POINTER	F. $ CHARGES	G. DAYS OR UNITS	H. EPSDT Family Plan	I. ID. QUAL.	J. RENDERING PROVIDER ID. #
From MM DD YY			To MM DD YY												
1														NPI	
2														NPI	
3														NPI	
4														NPI	
5														NPI	
6														NPI	

25. FEDERAL TAX I.D. NUMBER SSN EIN ☐☐	26. PATIENT'S ACCOUNT NO.	27. ACCEPT ASSIGNMENT? (For govt. claims, see back) ☐YES ☐NO	28. TOTAL CHARGE $	29. AMOUNT PAID $	30. BALANCE DUE $

31. SIGNATURE OF PHYSICIAN OR SUPPLIER INCLUDING DEGREES OR CREDENTIALS (I certify that the statements on the reverse apply to this bill and are made a part thereof.) SIGNED _____ DATE _____	32. SERVICE FACILITY LOCATION INFORMATION a. NPI b.	33. BILLING PROVIDER INFO & PH. # ( ) a. NPI b.

APPROVED OMB 0938-0999 FORM CMS-1500 (08/05)

SECOND FOLD

FIRST FOLD   WHCF-10-ENV / WHCF-10-ENV-SS

PATIENT AND INSURED INFORMATION

PHYSICIAN OR SUPPLIER INFORMATION

Figure 11-6

d. Using the given source documents, the Capital City Medical Fee Schedule (Figure 11-7), and the blank CMS-1500 form provided (Figure 11-8), complete the following case study for patient Rhianna Burley (Case 11.4):

CASE 11-4

Capital City Medical—123 Unknown Boulevard, Capital City, NY 12345-2222 (555) 555-1234	Patient Information Form
Phil Wells, MD, Mannie Mends, MD, Bette R. Soone, MD	Tax ID: 75-0246810
	Group NPI: 1513171216

Patient Information:

Name: (Last, First) Burley, Rhianna ☐ Male ☒ Female Birth Date: 10/15/1982

Address: 91 Harper Ln, Capital City, NY 12345 Phone: (555) 555-8881

Social Security Number: 642-89-8999 Full-Time Student: ☐ Yes ☒ No

Marital Status: ☐ Single ☒ Married ☐ Divorced ☐ Other

Employment:

Employer: _____ Phone: ( ) _____

Address: _____

Condition Related to: ☐ Auto Accident ☐ Employment ☐ Other Accident

Date of Accident: _____ State: _____

Emergency Contact: _____ **Phone: ( )** _____

Primary Insurance: Health America Phone: ( ) _____

Address: 2031 Healthica Center, Capital City, NY 12345

Insurance Policyholder's Name: Pat Burley ☒ M ☐ F DOB: 01/18/1982

Address: Same

Phone: ( ) _____ Relationship to Insured: ☐ Self ☒ Spouse ☐ Child ☐ Other

Employer: Capital Engineering Phone: (555) 555-7949

Employer's Address: 3605 Graph Rd, Capital City, NY 12345

Policy/ID No: 45753331 Group No: 594615 Percent Covered: ____% Copay Amt: $25.00

Secondary Insurance: _____ Phone: ( ) _____

Address: _____

Insurance Policyholder's Name: _____ ☐ M ☐ F DOB: _____

Address: _____

Phone: ( ) _____ Relationship to Insured: ☐ Self ☐ Spouse ☐ Child ☐ Other

Employer: _____ Phone: ( ) _____

Employer's Address: _____

Policy/ID No: _____ Group No: ____ Percent Covered: ___% Copay Amt: $____

Reason for Visit: I feel nauseated, and I think I have a fever.

Known Allergies: _____

Referred by: _____

CASE 11-4
SOAP

09/22/20XX
Assignment of Benefits: Y
Signature on File: Y
Referring Physician: N

S: Rhianna Burley is complaining of nausea and headache. She started feeling ill yesterday evening. During the day, she played paintball with her husband and a few friends in the woods behind her house.

O: On exam, pt. has a fever of 101.8°F. She denies vomiting or diarrhea. She does have a mosquito bite on her right calf. The area around the bite is red, swollen, and 2 in. in diameter. CBC and diff is negative. Sed rate presents as normal.

A: 1. West Nile Virus—066.40

P: 1. Take meds as directed.
   2. If symptoms worsen, go to the ER immediately.
   3. Return in 3 days.

_____

Phil Wells, MD
Family Practice
NPI: 1234567890

CASE 11-4

Patient Name Rhianna Burley

Capital City Medical
123 Unknown Boulevard, Capital City, NY 12345-2222

Date of Service
09-22-20XX

New Patient			Arthrocentesis/Aspiration/Injection			Laboratory		
Problem Focused	99201		Arthrocentesis/Aspiration/Injection			Amylase	82150	
Expanded Problem, Focused	99202		Small Joint		20600	B12	82607	
Detailed	99203		Interm Joint		20605	CBC & Diff	85025	X
Comprehensive	99204		Major Joint		20610	Comp Metabolic Panel	80053	
Comprehensive/High Complex	99205		**Other Invasive/Noninvasive**			Chlamydia Screen	87110	
Well Exam Infant (up to 12 mos.)	99381		Audiometry	92552		Cholesterol	82465	
Well Exam 1–4 yrs.	99382		Cast Application			Digoxin	80162	
Well Exam 5–11 yrs.	99383		Location Long Short			Electrolytes	80051	
Well Exam 12–17 yrs.	99384		Catheterization	51701		Ferritin	82728	
Well Exam 18–39 yrs.	99385		Circumcision	54150		Folate	82746	
Well Exam 40–64 yrs.	99386		Colposcopy	57452		GC Screen	87070	
			Colposcopy w/Biopsy	57454		Glucose	82947	
			Cryosurgery Premalignant Lesion			Glucose 1 HR	82950	
			Location (s):			Glycosylated HGB A1C	83036	
Established Patient			Cryosurgery Warts			HCT	85014	
Post-Op Follow Up Visit	99024		Location (s):			HDL	83718	
Minimum	99211		Curettement Lesion			Hep BSAG	87340	
Problem Focused	99212		Single	11055		Hepatitis panel, acute	80074	
Expanded Problem Focused	99213	X	2–4	11056		HGB	85018	
Detailed	99214		>4	11057		HIV	86703	
Comprehensive/High Complex	99215		Diaphragm Fitting	57170		Iron & TIBC	83550	
Well Exam Infant (up to 12 mos.)	99391		Ear Irrigation	69210		Kidney Profile	80069	
Well exam 1–4 yrs.	99392		ECG	93000		Lead	83655	
Well Exam 5–11 yrs.	99393		Endometrial Biopsy	58100		Liver Profile	80076	
Well Exam 12–17 yrs.	99394		Exc. Lesion Malignant			Mono Test	86308	
Well Exam 18–39 yrs.	99395		Benign			Pap Smear	88155	
Well Exam 40–64 yrs.	99396		Location			Pregnancy Test	84703	
Obstetrics			Exc. Skin Tags (1–15)	11200		Obstetric Panel	80055	
Total OB Care	59400		Each Additional 10	11201		Pro Time	85610	
Injections			Fracture Treatment			PSA	84153	
Administration Sub. / IM	90772		Loc			RPR	86592	
Drug			w/Reduc		w/o Reduc	Sed. Rate	85651	X
Dosage			I & D Abscess Single/Simple	10060		Stool Culture	87045	
Allergy	95115		Multiple or Comp	10061		Stool O & P	87177	
Cocci Skin Test	86490		I & D Pilonidal Cyst Simple	10080		Strep Screen	87880	
DPT	90701		Pilonidal Cyst Complex	10081		Theophylline	80198	
Hemophilus	90646		IV Therapy—To One Hour	90760		Thyroid Uptake	84479	
Influenza	90658		Each Additional Hour	90761		TSH	84443	
MMR	90707		Laceration Repair			Urinalysis	81000	
OPV	90712		Location Size Simp/Comp			Urine Culture	87088	
Pneumovax	90732		Laryngoscopy	31505		Drawing Fee	36415	X
TB Skin Test	86580		Oximetry	94760		Specimen Collection	99000	
TD	90718		Punch Biopsy			**Other:**		
Unlisted Immun	90749		Rhythm Strip	93040				
Tetanus Toxoid	90703		Treadmill	93015				
Vaccine/Toxoid Admin <8 Yr Old w/ Counseling	90465		Trigger Point or Tendon Sheath Inj.	20550				
Vaccine/Toxoid Administration for Adult	90471		Tympanometry	92567				

Diagnosis/ICD-9: **066.40**

I acknowledge receipt of medical services and authorize the release of any medical information necessary to process this claim for healthcare payment only. I do authorize payment to the provider.

Patient Signature Rhianna Burley

Total Estimated Charges: _____

Payment Amount: _____

Next Appointment: _____

Figure 11-7

Capital City Medical
Fee Schedule

New Patient OV	
Problem Focused 99201	$45
Expanded Problem Focused 99202	$65
Detailed 99203	$85
Comprehensive 99204	$105
Comprehensive/High Complex 99205	$115
Well Exam infant (less than 1 year) 99381	$45
Well Exam 1–4 yrs. 99382	$50
Well Exam 5–11 yrs. 99383	$55
Well Exam 12–17 yrs. 99384	$65
Well Exam 18–39 yrs. 99385	$85
Well Exam 40–64 yrs. 99386	$105
Established Patient OV	
Post Op Follow Up Visit 99024	$0
Minimum 99211	$35
Problem Focused 99212	$45
Expanded Problem Focused 99213	$55
Detailed 99214	$65
Comprehensive/High Complex 99215	$75
Well exam infant (less than 1 year) 99391	$35
Well Exam 1–4 yrs. 99392	$40
Well Exam 5–11 yrs. 99393	$45
Well Exam 12–17 yrs. 99394	$55
Well Exam 18–39 yrs. 99395	$65
Well Exam 40–64 yrs. 99396	$75
Obstetrics	
Total OB Care 59400	$1700
Injections	
Administration 90772	$10
Allergy 95115	$35
DPT 90701	$50
Drug various codes	$35
Influenza 90658	$25
MMR 90707	$50
OPV 90712	$40
Pneumovax 90732	$35
TB Skin Test 86580	$15
TD 90718	$40
Tetanus Toxoid 90703	$40
Vaccine/Toxoid Administration for Younger Than 8 Years Old w/ counseling 90465	$10
Vaccine/Toxoid Administration for Adult 90471	$10
Arthrocentesis/Aspiration/Injection	
Small Joint 20600	$50
Interm Joint 20605	$60
Major Joint 20610	$70
Trigger Point/Tendon Sheath Inj. 20550	$90
Other Invasive/Noninvasive Procedures	
Catheterization 51701	$55
Circumcision 54150	$150
Colposcopy 57452	$225
Colposcopy w/Biopsy 57454	$250
Cryosurgery Premalignant Lesion various codes	$160
Endometrial Biopsy 58100	$190
Excision Lesion Malignant various codes	$145
Excision Lesion Benign various codes	$125
Curettement Lesion	
Single 11055	$70
2–4 11056	$80
>4 11057	$90
Excision Skin Tags (1–15) 11200	$55
Each Additional 10 11201	$30
I & D Abscess Single/Simple 10060	$75
Multiple/Complex 10061	$95
I & D Pilonidal Cyst Simple 10080	$105
I & D Pilonidal Cyst Complex 10081	$130
Laceration Repair various codes	$60

Punch Biopsy various codes	$80
Nebulizer various codes	$45
Cast Application various codes	$85
Laryngoscopy 31505	$255
Audiometry 92552	$85
Tympanometry 92567	$85
Ear Irrigation 69210	$25
Diaphragm Fitting 57170	$30
IV Therapy (up to one hour) 90760	$65
Each additional hour 90761	$50
Oximetry 94760	$10
ECG 93000	$75
Holter Monitor various codes	$170
Rhythm Strip 93040	$60
Treadmill 93015	$375
Cocci Skin Test 86490	$20
X-ray, spine, chest, bone—any area various codes	$275
Avulsion Nail 11730	$200
Laboratory	
Amylase 82150	$40
B12 82607	$30
CBC & Diff 85025	$95
Comp Metabolic Panel 80053	$75
Chlamydia Screen 87110	$70
Cholestrerol 82465	$75
Digoxin 80162	$40
Electrolytes 80051	$70
Estrogen, Total 82672	$50
Ferritin 82728	$40
Folate 82746	$30
GC Screen 87070	$60
Glucose 82947	$35
Glycosylated HGB A1C 83036	$45
HCT 85014	$30
HDL 83718	$35
HGB 85018	$30
Hep BSAG 83740	$40
Hepatitis panel, acute 80074	$95
HIV 86703	$100
Iron & TIBC 83550	$45
Kidney Profile 80069	$95
Lead 83665	$55
Lipase 83690	$40
Lipid Panel 80061	$95
Liver Profile 80076	$95
Mono Test 86308	$30
Pap Smear 88155	$90
Pap Collection/Supervision 88142	$95
Pregnancy Test 84703	$90
Obstetric Panel 80055	$85
Pro Time 85610	$50
PSA 84153	$50
RPR 86592	$55
Sed. Rate 85651	$50
Stool Culture 87045	$80
Stool O & P 87177	$105
Strep Screen 87880	$35
Theophylline 80198	$40
Thyroid Uptake 84479	$75
TSH 84443	$50
Urinalysis 81000	$35
Urine Culture 87088	$80
Drawing Fee 36415	$15
Specimen Collection 99000	$10

HEALTH INSURANCE CLAIM FORM

APPROVED BY NATIONAL UNIFORM CLAIM COMMITTEE 08/05

Figure 11-8

e. Using the given source documents, the Capital City Medical Fee Schedule (Figure 11-9), and the blank CMS-1500 form provided (Figure 11-10), complete the following case study for patient Linda Freed (Case 11-5):

CASE 11-5

Capital City Medical—123 Unknown Boulevard, Capital City, NY 12345-2222 (555) 555-1234	Patient Information Form
	Tax ID: 75-0246810
Phil Wells, MD, Mannie Mends, MD, Bette R. Soone, MD	Group NPI: 1513171216

Patient Information:

Name: (Last, First) Freed, Linda _____ ☐ Male ☒ Female Birth Date: 04/06/1969

Address: 23 Penn Ave, Capital City, NY 12345 _____ Phone: (555) 555-6622 _____

Social Security Number: 402-31-1775 _____ Full-Time Student: ☐ Yes ☒ No

Marital Status: ☐ Single ☐ Married ☒ Divorced ☐ Other

Employment:

Employer: Extreme Hair, Ltd. _____ Phone: (555) 555-8220

Address: 333 Long Ave., Capital City, NY 12345 _____

Condition Related to: ☐ Auto Accident ☐ Employment ☐ Other Accident

Date of Accident: _____ State: _____

Emergency Contact: _____ **Phone: ( )** _____

Primary Insurance: Blue Cross Blue Shield _____ Phone: ( ) _____

Address: 379 Blue Plaza, Capital City, NY 12345 _____

Insurance Policyholder's Name: Same _____ ☐ M ☐ F DOB: _____

Address: _____

Phone: ( ) _____ Relationship to Insured: ☒ Self ☐ Spouse ☐ Child ☐ Other

Employer: _____ Phone: ( ) _____

Employer's Address: _____

Policy/ID No: YYJ288236692 _____ Group No: 023443 Percent Covered: ____% Copay Amt: $10.00

Secondary Insurance: _____ Phone: ( ) _____

Address: _____

Insurance Policyholder's Name: _____ ☐ M ☐ F DOB: _____

Address: _____

Phone: ( ) _____ Relationship to Insured: ☐ Self ☐ Spouse ☐ Child ☐ Other

Employer: _____ Phone: ( ) _____

Employer's Address: _____

Policy/ID No: _____ Group No: _____ Percent Covered: ____% Copay Amt: $_____

Reason for Visit: Check up on my diabetes, Type I _____

Known Allergies: _____

Referred by: _____

CASE 11-5
SOAP

02/16/20XX
Assignment of Benefits: Y
Signature on File: Y
Referring Physician: N

S: Linda Freed is in the office today for a checkup on her DMI. She says her sugar has been stable.

O: Pt. has lost a few pounds since her last visit. EENT: Clear. No edema of the lower extremities. Her glucose in the office today is 124.

A: 1. DMI, controlled—250.01

P: 1. Refill insulin and test strips.
   2. Return in 3 months.
   3. Continue testing 3×/day.

_____

Phil Wells, MD
Family Practice
NPI: 1234567890

CASE 11-5

Patient Name Linda Freed

Capital City Medical
123 Unknown Boulevard, Capital City, NY 12345-2222

Date of Service
02-16-200X

New Patient			Other Invasive/Noninvasive			Laboratory		
Problem Focused	99201		Arthrocentesis/Aspiration/Injection			Amylase	82150	
Expanded Problem, Focused	99202		Small Joint	20600		B12	82607	
Detailed	99203		Interm Joint	20605		CBC & Diff	85025	X
Comprehensive	99204		Major Joint	20610		Comp Metabolic Panel	80053	
Comprehensive/High Complex	99205		**Other Invasive/Noninvasive**			Chlamydia Screen	87110	
Well Exam Infant (up to 12 mos.)	99381		Audiometry	92552		Cholesterol	82465	
Well Exam 1–4 yrs.	99382		Cast Application			Digoxin	80162	
Well Exam 5–11 yrs.	99383		Location Long Short			Electrolytes	80051	
Well Exam 12–17 yrs.	99384		Catheterization	51701		Ferritin	82728	
Well Exam 18–39 yrs.	99385		Circumcision	54150		Folate	82746	
Well Exam 40–64 yrs.	99386		Colposcopy	57452		GC Screen	87070	
			Colposcopy w/Biopsy	57454		Glucose	82947	
			Cryosurgery Premalignant Lesion			Glucose 1 HR	82950	
			Location(s):			Glycosylated HGB A1C	83036	
Established Patient			Cryosurgery Warts			HCT	85014	
Post-Op Follow Up Visit	99024		Location(s):			HDL	83718	
Minimum	99211		Curettement Lesion			Hep BSAG	87340	
Problem Focused	99212		Single	11055		Hepatitis panel, acute	80074	
Expanded Problem Focused	99213	X	2–4	11056		HGB	85018	
Detailed	99214		>4	11057		HIV	86703	
Comprehensive/High Complex	99215		Diaphragm Fitting	57170		Iron & TIBC	83550	
Well Exam Infant (up to 12 mos.)	99391		Ear Irrigation	69210		Kidney Profile	80069	
Well exam 1–4 yrs.	99392		ECG	93000		Lead	83655	
Well Exam 5–11 yrs.	99393		Endometrial Biopsy	58100		Liver Profile	80076	
Well Exam 12–17 yrs.	99394		Exc. Lesion Malignant			Mono Test	86308	
Well Exam 18–39 yrs.	99395		Benign			Pap Smear	88155	
Well Exam 40–64 yrs.	99396		Location			Pregnancy Test	84703	
Obstetrics			Exc. Skin Tags (1–15)	11200		Obstetric Panel	80055	
Total OB Care	59400		Each Additional 10	11201		Pro Time	85610	
Injections			Fracture Treatment			PSA	84153	
Administration Sub. / IM	90772		Loc			RPR	86592	
Drug			w/Reduc w/o Reduc			Sed. Rate	85651	
Dosage			I & D Abscess Single/Simple	10060		Stool Culture	87045	
Allergy	95115		Multiple or Comp	10061		Stool O & P	87177	
Cocci Skin Test	86490		I & D Pilonidal Cyst Simple	10080		Strep Screen	87880	
DPT	90701		Pilonidal Cyst Complex	10081		Theophylline	80198	
Hemophilus	90646		IV Therapy—To One Hour	90760		Thyroid Uptake	84479	
Influenza	90658		Each Additional Hour	90761		TSH	84443	
MMR	90707		Laceration Repair			Urinalysis	81000	
OPV	90712		Location Size Simp/Comp			Urine Culture	87088	
Pneumovax	90732		Laryngoscopy	31505		Drawing Fee	36415	X
TB Skin Test	86580		Oximetry	94760		Specimen Collection	99000	
TD	90718		Punch Biopsy			**Other:**		
Unlisted Immun	90749		Rhythm Strip	93040				
Tetanus Toxoid	90703		Treadmill	93015				
Vaccine/Toxoid Admin <8 Yr Old w/ Counseling	90465		Trigger Point or Tendon Sheath Inj.	20550				
Vaccine/Toxoid Administration for Adult	90471		Tympanometry	92567				

Diagnosis/ICD-9: **250.01**

I acknowledge receipt of medical services and authorize the release of any medical information necessary to process this claim for healthcare payment only. I do authorize payment to the provider.

Patient Signature Linda Freed

Total Estimated Charges: _____

Payment Amount: _____

Next Appointment: _____

Figure 11-9

Capital City Medical
Fee Schedule

New Patient OV			Punch Biopsy various codes	$80
Problem Focused 99201	$45		Nebulizer various codes	$45
Expanded Problem Focused 99202	$65		Cast Application various codes	$85
Detailed 99203	$85		Laryngoscopy 31505	$255
Comprehensive 99204	$105		Audiometry 92552	$85
Comprehensive/High Complex 99205	$115		Tympanometry 92567	$85
Well Exam infant (less than 1 year) 99381	$45		Ear Irrigation 69210	$25
Well Exam 1–4 yrs. 99382	$50		Diaphragm Fitting 57170	$30
Well Exam 5–11 yrs. 99383	$55		IV Therapy (up to one hour) 90760	$65
Well Exam 12–17 yrs. 99384	$65		Each additional hour 90761	$50
Well Exam 18–39 yrs. 99385	$85		Oximetry 94760	$10
Well Exam 40–64 yrs. 99386	$105		ECG 93000	$75
Established Patient OV			Holter Monitor various codes	$170
Post Op Follow Up Visit 99024	$0		Rhythm Strip 93040	$60
Minimum 99211	$35		Treadmill 93015	$375
Problem Focused 99212	$45		Cocci Skin Test 86490	$20
Expanded Problem Focused 99213	$55		X-ray, spine, chest, bone—any area various codes	$275
Detailed 99214	$65		Avulsion Nail 11730	$200
Comprehensive/High Complex 99215	$75		**Laboratory**	
Well exam infant (less than 1 year) 99391	$35		Amylase 82150	$40
Well Exam 1–4 yrs. 99392	$40		B12 82607	$30
Well Exam 5–11 yrs. 99393	$45		CBC & Diff 85025	$95
Well Exam 12–17 yrs. 99394	$55		Comp Metabolic Panel 80053	$75
Well Exam 18–39 yrs. 99395	$65		Chlamydia Screen 87110	$70
Well Exam 40–64 yrs. 99396	$75		Cholestrerol 82465	$75
Obstetrics			Digoxin 80162	$40
Total OB Care 59400	$1700		Electrolytes 80051	$70
Injections			Estrogen, Total 82672	$50
Administration 90772	$10		Ferritin 82728	$40
Allergy 95115	$35		Folate 82746	$30
DPT 90701	$50		GC Screen 87070	$60
Drug various codes	$35		Glucose 82947	$35
Influenza 90658	$25		Glycosylated HGB A1C 83036	$45
MMR 90707	$50		HCT 85014	$30
OPV 90712	$40		HDL 83718	$35
Pneumovax 90732	$35		HGB 85018	$30
TB Skin Test 86580	$15		Hep BSAG 83740	$40
TD 90718	$40		Hepatitis panel, acute 80074	$95
Tetanus Toxoid 90703	$40		HIV 86703	$100
Vaccine/Toxoid Administration for Younger			Iron & TIBC 83550	$45
Than 8 Years Old w/ counseling 90465	$10		Kidney Profile 80069	$95
Vaccine/Toxoid Administration for Adult 90471	$10		Lead 83665	$55
Arthrocentesis/Aspiration/Injection			Lipase 83690	$40
Small Joint 20600	$50		Lipid Panel 80061	$95
Interm Joint 20605	$60		Liver Profile 80076	$95
Major Joint 20610	$70		Mono Test 86308	$30
Trigger Point/Tendon Sheath Inj. 20550	$90		Pap Smear 88155	$90
Other Invasive/Noninvasive Procedures			Pap Collection/Supervision 88142	$95
Catheterization 51701	$55		Pregnancy Test 84703	$90
Circumcision 54150	$150		Obstetric Panel 80055	$85
Colposcopy 57452	$225		Pro Time 85610	$50
Colposcopy w/Biopsy 57454	$250		PSA 84153	$50
Cryosurgery Premalignant Lesion various codes	$160		RPR 86592	$55
Endometrial Biopsy 58100	$190		Sed. Rate 85651	$50
Excision Lesion Malignant various codes	$145		Stool Culture 87045	$80
Excision Lesion Benign various codes	$125		Stool O & P 87177	$105
Curettement Lesion			Strep Screen 87880	$35
Single 11055	$70		Theophylline 80198	$40
2–4 11056	$80		Thyroid Uptake 84479	$75
>4 11057	$90		TSH 84443	$50
Excision Skin Tags (1–15) 11200	$55		Urinalysis 81000	$35
Each Additional 10 11201	$30		Urine Culture 87088	$80
I & D Abscess Single/Simple 10060	$75		Drawing Fee 36415	$15
Multiple/Complex 10061	$95		Specimen Collection 99000	$10
I & D Pilonidal Cyst Simple 10080	$105			
I & D Pilonidal Cyst Complex 10081	$130			
Laceration Repair various codes	$60			

1500

HEALTH INSURANCE CLAIM FORM

APPROVED BY NATIONAL UNIFORM CLAIM COMMITTEE 08/05

| | PICA | | | | | | | PICA | |

1. MEDICARE ☐ (Medicare #) **MEDICAID** ☐ (Medicaid #) **TRICARE CHAMPUS** ☐ (Sponsor's SSN) **CHAMPVA** ☐ (Member ID#) **GROUP HEALTH PLAN** ☐ (SSN or ID) **FECA BLK LUNG** ☐ (SSN) **OTHER** ☐ (ID)

1a. INSURED'S I.D. NUMBER (For Program in Item 1)

2. PATIENT'S NAME (Last Name, First Name, Middle Initial)

3. PATIENT'S BIRTH DATE MM | DD | YY **SEX** M ☐ F ☐

4. INSURED'S NAME (Last Name, First Name, Middle Initial)

5. PATIENT'S ADDRESS (No., Street)

6. PATIENT RELATIONSHIP TO INSURED Self ☐ Spouse ☐ Child ☐ Other ☐

7. INSURED'S ADDRESS (No, Street)

CITY | **STATE**

8. PATIENT STATUS Single ☐ Married ☐ Other ☐

CITY | **STATE**

ZIP CODE | **TELEPHONE** (Include Area Code) ( )

Employed ☐ Full-Time Student ☐ Part-Time Student ☐

ZIP CODE | **TELEPHONE** (Include Area Code) ( )

9. OTHER INSURED'S NAME (Last Name, First Name, Middle Initial)

10. IS PATIENT'S CONDITION RELATED TO:

11. INSURED'S POLICY GROUP OR FECA NUMBER

a. OTHER INSURED'S POLICY OR GROUP NUMBER

a. EMPLOYMENT? (Current or Previous) ☐ YES ☐ NO

a. INSURED'S DATE OF BIRTH MM | DD | YY **SEX** M ☐ F ☐

b. OTHER INSURED'S DATE OF BIRTH MM | DD | YY **SEX** M ☐ F ☐

b. AUTO ACCIDENT? PLACE (State) ☐ YES ☐ NO

b. EMPLOYER'S NAME OR SCHOOL NAME

c. EMPLOYER'S NAME OR SCHOOL NAME

c. OTHER ACCIDENT? ☐ YES ☐ NO

c. INSURANCE PLAN NAME OR PROGRAM NAME

d. INSURANCE PLAN NAME OR PROGRAM NAME

10d. RESERVED FOR LOCAL USE

d. IS THERE ANOTHER HEALTH BENEFIT PLAN? ☐ YES ☐ NO *If yes*, return to and complete item 9 a-d.

READ BACK OF FORM BEFORE COMPLETING & SIGNING THIS FORM.
12. PATIENT'S OR AUTHORIZED PERSON'S SIGNATURE I authorize the release of any medical or other information necessary to process this claim. I also request payment of government benefits either to myself or to the party who accepts assignment below.

SIGNED _____ DATE _____

13. INSURED'S OR AUTHORIZED PERSON'S SIGNATURE I authorize payment of medical benefits to the undersigned physician or supplier for services described below.

SIGNED _____

14. DATE OF CURRENT: MM | DD | YY ◄ ILLNESS (First symptom) OR INJURY (Accident) OR PREGNANCY (LMP)

15. IF PATIENT HAS HAD SAME OR SIMILAR ILLNESS, GIVE FIRST DATE MM | DD | YY

16. DATES PATIENT UNABLE TO WORK IN CURRENT OCCUPATION FROM MM | DD | YY TO MM | DD | YY

17. NAME OF REFERRING PHYSICIAN OR OTHER SOURCE

17a.
17b. NPI

18. HOSPITALIZATION DATES RELATED TO CURRENT SERVICES FROM MM | DD | YY TO MM | DD | YY

19. RESERVED FOR LOCAL USE

20. OUTSIDE LAB? ☐ YES ☐ NO **$ CHARGES**

21. DIAGNOSIS OR NATURE OF ILLNESS OR INJURY (Relate Items 1,2,3 or 4 to Item 24E by Line)

1. |_____._____| 3. |_____._____|
2. |_____._____| 4. |_____._____|

22. MEDICAID RESUBMISSION CODE | ORIGINAL REF. NO.

23. PRIOR AUTHORIZATION NUMBER

24. A. DATE(S) OF SERVICE						B. PLACE OF SERVICE	C. EMG	D. PROCEDURES, SERVICES, OR SUPPLIES (Explain Unusual Circumstances)		E. DIAGNOSIS POINTER	F. $ CHARGES	G. DAYS OR UNITS	H. EPSDT Family Plan	I. ID. QUAL.	J. RENDERING PROVIDER ID. #
From MM	DD	YY	To MM	DD	YY			CPT/HCPCS	MODIFIER						
1														NPI	
2														NPI	
3														NPI	
4														NPI	
5														NPI	
6														NPI	

25. FEDERAL TAX I.D. NUMBER SSN ☐ EIN ☐

26. PATIENT'S ACCOUNT NO.

27. ACCEPT ASSIGNMENT? (For govt. claims, see back) ☐ YES ☐ NO

28. TOTAL CHARGE $

29. AMOUNT PAID $

30. BALANCE DUE $

31. SIGNATURE OF PHYSICIAN OR SUPPLIER INCLUDING DEGREES OR CREDENTIALS (I certify that the statements on the reverse apply to this bill and are made a part thereof.)

SIGNED _____ DATE _____

32. SERVICE FACILITY LOCATION INFORMATION
a. NPI | b.

33. BILLING PROVIDER INFO & PH. # ( )
a. NPI | b.

NUCC Instruction Manual available at: www.nucc.org
WCMS-1500CS

APPROVED OMB 0938-0999 FORM CMS-1500 (08/05)

Vertical left margin text: SECOND FOLD — FIRST FOLD WHCF-10-ENV / WHCF-10-ENV-SS

Vertical right margin text: CARRIER ↕ — PATIENT AND INSURED INFORMATION — PHYSICIAN OR SUPPLIER INFORMATION

Figure 11-10

REVIEW QUESTIONS

MATCHING

Choose the correct answer, and write its corresponding letter in the space provided.

a. encryption
b. guarantor
c. release of information form
d. clearinghouse
e. EMCs

1. _____ The person financially responsible for medical services
2. _____ Electronic medical claims
3. _____ Written authorization by a patient to disclose personal information to a specifically named entity
4. _____ Scrambling of information during transmission so that the information cannot be intercepted and read by anyone other than the intended recipient
5. _____ A company that receives claims from medical facilities, audits the claims for errors, and then forwards clean claims to the insurance company for the purpose of reimbursement

MULTIPLE CHOICE

Circle the letter of the choice that best completes each statement or answers the question.

1. Which of the following is a disadvantage of electronic medical claims?
   a. They are more efficient.
   b. Claims can sometimes be slowed down.
   c. There are issues with claims attachments.
   d. None of the above

2. Which of the following is another name for a superbill?
   a. Encounter form
   b. Routing slip
   c. Charge slip
   d. All of the above

3. When is the amount paid filled in for FL 29?
   a. When submitting the primary claim
   b. After the primary insurance EOB has been received and the secondary claim is to be submitted
   c. Never
   d. When submitting both the primary and secondary claims

4. How much of the physician's income can be generated by insurance claims?
   a. 60 percent
   b. 70 percent
   c. 80 percent
   d. 75 percent

5. Which of the following is the definition of the birthday rule?

a. If a dependent child is covered by both parents' insurance plans, and the parents are not separated or divorced, the primary insurance plan is determined by the parent whose birthday is earlier in the calendar year.

b. If two or more plans cover a dependent child of separated or divorced parents

who do not have joint custody, the primary insurance plan is determined by the parent whose birthday is earlier in the calendar year.

c. Both a and b

d. None of the above

SHORT ANSWER

Provide the correct response to each question that follows.

1. a. What is the result of not acquiring a patient's signature on the assignment of benefits form?

_____

_____

_____

b. What is a signed assignment of benefits form called in most medical offices?

_____

c. If a signed assignment of benefits form is not on file, should you still submit a claim to the insurance carrier? Why or why not?

_____

_____

_____

2. a. What patient information is needed for a billing service to process claims?

_____

_____

b. If a medical office uses a billing service, where will the insurance payment be sent, and how will this payment be handled?

_____

_____

_____

3. What items does the patient information form include?

1. _____

2. _____

4. When an assignment of benefits form is signed, indicating "signature on file," can this form be used to release a patient's health care information to other entities other than the insurance carrier? Why or why not?

_____

_____

_____

5. HIPAA implemented the 10 Transaction Standards, which eliminated confusion when medical information is exchanged between the provider and the insurance carrier. What are the 10 Transaction Standards?

1. _____

2. _____

3. _____

4. _____

5. _____

6. _____

7. _____

8. _____

9. _____

10. _____

TRUE/FALSE

Identify each statement as true (T) or false (F).

1. _____ An incorrect claim must be corrected, but does not cost any additional fees each time it is returned for errors.

2. _____ Original CMS-1500 claim forms must be used for submittal; thus, copied claims cannot be submitted.

3. _____ Guidelines for completing the CMS-1500 form do not vary at state and local levels.

4. _____ When entering the amount of charges in FL 24, you must use a dollar sign and a decimal point.

5. _____ The term "signature on file" can be used in box 12.

CHAPTER 12
Hospital Medical Billing

CHAPTER OBJECTIVES

Upon completion of this chapter in your student text, you should be able to do the following:

1. Understand the inpatient billing process used by hospitals.
2. Submit accurate and timely hospital claims and practice good follow-up and collection techniques.
3. Identify the different types of facilities and differentiate between inpatient and outpatient services.
4. Understand that hospital billing and coding are based on revenue.
5. Recognize that hospital reimbursement is not a fee for service, but a fixed fee payment based on the diagnosis rather than on time or services rendered.
6. Complete the UB-04 hospital billing claim form.

CHAPTER OUTLINE

Inpatient Billing Process

Charge Description Master

Types of Payers

Coding and Reimbursement Methods

Diagnosis Related Group System
    Cost Outliers

UB-04 Hospital Billing Claim Form

Instructions for Completing the UB-04 Claim Form

Codes for Use on the UB-04 Claim Form
    Type of Bill Codes (Form Locator 4)
    Sex Codes (Form Locator 11)
    Admission/Discharge Hour Codes (Form Locators 13 and 16)
    Admission Type Codes (Form Locator 14)
    Source of Admission (Form Locator 15)
    Discharge Status Codes (Form Locator 17)
    Condition Codes (Form Locators 18–28)
    Occurrence Code Examples (Form Locators 31–34)
    Value Codes (Form Locators 39–41)
    Revenue Codes (Form Locator 42)
    Patient Relationship (Form Locator 59)
    Practice Exercises

KEY TERMS

Using the highlighted terms and glossary in the textbook, define the following terms:

1. admitting physician _____
_____

2. Ambulatory Payment Classification (APC) system _____
_____

3. ambulatory surgical center (ASC) _____
_____

4. ambulatory surgical unit (ASU) _____
_____

5. attending physician _____
_____

6. charge description master (CDM) _____
_____

7. comorbidity _____
_____

8. cost outlier _____
_____

9. Diagnosis Related Group (DRG) _____
_____

10. emergency care _____
_____

11. grouper _____
_____

12. hospice _____
_____

13. hospital acquired conditions (HAC) _____
_____

14. inpatient care _____
_____

15. master patient index _____
_____

16. Medicare DRG (CMS-DRG & MS-DRG) _____
_____

17. operating physician _____
_____

18. outpatient care _____
_____

19. Outpatient Prospective Payment System (OPPS) _____
_____

20. patient control number (PCN) _____
_____

21. present on admission (POA) _____

_____

22. principal diagnosis _____

_____

23. prospective payment system _____

_____

24. registration _____

_____

25. rendering physician _____

_____

26. skilled nursing facility (SNF) _____

_____

27. urgent care _____

_____

CRITICAL THINKING QUESTIONS

Using the knowledge you have gained from reading the textbook, apply critical thinking skills to answer the following questions:

1. Answer the following questions related to the Ambulatory Payment Classification (APC) system:
   a. In your own words, briefly describe the purpose of the APC.

   _____

   _____

   _____

   _____

   _____

   b. During billing, who assigns an APC?

   _____

   _____

   c. What 13 types of services are APCs applied to?
   1. _____
   2. _____
   3. _____
   4. _____
   5. _____
   6. _____
   7. _____
   8. _____
   9. _____
   10. _____
   11. _____
   12. _____
   13. _____

2. Answer the following questions related to Diagnosis Related Groups (DRGs) and case mixes:

a. In your own words, briefly describe the purpose of a DRG.

_____

_____

_____

_____

b. During billing, who assigns a DRG?

_____

_____

c. In what seven ways is a DRG classified?

1. _____
2. _____
3. _____
4. _____
5. _____
6. _____
7. _____

d. How can a hospital determine reimbursement for a DRG?

_____

_____

_____

e. How does a hospital determine its charges for a DRG?

_____

_____

_____

_____

_____

f. What are the five factors that contribute to a facility's case mix?

1. _____
2. _____
3. _____
4. _____
5. _____

g. In your own words, how has DRG reimbursement changed hospital reimbursement?

_____

_____

_____

_____

h. What are the eight situations that could cause a DRG cost outlier?

1. _____
2. _____
3. _____
4. _____
5. _____
6. _____
7. _____
8. _____

i. If a cost outlier occurs, how is it reimbursed by the insurance carrier?

_____

_____

_____

3. Answer the following questions related to ICD-10-PCS:

a. What type of medical facility uses ICD-10-PCS?

_____

b. Under what four circumstances should ICD-10-PCS be used?

1. _____
2. _____
3. _____
4. _____

4. Answer the following questions related to hospital billing and the UB-04 form:

a. What claim form is used for billing hospital services?

_____

b. Why is the UB-04 printed in red ink on white paper?

_____

_____

_____

c. What are revenue codes used for?

_____

_____

_____

d. What are value codes used for?

_____

_____

_____

e. What are type of bill codes used for?

_____

_____

_____

f. What are sex codes used for?

_____

_____

g. What are source of admission codes used for?

_____

_____

h. What are discharge codes used for?

_____

_____

i. What are condition codes used for?

_____

_____

j. What are occurrence codes used for?

_____

_____

k. What are patient relationship codes used for?

_____

_____

5. a. How would you show where the patient was discharged to?

_____

_____

b. What are some examples of discharge status codes with their descriptions?

_____

_____

c. What is discharge status, and why is accuracy important when entering the discharge status code?

_____

_____

_____

PRACTICE EXERCISES

1. Using the form locator information supplied in your textbook, write each form locator for the UB-04 along with the description for each. Add any notes you think will be helpful when filling out cases.

2. Using the ICD-9-CM Volume 3, code the following procedures:

Epiglottidectomy

Code _____

Secondary insertion of intraocular lens prosthesis

Code _____

Implantation of chemotherapy agent

Code _____

Laporascopically assisted vaginal hysterectomy

Code _____

Dilation of urethra

Code _____

Open repair of diaphragmatic hernia, abdominal approach

Code _____

Bone marrow aspiration from donor for transplant

Code _____

Bursotomy of left hand

Code _____

Indwelling urethral catheterization

Code _____

Classical Cesarean section

Code _____

Control of epistaxis by cauterization and packing

Code _____

Endoscopic destruction of lesion, left lung

Code _____

Drainage of popliteal space

Code _____

Retinal electrolysis for tear repair, right eye

Code _____

Microscopic examination of a vaginal culture

Code _____

Renal function study

Code _____

Skin graft of dermal layer for breast augmentation

Code _____

Insertion for drainage tube, right kidney

Code _____

Jones operation for hammer toe, left foot, 2nd digit

Code _____

Lengthening of right femur with bone graft

Code _____

Laparoscopic lysis of liver adhesions

Code _____

Systemic arterial blood gas measurement

Code _____

Nephrectomy for transplanted kidney

Code _____

Retrograde pyelogram

Code _____

X-ray of left knee

Code _____

Reattachment of left thumb

Code _____

PET scan of bone marrow

Code _____

Suture of right ear

Code _____

Denver developmental test

Code _____

Ultrasonic heat therapy

Code _____

Ultrasound of head and neck

Code _____

3. The case studies that follow are provided for additional practice in completing the UB-04 claim form for hospital billing. By applying what you have learned in your student text, accurately complete each case study. All the information you need is provided, including patient demographics, diagnostic and procedure codes, and a brief case history of each patient's health problem. Complete the cases based on the following criteria:

- All patients have release of information and assignment of benefit signatures on file.
- All physicians and hospitals participate in all the health care plans listed, and all physicians and hospitals accept assignment for these plans.
- The hospital is the billing entity.
- The national transition to NPI numbers is complete, and legacy PINs of individual payers are no longer used. If legacy PINs are still being used by selected payers in your region, your instructor may provide legacy PINs in addition to the NPI.
- 2012 ICD-9-CM and CPT codes are used.
- Use six-digit dates for *all* dates.

- All street names should be entered with standard postal abbreviations, even if they are spelled out on the source documents.

- Room charges reflect the daily rate and should be multiplied times the number of days to get the total room charge for the stay.

- All other services reflect the total charges for all units provided.

- Revenue codes should be entered in ascending order.

To complete each case study, use the blank UB-04 form provided after each case.

    a. Using the given source documents and the blank UB-04 form provided (Figure 12-1), complete the following case study for patient Cristal McLean (Case 12-1):

CASE 12-1

Capital City General Hospital
1000 Cherry Street
Capital City, NY 12345-2222
(555) 555-1000

Patient Information:	Cristal McLean
	921 Sweet Street, Capital City, NY 12345
	555-555-6644
DOB:	10-17-1982
Sex:	Female
SSN:	186-03-1982
Status:	Single **Student:** No
Employer:	Shopaholic's
	3829 Clearview Mall, Capital City, NY 12345
	555-555-7467
Responsible Party:	Cristal McLean
Responsible Party Address:	Same
Insurance Information:	Blue Cross Blue Shield
	379 Blue Plaza Capital City, NY 12345
ID #:	YYJ674976211 **Group #:** 10203
Insured's Name:	Same **Relationship to Patient:** Self
Insured's DOB:	
❏ **Male** ❏ **Female**	
Insured's Address:	
Insured's Employer:	
Authorization:	565688221 **Approved # of Days:** 2
Attending Physician:	Bette R. Soone, MD
Federal Tax ID #:	75-7654321
NPI:	0987654321

Reason for visit: I am having a lot of ankle swelling and headaches.

CASE 12-1

HPI: This is a white female admitted on August 2, 20XX, at 7:15 am for elevated BP: 140/88, B/L edema of lower extremities, and albuminuria. Pt. has pre-eclampsia. Pt. has no history of complications with previous pregnancy. She is $7^1/_2$ months pregnant. LMP 12/03/XX Pt. has healthy two-year-old boy at home. No effects to baby's health at this time. Her BP and albumin have stayed mildly elevated at this time. If no improvement within 1 week, we may have to induce labor. Pt. was discharged on August 5, 20XX, at 11:00 a.m.

Patient Control #:	658423	Type of Admission:	1
MR #:	0123573356	Source of Admission:	1
Hospital NPI:	1212121212	Discharge Status:	01
Hospital Tax ID:	75-7575757	Type of Bill Code:	111

Fees:

Revenue Codes	Units	Total Charges	Dates of Service
110 Room/Board/Semi	3	$ 400.00/day	08/02/20XX–08/04/20XX
250 Pharmacy	3	$ 300.00	08/02/20XX–08/04/20XX
260 IV Therapy	2	$ 550.00	08/02/20XX–08/03/20XX
270 Med/Surg Supplies	3	$ 450.00	08/02/20XX–08/04/20XX
320 Radiology	1	$ 250.00	08/02/20XX
001 TOTAL		$2350.00	

Principal DX:	642.43
Admitting DX:	642.43
Principal Procedure Code:	88.78, 38.99

1			2		3a PAT CNTL #			4 TYPE OF BILL
					b MED. REC #			
					5 FED. TAX NO.	6 STATEMENT COVERS PERIOD FROM THROUGH	7	

8 PATIENT NAME	a		9 PATIENT ADDRESS	a					
b			b			c	d		e

10 BIRTHDATE	11 SEX	12 DATE	ADMISSION 13 HR	14 TYPE	15 SRC	16 DHR	17 STAT	18	19	20	21	CONDITION CODES 22	23	24	25	26	27	28	29 ACDT STATE	30

31 CODE	OCCURRENCE DATE	32 CODE	OCCURRENCE DATE	33 CODE	OCCURRENCE DATE	34 CODE	OCCURRENCE DATE	35 CODE	OCCURRENCE SPAN FROM THROUGH	36 CODE	OCCURRENCE SPAN FROM THROUGH	37
a												
b												

38		39 CODE	VALUE CODES AMOUNT	40 CODE	VALUE CODES AMOUNT	41 CODE	VALUE CODES AMOUNT
		a					
		b					
		c					
		d					

42 REV.CD.	43 DESCRIPTION	44 HCPCS/RATE/HPPS CODE	45 SERV. DATE	46 SERV. UNITS	47 TOTAL CHARGES	48 NON-COVERED CHARGES	49	
1								1
2								2
3								3
4								4
5								5
6								6
7								7
8								8
9								9
10								10
11								11
12								12
13								13
14								14
15								15
16								16
17								17
18								18
19								19
20								20
21								21
22								22
23	PAGE ____ OF ____	CREATION DATE		TOTALS ➡				23

50 PAYER NAME		51 HEALTH PLAN ID	52 REL INFO	53 ASG. BEN.	54 PRIOR PAYMENTS	55 EST. AMOUNT DUE	56 NPI		
A							57 OTHER PRV ID		A
B									B
C									C

58 INSURED'S NAME		59 P. REL	60 INSURED'S UNIQUE ID	61 GROUP NAME	62 INSURANCE GROUP NO.	
A						A
B						B
C						C

63 TREATMENT AUTHORIZATION CODES	64 DOCUMENT CONTROL NUMBER	65 EMPLOYER NAME	
A			A
B			B
C			C

66 DX	67	A	B	C	D	E	F	G	H	68
	I	J	K	L	M	N	O	P	Q	

69 ADMIT DX	70 PATIENT REASON DX	a	b	c	71 PPS CODE	72 ECI	a	b	c	73

74 PRINCIPAL PROCEDURE CODE DATE	a. OTHER PROCEDURE CODE DATE	b. OTHER PROCEDURE CODE DATE	75	76 ATTENDING	NPI		QUAL	
				LAST		FIRST		
c. OTHER PROCEDURE CODE DATE	d. OTHER PROCEDURE CODE DATE	e. OTHER PROCEDURE CODE DATE		77 OPERATING	NPI		QUAL	
				LAST		FIRST		
80 REMARKS		81CC a		78 OTHER	NPI		QUAL	
		b		LAST		FIRST		
		c		79 OTHER	NPI		QUAL	
		d		LAST		FIRST		

UB-04 CMS-1450   NLCF-UB04-1   APPROVED OMB NO. 0938-0997 OCR/Original   **NUBC** National Uniform Billing Committee   THE CERTIFICATIONS ON THE REVERSE APPLY TO THIS BILL AND ARE MADE A PART HEREOF.

Figure 12-1

b. Using the given source documents and the blank UB-04 form provided (Figure 12-2), complete the following case study for patient Raquel Freeman (Case 12-2):

CASE 12-2

Capital City General Hospital
1000 Cherry Street
Capital City, NY 12345-2222
(555) 555-1000

Patient Information:	Raquel Freeman
	22 Lock Drive, Capital City, NY 12345
	555-555-9924
DOB:	09-20-1995
Sex:	Female
SSN:	810-10-2240
Status:	Single **Student:** Yes
Employer:	

Responsible Party:	Seth Freeman
Responsible Party Address:	Same
Insurance Information:	Blue Cross Blue Shield
	379 Blue Plaza Capital City, NY 12345
ID #:	YYZ546676122 **Group #:** 9001
Insured's Name:	Seth Freeman **Relationship to Patient:** Father
Insured's DOB:	10/03/1972
☒ Male ☐ Female	
Insured's Address:	Same
Insured's Employer:	Private Investivations, Inc.
	62 Catch Way
	Capital City, NY 12345
Authorization:	565688221 **Approved # of Days:** 4
Attending Physician:	Phil Wells, MD
Federal Tax ID #:	75-0246810
NPI:	1234567890

Reason for visit: My daughter is running a high fever and her head hurts.

CASE 12-2

HPI: This is an African American female admitted on September 4, 20XX, at 8:00 am for bacterial meningitis. The patient has a severe headache that is accompanied by a fever of 102.4°F. Over the course of treatment, the pt. improved remarkably with current treatment. Pt. was discharged on September 8, 20XX, at 9:30 a.m.

Patient Control #:	135535	Type of Admission:	1
MR #:	85735681	Source of Admission:	1
Hospital NPI:	1212121212	Discharge Status:	01
Hospital Tax ID:	75-7575757	Type of Bill Code:	111

Fees:

Revenue Codes	Units	Total Charges	Dates of Service
110 Room/Board/Semi	4	$ 400.00/day	09/04/20XX–09/08/20XX
250 Pharmacy	5	$ 450.00	09/04/20XX–09/08/20XX
260 IV Therapy	4	$ 400.00	09/04/20XX–09/07/20XX
270 Med/Surg Supplies	4	$ 480.00	09/04/20XX–09/07/20XX
300 Pathology	1	$ 450.00	09/04/20XX
001 TOTAL		$3380.00	

Principal DX:	320.82	
Admitting DX:	320.82	
Principal Procedure Code:	03.31	

1			2		3a PAT CNTL #		4 TYPE OF BILL
					b MED. REC #		
					5 FED. TAX NO.	6 STATEMENT COVERS PERIOD FROM THROUGH	7

8 PATIENT NAME	a		9 PATIENT ADDRESS	a				
b			b			c	d	e

| 10 BIRTHDATE | 11 SEX | 12 DATE | ADMISSION 13 HR | 14 TYPE | 15 SRC | 16 DHR | 17 STAT | 18 | 19 | 20 | 21 | CONDITION CODES 22 23 24 25 26 27 28 | 29 ACDT STATE | 30 |

| 31 OCCURRENCE CODE   DATE | 32 OCCURRENCE CODE   DATE | 33 OCCURRENCE CODE   DATE | 34 OCCURRENCE CODE   DATE | 35 OCCURRENCE SPAN CODE   FROM   THROUGH | 36 OCCURRENCE SPAN CODE   FROM   THROUGH | 37 |

a
b

38		39 CODE VALUE CODES AMOUNT	40 CODE VALUE CODES AMOUNT	41 CODE VALUE CODES AMOUNT
		a		
		b		
		c		
		d		

42 REV.CD.	43 DESCRIPTION	44 HCPCS/RATE/HPPS CODE	45 SERV. DATE	46 SERV. UNITS	47 TOTAL CHARGES	48 NON-COVERED CHARGES	49
1							1
2							2
3							3
4							4
5							5
6							6
7							7
8							8
9							9
10							10
11							11
12							12
13							13
14							14
15							15
16							16
17							17
18							18
19							19
20							20
21							21
22							22
23	PAGE ____ OF ____	CREATION DATE		TOTALS ➤			23

50 PAYER NAME	51 HEALTH PLAN ID	52 REL INFO	53 ASG. BEN.	54 PRIOR PAYMENTS	55 EST. AMOUNT DUE	56 NPI	
A							A
B						57 OTHER PRV ID	B
C							C

58 INSURED'S NAME	59 P. REL	60 INSURED'S UNIQUE ID	61 GROUP NAME	62 INSURANCE GROUP NO.	
A					A
B					B
C					C

63 TREATMENT AUTHORIZATION CODES	64 DOCUMENT CONTROL NUMBER	65 EMPLOYER NAME	
A			A
B			B
C			C

66 DX	67	A	B	C	D	E	F	G	H	68
	I	J	K	L	M	N	O	P	Q	

| 69 ADMIT DX | 70 PATIENT REASON DX   a   b   c | 71 PPS CODE | 72 ECI   a   b   c | 73 |

74 PRINCIPAL PROCEDURE CODE DATE	a. OTHER PROCEDURE CODE DATE	b. OTHER PROCEDURE CODE DATE	75	76 ATTENDING NPI QUAL
				LAST FIRST
c. OTHER PROCEDURE CODE DATE	d. OTHER PROCEDURE CODE DATE	e. OTHER PROCEDURE CODE DATE		77 OPERATING NPI QUAL
				LAST FIRST

80 REMARKS	81CC a		78 OTHER NPI QUAL
	b		LAST FIRST
	c		79 OTHER NPI QUAL
	d		LAST FIRST

UB-04 CMS-1450   NLCF-UB04-1   APPROVED OMB NO. 0938-0997 OCR/Original   **NUBC** National Uniform Billing Committee   THE CERTIFICATIONS ON THE REVERSE APPLY TO THIS BILL AND ARE MADE A PART HEREOF.

Figure 12-2

c. Using the given source documents and the blank UB-04 form provided (Figure 12-3), complete the following case study for patient Jamal Clinton (Case 12-3):

CASE 12-3

Capital City General Hospital
1000 Cherry Street
Capital City, NY 12345-2222
(555) 555-1000

Patient Information: Jamal Clinton
189 Maryland Avenue, Capital City, NY 12345
555-555-1456

DOB: 05-19-1962

Sex: Male

SSN: 727-22-1581

Status: Divorced   **Student:** No

Employer: Capital City College
400 College Road, Capital City, NY 12345
555-555-4001

Responsible Party: Jamal Clinton

Responsible Party Address: Same

Insurance Information: Aetna
1625 Healthcare Bldg., Capital City, NY 12345

ID #:   300265   **Group #:** 7224

Insured's Name: Same   **Relationship to Patient:** Self

Insured's DOB:

❏ **Male**   ❏ **Female**

Insured's Address:

Insured's Employer:

Authorization: 8630656131   **Approved # of Days:** 2

Attending Physician: Phil Wells, MD

Federal Tax ID #:   75-0246810

NPI: 1234567890

Reason for visit: Kidney infection.

CASE 12-3

HPI: This is an African American male admitted on December 12, 20XX, at 10:15 a.m. for a kidney infection. Pt. has a history of kidney infections. There is no evidence of damage to the kidneys. Pt. was discharged on December 14, 20XX, at 10:00 a.m.

Patient Control #:	523523	Type of Admission:	1
MR #:	2563216841	Source of Admission:	1
Hospital NPI:	1212121212	Discharge Status:	01
Hospital Tax ID:	75-7575757	Type of Bill Code:	111

Fees:

Revenue Codes	Units	Total Charges	Dates of Service
110 Room/Board/Semi	2	$ 400.00/day	12/12/20XX–12/14/20XX
250 Pharmacy	3	$ 300.00	12/12/20XX–12/14/20XX
260 IV Therapy	2	$ 500.00	12/12/20XX–12/13/20XX
270 Med/Surg Supplies	2	$ 200.00	12/12/20XX–12/13/20XX
320 Radiology	2	$ 500.00	12/13/20XX
001 TOTAL		$2300.00	

Principal DX:	590.10, 041.40
Admitting DX:	590.10
Principal Procedure Code:	92.03, 87.79

1		2		3a PAT CNTL #			4 TYPE OF BILL
				b MED. REC #			
				5 FED. TAX NO.	6 STATEMENT COVERS PERIOD FROM THROUGH		7

8 PATIENT NAME	a		9 PATIENT ADDRESS	a				
b			b			c	d	e

| 10 BIRTHDATE | 11 SEX | 12 DATE | ADMISSION 13 HR | 14 TYPE | 15 SRC | 16 DHR | 17 STAT | 18 | 19 | 20 | 21 | CONDITION CODES 22 23 24 25 26 27 28 | 29 ACDT STATE | 30 |

31 OCCURRENCE CODE DATE	32 OCCURRENCE CODE DATE	33 OCCURRENCE CODE DATE	34 OCCURRENCE CODE DATE	35 OCCURRENCE SPAN CODE FROM THROUGH	36 OCCURRENCE SPAN CODE FROM THROUGH	37

a
b

38		39 VALUE CODES CODE AMOUNT	40 VALUE CODES CODE AMOUNT	41 VALUE CODES CODE AMOUNT
	a			
	b			
	c			
	d			

42 REV.CD.	43 DESCRIPTION	44 HCPCS/RATE/HPPS CODE	45 SERV. DATE	46 SERV. UNITS	47 TOTAL CHARGES	48 NON-COVERED CHARGES	49
1							1
2							2
3							3
4							4
5							5
6							6
7							7
8							8
9							9
10							10
11							11
12							12
13							13
14							14
15							15
16							16
17							17
18							18
19							19
20							20
21							21
22							22
23	PAGE ____ OF ____	CREATION DATE	TOTALS ▶				23

50 PAYER NAME	51 HEALTH PLAN ID	52 REL INFO	53 ASG. BEN.	54 PRIOR PAYMENTS	55 EST. AMOUNT DUE	56 NPI	
A							57	A
B							OTHER	B
C							PRV ID	C

58 INSURED'S NAME	59 P. REL	60 INSURED'S UNIQUE ID	61 GROUP NAME	62 INSURANCE GROUP NO.	
A					A
B					B
C					C

63 TREATMENT AUTHORIZATION CODES	64 DOCUMENT CONTROL NUMBER	65 EMPLOYER NAME	
A			A
B			B
C			C

66 DX	67	A	B	C	D	E	F	G	H	68
	I	J	K	L	M	N	O	P	Q	

69 ADMIT DX	70 PATIENT REASON DX a b c	71 PPS CODE	72 ECI a b c	73

74 PRINCIPAL PROCEDURE CODE DATE	a. OTHER PROCEDURE CODE DATE	b. OTHER PROCEDURE CODE DATE	75	76 ATTENDING NPI QUAL
				LAST FIRST
c. OTHER PROCEDURE CODE DATE	d. OTHER PROCEDURE CODE DATE	e. OTHER PROCEDURE CODE DATE		77 OPERATING NPI QUAL
				LAST FIRST

80 REMARKS	81CC a	78 OTHER NPI QUAL
	b	LAST FIRST
	c	79 OTHER NPI QUAL
	d	LAST FIRST

UB-04 CMS-1450 NLCF-UB04-1   APPROVED OMB NO. 0938-0997 OCR/Original   **NUBC** National Uniform Billing Committee   THE CERTIFICATIONS ON THE REVERSE APPLY TO THIS BILL AND ARE MADE A PART HEREOF.

Figure 12-3

d. Using the given source documents and the blank UB-04 form provided (Figure 12-4), complete the following case study for patient Dalton Sizer (Case 12-4):

CASE 12-4

Capital City General Hospital
1000 Cherry Street
Capital City, NY 12345-2222
(555) 555-1000

Patient Information: Dalton Sizer
16 Marigold Lane, Capital City, NY 12345
555-555-3007

DOB: 01-20-1970

Sex: Male

SSN: 301-19-0431

Status: Married   **Student:** No

Employer: Woodlands Excavating Co.
2112 Sycamore Drive, Capital City, NY 12345
555-555-1887

Responsible Party: Dalton Sizer

Responsible Party Address: Same

Insurance Information: Aetna
1625 Healthcare Bldg., Capital City NY 12345

ID #:   6543684   **Group #:** 5493

Insured's Name: Same   **Relationship to Patient:** Self

Insured's DOB:

❏ Male   ❏ Female

Insured's Address:

Insured's Employer:

Authorization: **Approved # of Days:** 2

Attending Physician: Elby Alright, MD

Federal Tax ID #:   75-7654321

NPI: 9876543210

Reason for visit: I hit the back of my head on the corner of the bathroom sink counter while standing up from bending over in the bathroom.

CASE 12-4

Capital City General Hospital Outpatient Radiology

Patient's Name: Dalton Sizer   **DOB:** 01/20/1970

Date of Procedure: 11/08/20XX   **PCP:** Elby Alright, MD

Ordering Physician: Elby Alright, MD   **MR #:** DS163540

Report #: DS-01907

Diagnosis: Wound, posterior scalp, open due to striking head against bathroom counter

Procedure: MRI OF BRAIN

Exam is performed with the administration of IV contrast. Study reveals a wound on the posterior portion of the scalp that is consistent with recent trauma. This wound measures 2 × 0.2 in.

The brain presents normal in size without any hematoma, hemorrhage, laceration, or lesion. There is no evidence of disease at this time.

DX Code: 873.0, E917.3   **Source of Admission:**   1

CPT Procedure Code: 70552   **Discharge Status:**   01

Hospital NPI:	6767676767	**Type of Bill Code:**	131
Hospital Tax ID:	75-7575757	**Patient Control #:**	006314

Fees:

Revenue Codes	Units	Total Charges	Dates of Service
250 Pharmacy	1	$ 90.00	11/08/20XX
260 IV Therapy	1	$ 375.00	11/08/20XX
320 Radiology	1	$ 920.00	11/08/20XX
001 TOTAL		$1385.00	

1		2			3a PAT CNTL #		4 TYPE OF BILL
					b MED. REC #		
				5 FED. TAX NO.	6 STATEMENT COVERS PERIOD FROM THROUGH	7	

8 PATIENT NAME	a		9 PATIENT ADDRESS	a				
b			b			c	d	e

| 10 BIRTHDATE | 11 SEX | 12 DATE | ADMISSION 13 HR | 14 TYPE | 15 SRC | 16 DHR | 17 STAT | CONDITION CODES 18 19 20 21 22 23 24 25 26 27 28 | 29 ACDT STATE | 30 |

31 OCCURRENCE CODE DATE	32 OCCURRENCE CODE DATE	33 OCCURRENCE CODE DATE	34 OCCURRENCE CODE DATE	35 OCCURRENCE SPAN CODE FROM THROUGH	36 OCCURRENCE SPAN CODE FROM THROUGH	37
a						
b						

38		39 CODE VALUE CODES AMOUNT	40 CODE VALUE CODES AMOUNT	41 CODE VALUE CODES AMOUNT
	a			
	b			
	c			
	d			

	42 REV.CD.	43 DESCRIPTION	44 HCPCS/RATE/HPPS CODE	45 SERV. DATE	46 SERV. UNITS	47 TOTAL CHARGES	48 NON-COVERED CHARGES	49	
1									1
2									2
3									3
4									4
5									5
6									6
7									7
8									8
9									9
10									10
11									11
12									12
13									13
14									14
15									15
16									16
17									17
18									18
19									19
20									20
21									21
22									22
23	PAGE ___ OF ___		CREATION DATE		TOTALS ➡				23

50 PAYER NAME	51 HEALTH PLAN ID	52 REL INFO	53 ASG. BEN.	54 PRIOR PAYMENTS	55 EST. AMOUNT DUE	56 NPI	
A							A
B						57 OTHER	B
C						PRV ID	C

58 INSURED'S NAME	59 P. REL	60 INSURED'S UNIQUE ID	61 GROUP NAME	62 INSURANCE GROUP NO.	
A					A
B					B
C					C

63 TREATMENT AUTHORIZATION CODES	64 DOCUMENT CONTROL NUMBER	65 EMPLOYER NAME	
A			A
B			B
C			C

66 DX	67	A	B	C	D	E	F	G	H	68
	I	J	K	L	M	N	O	P	Q	

69 ADMIT DX	70 PATIENT REASON DX a b c	71 PPS CODE	72 ECI a b c	73

74 PRINCIPAL PROCEDURE CODE DATE	a. OTHER PROCEDURE CODE DATE	b. OTHER PROCEDURE CODE DATE	75	76 ATTENDING NPI	QUAL
				LAST FIRST	
c. OTHER PROCEDURE CODE DATE	d. OTHER PROCEDURE CODE DATE	e. OTHER PROCEDURE CODE DATE		77 OPERATING NPI	QUAL
				LAST FIRST	

80 REMARKS	81CC a	78 OTHER NPI	QUAL
	b	LAST	FIRST
	c	79 OTHER NPI	QUAL
	d	LAST	FIRST

UB-04 CMS-1450 NLCF-UB04-1   APPROVED OMB NO. 0938-0997 OCR/Original   **NUBC** National Uniform Billing Committee   THE CERTIFICATIONS ON THE REVERSE APPLY TO THIS BILL AND ARE MADE A PART HEREOF.

Figure 12-4

e. Using the given source documents and the blank UB-04 form provided (Figure 12-5), complete the following case study for patient Marvin Hall (Case 12-5):

CASE 12-5

Capital City General Hospital
1000 Cherry Street
Capital City, NY 12345-2222
(555) 555-1000

Patient Information: Marvin Hall
510 County Line Road, Capital City, NY 12345
555-555-2505

DOB: 05-29-1943

Sex: Male

SSN: 625-44-0827

Status: Married   **Student:** No

Employer: Retired

Responsible Party: Marvin Hall

Responsible Party Address: Same

Insurance Information: Medicare
P.O. Box 9834, Capital City, NY 12345

ID #: 564695238A   **Group #:**

Insured's Name: Same   **Relationship to Patient:** Self

Insured's DOB:

❏ Male   ❏ Female

Insured's Address:

Insured's Employer:

Authorization: **Approved # of Days:**

Attending Physician: Elby Alright, MD

Federal Tax ID #: 75-7654321

NPI: 9876543210

Reason for visit: My doctor sent me to get a chest X-ray to see whether I have pleurisy.

CASE 12-5

Capital City General Hospital Outpatient Radiology

Patient's Name: Marvin Hall

Date of Procedure: 01/07/20XX

Ordering Physician: Elby Alright, MD

Report #: MH-624702

Diagnosis: Pleurisy

Procedure: X-ray of chest

DOB: 05/29/1943

PCP: Elby Alright, MD

MR #: 22668874

Study compared with previous CXR. The pleural membrane shows evidence of inflammation and infection. Films are consistent with diagnosis.

DX Code: 511.0

CPT Procedure Code: 71030

Source of Admission: 1

Discharge Status: 01

| Hospital NPI: | 6767676767 | Type of Bill Code: | 132 |
| Hospital Tax ID: | 75-7575757 | Patient Control #: | 883070 |

Fees:

Revenue Codes	Units	Total Charges	Dates of Service
972 Radiologist	1	$250.00	01/07/20XX
320 Radiology	1	$280.00	01/07/20XX
001 TOTAL		$530.00	

1			2		3a PAT CNTL #				4 TYPE OF BILL
					b MED. REC #				
					5 FED. TAX NO.		6 STATEMENT COVERS PERIOD FROM THROUGH	7	

8 PATIENT NAME	a	9 PATIENT ADDRESS	a			
b		b		c	d	e

10 BIRTHDATE	11 SEX	12 DATE	ADMISSION 13 HR	14 TYPE	15 SRC	16 DHR	17 STAT	18	19	20	21	CONDITION CODES 22 23 24 25 26 27 28	29 ACDT STATE	30

31 OCCURRENCE CODE DATE	32 OCCURRENCE CODE DATE	33 OCCURRENCE CODE DATE	34 OCCURRENCE CODE DATE	35 OCCURRENCE SPAN CODE FROM THROUGH	36 OCCURRENCE SPAN CODE FROM THROUGH	37
a						
b						

38		39 VALUE CODES CODE AMOUNT	40 VALUE CODES CODE AMOUNT	41 VALUE CODES CODE AMOUNT
	a			
	b			
	c			
	d			

42 REV.CD.	43 DESCRIPTION	44 HCPCS/RATE/HPPS CODE	45 SERV. DATE	46 SERV. UNITS	47 TOTAL CHARGES	48 NON-COVERED CHARGES	49
1							1
2							2
3							3
4							4
5							5
6							6
7							7
8							8
9							9
10							10
11							11
12							12
13							13
14							14
15							15
16							16
17							17
18							18
19							19
20							20
21							21
22							22
23	PAGE ____ OF ____	CREATION DATE		TOTALS ➡			23

50 PAYER NAME	51 HEALTH PLAN ID	52 REL INFO	53 ASG BEN	54 PRIOR PAYMENTS	55 EST. AMOUNT DUE	56 NPI	
A							57 OTHER PRV ID
B							
C							

58 INSURED'S NAME	59 P. REL	60 INSURED'S UNIQUE ID	61 GROUP NAME	62 INSURANCE GROUP NO.
A				
B				
C				

63 TREATMENT AUTHORIZATION CODES	64 DOCUMENT CONTROL NUMBER	65 EMPLOYER NAME
A		
B		
C		

66 DX	67	A	B	C	D	E	F	G	H	68
	I	J	K	L	M	N	O	P	Q	

69 ADMIT DX	70 PATIENT REASON DX a b c	71 PPS CODE	72 ECI a b c	73

74 PRINCIPAL PROCEDURE CODE DATE	a. OTHER PROCEDURE CODE DATE	b. OTHER PROCEDURE CODE DATE	75	76 ATTENDING NPI	QUAL
				LAST FIRST	
c. OTHER PROCEDURE CODE DATE	d. OTHER PROCEDURE CODE DATE	e. OTHER PROCEDURE CODE DATE		77 OPERATING NPI	QUAL
				LAST FIRST	

80 REMARKS	81 CC a	78 OTHER NPI	QUAL
	b	LAST FIRST	
	c	79 OTHER NPI	QUAL
	d	LAST FIRST	

UB-04 CMS-1450   NLCF-UB04-1   APPROVED OMB NO. 0938-0997 OCR/Original   **NUBC** National Uniform Billing Committee   THE CERTIFICATIONS ON THE REVERSE APPLY TO THIS BILL AND ARE MADE A PART HEREOF.

Figure 12-5

REVIEW QUESTIONS

MATCHING

Choose the correct answer, and write its corresponding letter in the space provided.

a. Master Patient Index
b. discharge analyst
c. chargemaster
d. inlier
e. outlier

1. _____ The main database for all of a hospital's patients
2. _____ A hospital case that exceeds a specific DRG length of stay
3. _____ A hospital case that falls below the mean average or expected length of stay for a specific DRG
4. _____ Organizes revenue codes, procedures codes, descriptions, and charges
5. _____ Used to check the completeness of a patient's medical record for dictated reports and signatures

MULTIPLE CHOICE

Circle the letter of the choice that best completes each statement or answers the question.

1. When does a hospital submit a bill for its services for an inpatient case?
    a. Every day of the hospital stay
    b. After the admission sheet is completed and signed by the physician
    c. After the discharge summary is completed and signed by the physician
    d. At the end of the month

2. What is the term for the process of a grouper searching all listed diagnoses, comorbidities, complications, and procedures to assign and calculate a DRG for a patient's case?
    a. Analyzing
    b. Grouping
    c. Looping
    d. All of the above

3. What is a cost outlier?
    a. When the hospital has to cut costs
    b. Upcoding a patient's case
    c. A DRG cannot be assigned due to an atypical situation
    d. None of the above

4. Which of the following is *not* considered inpatient care?
    a. Ambulatory Surgical Unit in the hospital
    b. Skilled nursing facility
    c. Hospice
    d. Rehabilitation Center

5. Which of the following medical facilities does *not* utilize the UB-04 for billing purposes?
    a. A physician's office
    b. Hospital outpatient departments and rural health clinics
    c. Hospital inpatient departments
    d. Both a and b

SHORT ANSWER

Provide the correct response to each question that follows.

1. What are the discharge analyst's duties?

   _____

2. What are the three sex codes? List and define each.

   1. _____

      _____

      _____

   2. _____

      _____

      _____

   3. _____

      _____

      _____

3. Where is a hospital's Patient Account Service Department (PAS) usually located?

   _____

4. What is the purpose of the PAS?

   _____

   _____

   _____

5. What five pieces of information are included in the charge master that is printed out on the UB-04 for reimbursement? Briefly explain each.

   1. _____

      _____

      _____

   2. _____

      _____

      _____

   3. _____

      _____

      _____

   4. _____

      _____

      _____

   5. _____

      _____

      _____

TRUE/FALSE

Identify each statement as true (T) or false (F).

1. _____ With APCs, services often rendered with a procedure are often unbundled.

2. _____ A grouper cannot determine the difference between an acute and chronic condition.

3. _____ When referring to DRGs, the abbreviation C&C is used to identify complications or comorbidities.

4. _____ More than one APC or DRG can be assigned to one specific patient.

5. _____ Admission and discharge hour codes are listed in military time.

CHAPTER 13
Medicare Medical Billing

CHAPTER OBJECTIVES

Upon completion of this chapter in your student text, you should be able to do the following:

1. Discuss government billing guidelines.
2. Determine the amount due from the patient for a participating provider.
3. Understand the different Medicare fee schedules.
4. Examine and complete accurate Medicare claims forms.
5. Identify the types of Medicare fraud and abuse that can occur.

CHAPTER OUTLINE

Medicare History
    Medicare Administration

Medicare Part A Coverage and Eligibility Requirements
    Inpatient Hospital Care
    Skilled Nursing Facility
    Home Health Care
    Hospice Care
    Blood
    Organ Transplants
    Inpatient Benefit Days

Medicare Part B Coverage and Eligibility Requirements

Medicare Part C

Medicare Part D

Services Not Covered by Medicare Parts A and B

Medigap, Medicaid, and Supplemental Insurance

Requirements for Medical Necessity

Medicare Coverage Plans
    Fee-for-Service: The Original Medicare Plan
    Medicare Advantage Plans or Medicare Part C

Medicare Providers
    Part A Providers
    Part B Providers
    Participating versus Nonparticipating Medicare Part B Providers

Limiting Charge
    Patient's Financial Responsibility
    Determining the Medicare Fee and Limiting Charge

Patient Registration
    Copying the Medicare Card
    Copying the Driver's License
    Obtaining Patient Signatures
    Determining Primary and Secondary Payers
    Plans Primary to Medicare
    Consolidated Omnibus Budget Reconciliation Act of 1985
    People with Disabilities
    People with End-Stage Renal Disease
    Workers' Compensation
    Automobile, No-Fault, and Liability Insurance
    Veteran Benefits
    Medicare Coordination
    Medicare as the Secondary Payer
    Conditional Payment

Medicare Documents

Medicare Development Letter

Medicare Insurance Billing Requirements

Completing Medicare Part B Claims
    Form Locators 1 through 13 for Medicare Part B Claims
    Form Locators 14 through 33 for Medicare Part B Claims
    Filing Guidelines
    Local Coverage Determination

Medicare Remittance Notice

Medicare Fraud and Abuse
    Medicare Fraud
    Medicare Abuse
    Protecting against Medicare Fraud and Abuse

KEY TERMS

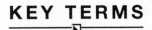

Using the highlighted terms and glossary in the textbook, define the following terms:

1. benefit period _____
_____

2. Consolidated Omnibus Budget Reconciliation Act of 1985 (COBRA) _____
_____

3. crossover _____
_____

4. end-stage renal disease (ESRD) _____
_____

5. Electronic Remittance Advice (ERA) _____
_____

6. Healthcare Common Procedure Coding System (HCPCS) _____
_____

7. intermediaries _____
_____

8. limiting charge _____

_____

9. Local coverage determination (LCDs) _____

_____

10. Medicare abuse _____

_____

11. Medicare Advantage (MA) _____

_____

12. Medicare Administrative Contractor (MAC) _____

_____

13. Medicare Development Letter _____

_____

14. Medicare fraud _____

_____

15. Medicare Part A _____

_____

16. Medicare Part B _____

_____

17. Medicare Part C _____

_____

18. Medicare Part D _____

_____

19. Medicare Remittance Notice (MRN) _____

_____

20. Medicare Secondary Payer (MSP) _____

_____

21. Medicare Summary Notice (MSN) _____

_____

22. Medigap_____

_____

23. non-par MFS _____

_____

24. Office of Inspector General (OIG) _____

_____

25. Program of All-Inclusive Care for the Elderly (PACE)_____

_____

26. Recovery Audit Contractor (RAC)_____

_____

27. scrubbing _____

_____

28. Tax Relief and Health Care Act (TRHCA) _____

_____

CRITICAL THINKING QUESTIONS

Using the knowledge you have gained from reading the textbook, apply critical thinking skills to answer the following questions.

1. a. In your own words, briefly explain the history of Medicare.

    _____
    _____
    _____
    _____

    b. How has Medicare changed the business of health care and health insurance?

    _____
    _____
    _____
    _____
    _____

    c. What will the future of Medicare likely be in 10 years?

    _____
    _____
    _____
    _____
    _____

2. Answer the following questions related to the administration of Medicare:
    a. Who directs Medicare?

    _____
    _____
    _____

    b. What U.S. department is CMS a division of?

    _____
    _____

    c. In your own words, what are the three roles of CMS?
        1. _____
        _____
        2. _____
        _____
        3. _____
        _____

    d. What is the primary function of CMS?

    _____
    _____
    _____

e. In your own words, what is a Medicare contractor, and what is its function?

_____

_____

_____

_____

3. Answer the following questions related to the different parts of Medicare:

a. What are seven roles and responsibilities of Medicare Part A: Intermediaries?

1. _____

2. _____

3. _____

4. _____

5. _____

6. _____

7. _____

b. What six groups of people qualify for Medicare Part A benefits?

1. _____

2. _____

3. _____

4. _____

5. _____

6. _____

c. What are the five roles and responsibilities of Medicare Part B: Carriers?

1. _____

2. _____

3. _____

4. _____

5. _____

d. In your own words, what is the primary function of Medicare intermediaries and carriers?

_____

_____

_____

_____

4. Answer the following questions related to Medicare coverage and claim processing:

a. Patient Jon Yates would like to know what his Medicare Part B will cover.

1. _____

2. _____

3. _____

4. _____

b. Briefly explain to your patient what eligibility requirements must be met to enroll in Medicare Part B.

_____

_____

_____

c. What is the contingency margin for?

1. _____

2. _____

3. _____

4. _____

d. How is the Medicare Part B premium determined?

_____

_____

_____

e. What are the two types of plans that a Medicare Advantage Plan beneficiary can choose from?

1. _____

2. _____

f. What seven benefits are covered under patient Perry Austin's Medicare Part C benefits?

1. _____

2. _____

3. _____

4. _____

5. _____

6. _____

7. _____

g. What is Medicare Part D used for?

_____

h. Who is eligible for Medicare Part D?

_____

_____

5. Answer the following questions related to Medicare fraud and abuse:

a. What are four sanctions that the DHHS will impose on individuals who consistently fail to comply with Medicare law or are deemed abusive to the Medicare program?

1. _____

2. _____

3. _____

4. _____

b. What are the penalties that can be imposed on those convicted of Medicare fraud and/or abuse?

_____

_____

_____

_____

c. As a health care professional, how can you avoid committing Medicare fraud and/or abuse?

_____

_____

_____

_____

_____

PRACTICE EXERCISES

1. Using the form locator information written out on your index cards from a prior chapter complete the following activity. Flag those FLs that would be filled out differently for Medicare patients.

2. Determine the amount owed by the patient.

   A. Participating physician's standard fee: $300.00

      Allowed amount $200.00

      Medicare pays 80%:   _____

      Patient or supplemental plan pays 20%:   _____

      Provider adjustment (write-off):   _____

   B. Non-par physician's standard fee (accepts assignment): $250.00

      Medicare non-par fee: _____

      Medicare pays 80%:   _____

      Patient or supplemental plan pays 20%:   _____

      Provider adjustment (write-off):   _____

   C. Non-par physician's standard fee (does not accept assignment): $250.00

      Medicare non-par fee: _____

      Limiting charge: _____

      Patient billed: _____

      Medicare pays patient: _____

      Total provider can collect: _____

      Patient out-of-pocket expense: _____

      Provider adjustment (write-off):   _____

3. The following case studies are provided for additional practice in completing the CMS-1500 claim form for Medicare physician outpatient billing. By applying what you have learned in your student text, accurately code and complete each case study. Patient demographics and a brief case history are provided. Complete the cases based on the following criteria:

- All patients have release of information and assignment of benefit signatures on file.

- All providers are participating and accept assignment.

- The group practice is the billing entity.

- The national transition to NPI numbers is complete, and legacy PINs and UPINs are no longer used.

- 2012 ICD-9-CM and CPT codes are used.

- Use eight-digit dates for birthdates. Use six-digit dates for all other dates.

- All street names should be entered with standard postal abbreviations, even if they are spelled out on the source documents.

- Enter ICD-9 codes in the order they are listed on the encounter form.

- When entering CPT codes, enter the E/M code first. Enter remaining codes in descending price order.

To determine the correct fees, refer to the Capital City Medical Fee Schedule, which is located after each case's source documents. Use the blank CMS-1500 form provided after each case.

a. Using the source documents, the Capital City Medical Fee Schedule (Figure 13-1), and the blank CMS-1500 form provided (Figure 13-2), complete the following case study for patient Bernard Ward (Case 13-1):

CASE 13-1

Patient Information:

Name: (Last, First) Ward, Bernard   ☒ Male   ☐ Female   Birth Date: 03/20/1957

Address: 420 Cardinal Ct, Township, NY 12345   Phone: (555) 555-2534

Social Security Number: 896-80-2944   Full-Time Student: ☐ Yes   ☒ No

Marital Status: ☐ Single   ☒ Married   ☐ Divorced   ☐ Other

Employment:

Employer: Retired   Phone: ( )

Address:

Condition Related to: ☐ Auto Accident   ☐ Employment   ☐ Other Accident

Date of Accident: State:

Emergency Contact: Phone: ( )

Primary Insurance: Medicaid   Phone: ( )

Address: P O. Box , 9834, Capital City, NY 12345

Insurance Policyholder's Name: Same   ☐ M ☐ F DOB:

Address:

Phone: Relationship to Insured: ☒ Self ☐ Spouse ☐ Child ☐ Other

Employer: Phone: ( )

Employer's Address:

Policy/ID No: 366736530A   Group No: Percent Covered: 80 % Copay Amt: $

Secondary Insurance: Phone: ( )

Address:

Insurance Policyholder's Name: ☐ M ☐ F DOB:

Address:

Phone: Relationship to Insured: ☐ Self ☐ Spouse ☐ Child ☐ Other

Employer: Phone: ( )

Employer's Address:

Policy/ID No: Group No: Percent Covered: % Copay Amt: $

Reason for Visit: I am here for a checkup on my MS.

Known Allergies:

Referred by:

CASE 13-1
SOAP

01/06/20XX
Assignment of Benefits: Y
Signature on File: Y
Referring Physician: N

S: Bernard Ward is here for a checkup on his multiple sclerosis. He has no recent complaints.

O: He denies any numbness, weakness, or stiffness. ROM is full.

A: 1. Multiple sclerosis in remission—340

P: 1. Continue medications.

    2. Keep appointment with neurologist.

    3. Return in 3 months, unless relapse occurs.

_____

Phil Wells, MD
Family Practice
NPI: 1234567890

CASE 13-1

Patient Name Bernard Ward

Capital City Medical
123 Unknown Boulevard, Capital City, NY 12345-2222

Date of Service
01-06-20XX

New Patient						Laboratory	
Problem Focused	99201	Arthrocentesis/Aspiration/Injection				Amylase	82150
Expanded Problem, Focused	99202	Small Joint		20600		B12	82607
Detailed	99203	Interm Joint		20605		CBC & Diff	85025
Comprehensive	99204	Major Joint		20610		Comp Metabolic Panel	80053
Comprehensive/High Complex	99205	**Other Invasive/Noninvasive**				Chlamydia Screen	87110
Well Exam Infant (up to 12 mos.)	99381	Audiometry		92552		Cholesterol	82465
Well Exam 1–4 yrs.	99382	Cast Application				Digoxin	80162
Well Exam 5–11 yrs.	99383	Location Long Short				Electrolytes	80051
Well Exam 12–17 yrs.	99384	Catheterization		51701		Ferritin	82728
Well Exam 18–39 yrs.	99385	Circumcision		54150		Folate	82746
Well Exam 40–64 yrs.	99386	Colposcopy		57452		GC Screen	87070
		Colposcopy w/Biopsy		57454		Glucose	82947
		Cryosurgery Premalignant Lesion				Glucose 1 HR	82950
		Location (s):				Glycosylated HGB A1C	83036
Established Patient		Cryosurgery Warts				HCT	85014
Post-Op Follow Up Visit	99024	Location (s):				HDL	83718
Minimum	99211	Curettement Lesion				Hep BSAG	87340
Problem Focused	99212	Single		11055		Hepatitis panel, acute	80074
Expanded Problem Focused	99213 X	2–4		11056		HGB	85018
Detailed	99214	>4		11057		HIV	86703
Comprehensive/High Complex	99215	Diaphragm Fitting		57170		Iron & TIBC	83550
Well Exam Infant (up to 12 mos.)	99391	Ear Irrigation		69210		Kidney Profile	80069
Well exam 1–4 yrs.	99392	ECG		93000		Lead	83655
Well Exam 5–11 yrs.	99393	Endometrial Biopsy		58100		Liver Profile	80076
Well Exam 12–17 yrs.	99394	Exc. Lesion Malignant				Mono Test	86308
Well Exam 18–39 yrs.	99395	Benign				Pap Smear	88155
Well Exam 40–64 yrs.	99396	Location				Pregnancy Test	84703
Obstetrics		Exc. Skin Tags (1–15)		11200		Obstetric Panel	80055
Total OB Care	59400	Each Additional 10		11201		Pro Time	85610
Injections		Fracture Treatment				PSA	84153
Administration Sub. / IM	90772	Loc				RPR	86592
Drug		w/Reduc		w/o Reduc		Sed. Rate	85651
Dosage		I & D Abscess Single/Simple		10060		Stool Culture	87045
Allergy	95115	Multiple or Comp		10061		Stool O & P	87177
Cocci Skin Test	86490	I & D Pilonidal Cyst Simple		10080		Strep Screen	87880
DPT	90701	Pilonidal Cyst Complex		10081		Theophylline	80198
Hemophilus	90646	IV Therapy—To One Hour		90760		Thyroid Uptake	84479
Influenza	90658	Each Additional Hour		90761		TSH	84443
MMR	90707	Laceration Repair				Urinalysis	81000
OPV	90712	Location Size Simp/Comp				Urine Culture	87088
Pneumovax	90732	Laryngoscopy		31505		Drawing Fee	36415
TB Skin Test	86580	Oximetry		94760		Specimen Collection	99000
TD	90718	Punch Biopsy				**Other:**	
Unlisted Immun	90749	Rhythm Strip		93040			
Tetanus Toxoid	90703	Treadmill		93015			
Vaccine/Toxoid Admin <8 Yr Old w/ Counseling	90465	Trigger Point or Tendon Sheath Inj.		20550			
Vaccine/Toxoid Administration for Adult	90471	Tympanometry		92567			

Diagnosis/ICD-9: **340**

I acknowledge receipt of medical services and authorize the release of any medical information necessary to process this claim for healthcare payment only. I do authorize payment to the provider.

Patient Signature _Bernard Ward_

Total Estimated Charges: _____

Payment Amount: _____

Next Appointment:

Figure 13-1

Capital City Medical
Fee Schedule

New Patient OV		Punch Biopsy various codes	$80
Problem Focused 99201	$45	Nebulizer various codes	$45
Expanded Problem Focused 99202	$65	Cast Application various codes	$85
Detailed 99203	$85	Laryngoscopy 31505	$255
Comprehensive 99204	$105	Audiometry 92552	$85
Comprehensive/High Complex 99205	$115	Tympanometry 92567	$85
Well Exam infant (less than 1 year) 99381	$45	Ear Irrigation 69210	$25
Well Exam 1–4 yrs. 99382	$50	Diaphragm Fitting 57170	$30
Well Exam 5–11 yrs. 99383	$55	IV Therapy (up to one hour) 90760	$65
Well Exam 12–17 yrs. 99384	$65	Each additional hour 90761	$50
Well Exam 18–39 yrs. 99385	$85	Oximetry 94760	$10
Well Exam 40–64 yrs. 99386	$105	ECG 93000	$75
Established Patient OV		Holter Monitor various codes	$170
Post Op Follow Up Visit 99024	$0	Rhythm Strip 93040	$60
Minimum 99211	$35	Treadmill 93015	$375
Problem Focused 99212	$45	Cocci Skin Test 86490	$20
Expanded Problem Focused 99213	$55	X-ray, spine, chest, bone—any area various codes	$275
Detailed 99214	$65	Avulsion Nail 11730	$200
Comprehensive/High Complex 99215	$75	**Laboratory**	
Well exam infant (less than 1 year) 99391	$35	Amylase 82150	$40
Well Exam 1–4 yrs. 99392	$40	B12 82607	$30
Well Exam 5–11 yrs. 99393	$45	CBC & Diff 85025	$95
Well Exam 12–17 yrs. 99394	$55	Comp Metabolic Panel 80053	$75
Well Exam 18–39 yrs. 99395	$65	Chlamydia Screen 87110	$70
Well Exam 40–64 yrs. 99396	$75	Cholestrerol 82465	$75
Obstetrics		Digoxin 80162	$40
Total OB Care 59400	$1700	Electrolytes 80051	$70
Injections		Estrogen, Total 82672	$50
Administration 90772	$10	Ferritin 82728	$40
Allergy 95115	$35	Folate 82746	$30
DPT 90701	$50	GC Screen 87070	$60
Drug various codes	$35	Glucose 82947	$35
Influenza 90658	$25	Glycosylated HGB A1C 83036	$45
MMR 90707	$50	HCT 85014	$30
OPV 90712	$40	HDL 83718	$35
Pneumovax 90732	$35	HGB 85018	$30
TB Skin Test 86580	$15	Hep BSAG 83740	$40
TD 90718	$40	Hepatitis panel, acute 80074	$95
Tetanus Toxoid 90703	$40	HIV 86703	$100
Vaccine/Toxoid Administration for Younger		Iron & TIBC 83550	$45
Than 8 Years Old w/ counseling 90465	$10	Kidney Profile 80069	$95
Vaccine/Toxoid Administration for Adult 90471	$10	Lead 83665	$55
Arthrocentesis/Aspiration/Injection		Lipase 83690	$40
Small Joint 20600	$50	Lipid Panel 80061	$95
Interm Joint 20605	$60	Liver Profile 80076	$95
Major Joint 20610	$70	Mono Test 86308	$30
Trigger Point/Tendon Sheath Inj. 20550	$90	Pap Smear 88155	$90
Other Invasive/Noninvasive Procedures		Pap Collection/Supervision 88142	$95
Catheterization 51701	$55	Pregnancy Test 84703	$90
Circumcision 54150	$150	Obstetric Panel 80055	$85
Colposcopy 57452	$225	Pro Time 85610	$50
Colposcopy w/Biopsy 57454	$250	PSA 84153	$50
Cryosurgery Premalignant Lesion various codes	$160	RPR 86592	$55
Endometrial Biopsy 58100	$190	Sed. Rate 85651	$50
Excision Lesion Malignant various codes	$145	Stool Culture 87045	$80
Excision Lesion Benign various codes	$125	Stool O & P 87177	$105
Curettement Lesion		Strep Screen 87880	$35
Single 11055	$70	Theophylline 80198	$40
2–4 11056	$80	Thyroid Uptake 84479	$75
>4 11057	$90	TSH 84443	$50
Excision Skin Tags (1–15) 11200	$55	Urinalysis 81000	$35
Each Additional 10 11201	$30	Urine Culture 87088	$80
I & D Abscess Single/Simple 10060	$75	Drawing Fee 36415	$15
Multiple/Complex 10061	$95	Specimen Collection 99000	$10
I & D Pilonidal Cyst Simple 10080	$105		
I & D Pilonidal Cyst Complex 10081	$130		
Laceration Repair various codes	$60		

HEALTH INSURANCE CLAIM FORM
APPROVED BY NATIONAL UNIFORM CLAIM COMMITTEE 08/05

| 1. MEDICARE MEDICAID TRICARE CHAMPVA GROUP FECA OTHER CHAMPUS HEALTH PLAN BLK LUNG | 1a. INSURED'S I.D. NUMBER (For Program in Item 1) |

☐(Medicare #) ☐(Medicaid #) ☐(Sponsor's SSN) ☐(Member ID#) ☐(SSN or ID) ☐(SSN) ☐(ID)

PICA ▢▢▢

2. PATIENT'S NAME (Last Name, First Name, Middle Initial)

3. PATIENT'S BIRTH DATE   SEX
MM   DD   YY
M☐   F☐

4. INSURED'S NAME (Last Name, First Name, Middle Initial)

5. PATIENT'S ADDRESS (No., Street)

6. PATIENT RELATIONSHIP TO INSURED
Self☐   Spouse☐   Child☐   Other☐

7. INSURED'S ADDRESS (No, Street)

CITY   STATE

8. PATIENT STATUS
Single☐   Married☐   Other☐

Full-Time   Part-Time
Employed☐ Student☐   Student☐

CITY   STATE

ZIP CODE   TELEPHONE (Include Area Code)
(   )

ZIP CODE   TELEPHONE (Include Area Code)
(   )

9. OTHER INSURED'S NAME (Last Name, First Name, Middle Initial)

10. IS PATIENT'S CONDITION RELATED TO:

11. INSURED'S POLICY GROUP OR FECA NUMBER

a. OTHER INSURED'S POLICY OR GROUP NUMBER

a. EMPLOYMENT? (Current or Previous)
☐YES   ☐NO

a. INSURED'S DATE OF BIRTH   SEX
MM   DD   YY
M☐   F☐

b. OTHER INSURED'S DATE OF BIRTH   SEX
MM   DD   YY
M☐   F☐

b. AUTO ACCIDENT?   PLACE (State)
☐YES   ☐NO

b. EMPLOYER'S NAME OR SCHOOL NAME

c. EMPLOYER'S NAME OR SCHOOL NAME

c. OTHER ACCIDENT?
☐YES   ☐NO

c. INSURANCE PLAN NAME OR PROGRAM NAME

d. INSURANCE PLAN NAME OR PROGRAM NAME

10d. RESERVED FOR LOCAL USE

d. IS THERE ANOTHER HEALTH BENEFIT PLAN?
☐YES   ☐NO   If yes, return to and complete item 9 a-d.

READ BACK OF FORM BEFORE COMPLETING & SIGNING THIS FORM.
12. PATIENT'S OR AUTHORIZED PERSON'S SIGNATURE I authorize the release of any medical or other information necessary to process this claim. I also request payment of government benefits either to myself or to the party who accepts assignment below.

SIGNED _____   DATE _____

13. INSURED'S OR AUTHORIZED PERSON'S SIGNATURE I authorize payment of medical benefits to the undersigned physician or supplier for services described below.

SIGNED _____

14. DATE OF CURRENT: ILLNESS (First symptom) OR INJURY (Accident) OR PREGNANCY (LMP)
MM   DD   YY

15. IF PATIENT HAS HAD SAME OR SIMILAR ILLNESS. GIVE FIRST DATE   MM   DD   YY

16. DATES PATIENT UNABLE TO WORK IN CURRENT OCCUPATION
MM   DD   YY   MM   DD   YY
FROM   TO

17. NAME OF REFERRING PHYSICIAN OR OTHER SOURCE

17a.
17b. NPI

18. HOSPITALIZATION DATES RELATED TO CURRENT SERVICES
MM   DD   YY   MM   DD   YY
FROM   TO

19. RESERVED FOR LOCAL USE

20. OUTSIDE LAB? $ CHARGES
☐YES   ☐NO

21. DIAGNOSIS OR NATURE OF ILLNESS OR INJURY (Relate Items 1,2,3 or 4 to Item 24E by Line)
1. |___.___| 3. |___.___|
2. |___.___| 4. |___.___|

22. MEDICAID RESUBMISSION
CODE   ORIGINAL REF. NO.

23. PRIOR AUTHORIZATION NUMBER

24. A. DATE(S) OF SERVICE		B. PLACE OF SERVICE	C. EMG	D. PROCEDURES, SERVICES, OR SUPPLIES (Explain Unusual Circumstances)		E. DIAGNOSIS POINTER	F. $ CHARGES	G. DAYS OR UNITS	H. EPSDT Family Plan	I. ID. QUAL.	J. RENDERING PROVIDER ID. #
From	To			CPT/HCPCS	MODIFIER						
MM DD YY	MM DD YY										
1											NPI
2											NPI
3											NPI
4											NPI
5											NPI
6											NPI

25. FEDERAL TAX I.D. NUMBER   SSN EIN
☐☐

26. PATIENT'S ACCOUNT NO.

27. ACCEPT ASSIGNMENT? (For govt. claims, see back)
☐YES   ☐NO

28. TOTAL CHARGE
$

29. AMOUNT PAID
$

30. BALANCE DUE
$

31. SIGNATURE OF PHYSICIAN OR SUPPLIER INCLUDING DEGREES OR CREDENTIALS (I certify that the statements on the reverse apply to this bill and are made a part thereof.)

SIGNED _____   DATE _____

32. SERVICE FACILITY LOCATION INFORMATION

a. NPI   b.

33. BILLING PROVIDER INFO & PH. # (   )

a. NPI   b.

Figure 13-2

b. Using the source documents, the Capital City Medical Fee Schedule (Figure 13-3), and the blank CMS-1500 form provided (Figure 13-4), complete the following case study for patient Bradley Hasson (Case 13-2):

CASE 13-2

Capital City Medical—123 Unknown Boulevard, Capital City, NY 12345-2222 (555) 555-1234	Patient Information Form
Phil Wells, MD, Mannie Mends, MD, Bette R. Soone, MD	Tax ID: 75-0246810
	Group NPI: 1513171216

Patient Information:

Name: (Last, First) Hasson, Bradley   ☒ Male ☐ Female   Birth Date: 08/11/1940

Address: 37 Mallow Ave, Capital City, NY 12345   Phone: (555) 555-6187

Social Security Number: 624-90-3754   Full-Time Student: ☐ Yes ☒ No

Marital Status: ☐ Single ☒ Married ☐ Divorced ☐ Other

Employment:

Employer: Retired   Phone: ( )

Address:

Condition Related to: ☐ Auto Accident ☐ Employment ☐ Other Accident

Date of Accident: _____ State: _____

Emergency Contact: _____ **Phone: ( )** _____

Primary Insurance: Medicare   Phone: ( )

Address: P O. Box, 9834, Capital City, NY 12345

Insurance Policyholder's Name: Same   ☐ M ☐ F DOB: _____

Address:

Phone: _____ Relationship to Insured: ☒ Self ☐ Spouse ☐ Child ☐ Other

Employer: _____ Phone: ( ) _____

Employer's Address:

Policy/ID No: 653524444A   Group No: _____ Percent Covered: 80 % Copay Amt: $____

Secondary Insurance: Blue Cross Blue Shield, Medigap   Phone: ( )

Address: 379 Blue Plaza, Capital City, NY 12345

Insurance Policyholder's Name: Same   ☐ M ☐ F DOB: _____

Address:

Phone: _____ Relationship to Insured: ☒ Self ☐ Spouse ☐ Child ☐ Other

Employer: _____ Phone: ( ) _____

Employer's Address:

Policy/ID No: YYZ6981399   Group No: _____ Percent Covered: ___% Copay Amt: $20.00

Reason for Visit: Follow-up on my Leukemia

Known Allergies: _____

Referred by: _____

CASE 13-2
SOAP

04/17/20XX
Assignment of Benefits: Y
Signature on File: Y
Referring Physician: N

S: Bradley Hasson is here today for a regular checkup on his leukemia. He presents with no complaints.

O: Pt. is responding well to recent therapy regimen. He denies weakness and tiredness.

A: 1. Chronic leukemia in remission—208.11

P: 1. Continue current therapy.
2. Keep appointment with oncologist.
3. Return in 2 months unless relapse or other illness occurs.

_____

Phil Wells, MD
Family Practice
NPI: 1234567890

CASE 13-2

Patient Name <u>Bradley Hasson</u>

Capital City Medical
123 Unknown Boulevard, Capital City, NY 12345-2222

Date of Service
<u>04-17-20XX</u>

New Patient			Other Invasive/Noninvasive			Laboratory	
Problem Focused	99201		Arthrocentesis/Aspiration/Injection			Amylase	82150
Expanded Problem, Focused	99202		Small Joint	20600		B12	82607
Detailed	99203		Interm Joint	20605		CBC & Diff	85025
Comprehensive	99204		Major Joint	20610		Comp Metabolic Panel	80053
Comprehensive/High Complex	99205		**Other Invasive/Noninvasive**			Chlamydia Screen	87110
Well Exam Infant (up to 12 mos.)	99381		Audiometry	92552		Cholesterol	82465
Well Exam 1–4 yrs.	99382		Cast Application			Digoxin	80162
Well Exam 5–11 yrs.	99383		Location Long Short			Electrolytes	80051
Well Exam 12–17 yrs.	99384		Catheterization	51701		Ferritin	82728
Well Exam 18–39 yrs.	99385		Circumcision	54150		Folate	82746
Well Exam 40–64 yrs.	99386		Colposcopy	57452		GC Screen	87070
			Colposcopy w/Biopsy	57454		Glucose	82947
			Cryosurgery Premalignant Lesion			Glucose 1 HR	82950
			Location (s):			Glycosylated HGB A1C	83036
Established Patient			Cryosurgery Warts			HCT	85014
Post-Op Follow Up Visit	99024		Location (s):			HDL	83718
Minimum	99211		Curettement Lesion			Hep BSAG	87340
Problem Focused	99212		Single	11055		Hepatitis panel, acute	80074
Expanded Problem Focused	99213	X	2–4	11056		HGB	85018
Detailed	99214		>4	11057		HIV	86703
Comprehensive/High Complex	99215		Diaphragm Fitting	57170		Iron & TIBC	83550
Well Exam Infant (up to 12 mos.)	99391		Ear Irrigation	69210		Kidney Profile	80069
Well exam 1–4 yrs.	99392		ECG	93000		Lead	83655
Well Exam 5–11 yrs.	99393		Endometrial Biopsy	58100		Liver Profile	80076
Well Exam 12–17 yrs.	99394		Exc. Lesion Malignant			Mono Test	86308
Well Exam 18–39 yrs.	99395		Benign			Pap Smear	88155
Well Exam 40–64 yrs.	99396		Location			Pregnancy Test	84703
Obstetrics			Exc. Skin Tags (1–15)	11200		Obstetric Panel	80055
Total OB Care	59400		Each Additional 10	11201		Pro Time	85610
Injections			Fracture Treatment			PSA	84153
Administration Sub. / IM	90772		Loc			RPR	86592
Drug			w/Reduc w/o Reduc			Sed. Rate	85651
Dosage			I & D Abscess Single/Simple	10060		Stool Culture	87045
Allergy	95115		Multiple or Comp	10061		Stool O & P	87177
Cocci Skin Test	86490		I & D Pilonidal Cyst Simple	10080		Strep Screen	87880
DPT	90701		Pilonidal Cyst Complex	10081		Theophylline	80198
Hemophilus	90646		IV Therapy—To One Hour	90760		Thyroid Uptake	84479
Influenza	90658		Each Additional Hour	90761		TSH	84443
MMR	90707		Laceration Repair			Urinalysis	81000
OPV	90712		Location Size Simp/Comp			Urine Culture	87088
Pneumovax	90732		Laryngoscopy	31505		Drawing Fee	36415
TB Skin Test	86580		Oximetry	94760		Specimen Collection	99000
TD	90718		Punch Biopsy			**Other:**	
Unlisted Immun	90749		Rhythm Strip	93040			
Tetanus Toxoid	90703		Treadmill	93015			
Vaccine/Toxoid Admin <8 Yr Old w/ Counseling	90465		Trigger Point or Tendon Sheath Inj.	20550			
Vaccine/Toxoid Administration for Adult	90471		Tympanometry	92567			

Diagnosis/ICD-9: **208.11**

I acknowledge receipt of medical services and authorize the release of any medical information necessary to process this claim for healthcare payment only. I do authorize payment to the provider.

Patient Signature <u>Bradley Hasson</u>

Total Estimated Charges: _____

Payment Amount: _____

Next Appointment: _____

Figure 13-3

Figure 13-3

Capital City Medical
Fee Schedule

New Patient OV			Punch Biopsy various codes	$80
Problem Focused 99201	$45		Nebulizer various codes	$45
Expanded Problem Focused 99202	$65		Cast Application various codes	$85
Detailed 99203	$85		Laryngoscopy 31505	$255
Comprehensive 99204	$105		Audiometry 92552	$85
Comprehensive/High Complex 99205	$115		Tympanometry 92567	$85
Well Exam infant (less than 1 year) 99381	$45		Ear Irrigation 69210	$25
Well Exam 1–4 yrs. 99382	$50		Diaphragm Fitting 57170	$30
Well Exam 5–11 yrs. 99383	$55		IV Therapy (up to one hour) 90760	$65
Well Exam 12–17 yrs. 99384	$65		Each additional hour 90761	$50
Well Exam 18–39 yrs. 99385	$85		Oximetry 94760	$10
Well Exam 40–64 yrs. 99386	$105		ECG 93000	$75
Established Patient OV			Holter Monitor various codes	$170
Post Op Follow Up Visit 99024	$0		Rhythm Strip 93040	$60
Minimum 99211	$35		Treadmill 93015	$375
Problem Focused 99212	$45		Cocci Skin Test 86490	$20
Expanded Problem Focused 99213	$55		X-ray, spine, chest, bone—any area various codes	$275
Detailed 99214	$65		Avulsion Nail 11730	$200
Comprehensive/High Complex 99215	$75		**Laboratory**	
Well exam infant (less than 1 year) 99391	$35		Amylase 82150	$40
Well Exam 1–4 yrs. 99392	$40		B12 82607	$30
Well Exam 5–11 yrs. 99393	$45		CBC & Diff 85025	$95
Well Exam 12–17 yrs. 99394	$55		Comp Metabolic Panel 80053	$75
Well Exam 18–39 yrs. 99395	$65		Chlamydia Screen 87110	$70
Well Exam 40–64 yrs. 99396	$75		Cholestrerol 82465	$75
Obstetrics			Digoxin 80162	$40
Total OB Care 59400	$1700		Electrolytes 80051	$70
Injections			Estrogen, Total 82672	$50
Administration 90772	$10		Ferritin 82728	$40
Allergy 95115	$35		Folate 82746	$30
DPT 90701	$50		GC Screen 87070	$60
Drug various codes	$35		Glucose 82947	$35
Influenza 90658	$25		Glycosylated HGB A1C 83036	$45
MMR 90707	$50		HCT 85014	$30
OPV 90712	$40		HDL 83718	$35
Pneumovax 90732	$35		HGB 85018	$30
TB Skin Test 86580	$15		Hep BSAG 83740	$40
TD 90718	$40		Hepatitis panel, acute 80074	$95
Tetanus Toxoid 90703	$40		HIV 86703	$100
Vaccine/Toxoid Administration for Younger Than 8 Years Old w/ counseling 90465	$10		Iron & TIBC 83550	$45
			Kidney Profile 80069	$95
Vaccine/Toxoid Administration for Adult 90471	$10		Lead 83665	$55
Arthrocentesis/Aspiration/Injection			Lipase 83690	$40
Small Joint 20600	$50		Lipid Panel 80061	$95
Interm Joint 20605	$60		Liver Profile 80076	$95
Major Joint 20610	$70		Mono Test 86308	$30
Trigger Point/Tendon Sheath Inj. 20550	$90		Pap Smear 88155	$90
Other Invasive/Noninvasive Procedures			Pap Collection/Supervision 88142	$95
Catheterization 51701	$55		Pregnancy Test 84703	$90
Circumcision 54150	$150		Obstetric Panel 80055	$85
Colposcopy 57452	$225		Pro Time 85610	$50
Colposcopy w/Biopsy 57454	$250		PSA 84153	$50
Cryosurgery Premalignant Lesion various codes	$160		RPR 86592	$55
Endometrial Biopsy 58100	$190		Sed. Rate 85651	$50
Excision Lesion Malignant various codes	$145		Stool Culture 87045	$80
Excision Lesion Benign various codes	$125		Stool O & P 87177	$105
Curettement Lesion			Strep Screen 87880	$35
Single 11055	$70		Theophylline 80198	$40
2–4 11056	$80		Thyroid Uptake 84479	$75
>4 11057	$90		TSH 84443	$50
Excision Skin Tags (1–15) 11200	$55		Urinalysis 81000	$35
Each Additional 10 11201	$30		Urine Culture 87088	$80
I & D Abscess Single/Simple 10060	$75		Drawing Fee 36415	$15
Multiple/Complex 10061	$95		Specimen Collection 99000	$10
I & D Pilonidal Cyst Simple 10080	$105			
I & D Pilonidal Cyst Complex 10081	$130			
Laceration Repair various codes	$60			

1500

HEALTH INSURANCE CLAIM FORM

APPROVED BY NATIONAL UNIFORM CLAIM COMMITTEE 08/05

☐☐☐ PICA   PICA ☐☐☐

| 1. MEDICARE | MEDICAID | TRICARE CHAMPUS | CHAMPVA | GROUP HEALTH PLAN | FECA BLK LUNG | OTHER | 1a. INSURED'S I.D. NUMBER | (For Program in Item 1) |

☐ (Medicare #) ☐ (Medicaid #) ☐ (Sponsor's SSN) ☐ (Member ID#) ☐ (SSN or ID) ☐ (SSN) ☐ (ID)

2. PATIENT'S NAME (Last Name, First Name, Middle Initial)

3. PATIENT'S BIRTH DATE   SEX
MM   DD   YY   M☐ F☐

4. INSURED'S NAME (Last Name, First Name, Middle Initial)

5. PATIENT'S ADDRESS (No., Street)

6. PATIENT RELATIONSHIP TO INSURED
Self☐ Spouse☐ Child☐ Other☐

7. INSURED'S ADDRESS (No, Street)

CITY   STATE

8. PATIENT STATUS
Single☐ Married☐ Other☐

CITY   STATE

ZIP CODE   TELEPHONE (Include Area Code)
(   )

Full-Time Part-Time
Employed☐ Student☐ Student☐

ZIP CODE   TELEPHONE (Include Area Code)
(   )

9. OTHER INSURED'S NAME (Last Name, First Name, Middle Initial)

10. IS PATIENT'S CONDITION RELATED TO:

11. INSURED'S POLICY GROUP OR FECA NUMBER

a. OTHER INSURED'S POLICY OR GROUP NUMBER

a. EMPLOYMENT? (Current or Previous)
☐ YES   ☐ NO

a. INSURED'S DATE OF BIRTH   SEX
MM   DD   YY   M☐   F☐

b. OTHER INSURED'S DATE OF BIRTH   SEX
MM   DD   YY   M☐   F☐

b. AUTO ACCIDENT?   PLACE (State)
☐ YES   ☐ NO

b. EMPLOYER'S NAME OR SCHOOL NAME

c. EMPLOYER'S NAME OR SCHOOL NAME

c. OTHER ACCIDENT?
☐ YES   ☐ NO

c. INSURANCE PLAN NAME OR PROGRAM NAME

d. INSURANCE PLAN NAME OR PROGRAM NAME

10d. RESERVED FOR LOCAL USE

d. IS THERE ANOTHER HEALTH BENEFIT PLAN?
☐ YES   ☐ NO   If yes, return to and complete item 9 a-d.

READ BACK OF FORM BEFORE COMPLETING & SIGNING THIS FORM.
12. PATIENT'S OR AUTHORIZED PERSON'S SIGNATURE I authorize the release of any medical or other information necessary to process this claim. I also request payment of government benefits either to myself or to the party who accepts assignment below.

SIGNED _____   DATE _____

13. INSURED'S OR AUTHORIZED PERSON'S SIGNATURE I authorize payment of medical benefits to the undersigned physician or supplier for services described below.

SIGNED _____

14. DATE OF CURRENT: ◄ ILLNESS (First symptom) OR
MM DD YY   INJURY (Accident) OR
                 PREGNANCY (LMP)

15. IF PATIENT HAS HAD SAME OR SIMILAR ILLNESS,
GIVE FIRST DATE   MM DD YY

16. DATES PATIENT UNABLE TO WORK IN CURRENT OCCUPATION
MM DD YY   MM DD YY
FROM   TO

17. NAME OF REFERRING PHYSICIAN OR OTHER SOURCE

17a.
17b. NPI

18. HOSPITALIZATION DATES RELATED TO CURRENT SERVICES
MM DD YY   MM DD YY
FROM   TO

19. RESERVED FOR LOCAL USE

20. OUTSIDE LAB? $ CHARGES
☐ YES   ☐ NO

21. DIAGNOSIS OR NATURE OF ILLNESS OR INJURY (Relate Items 1,2,3 or 4 to Item 24E by Line)
1. ____.____   3. ____.____
2. ____.____   4. ____.____

22. MEDICAID RESUBMISSION
CODE   ORIGINAL REF. NO.

23. PRIOR AUTHORIZATION NUMBER

24. A. DATE(S) OF SERVICE		B. PLACE OF SERVICE	C. EMG	D. PROCEDURES, SERVICES, OR SUPPLIES (Explain Unusual Circumstances)		E. DIAGNOSIS POINTER	F. $ CHARGES	G. DAYS OR UNITS	H. EPSDT Family Plan	I. ID. QUAL.	J. RENDERING PROVIDER ID. #
From MM DD YY	To MM DD YY			CPT/HCPCS	MODIFIER						
1										NPI	
2										NPI	
3										NPI	
4										NPI	
5										NPI	
6										NPI	

25. FEDERAL TAX I.D. NUMBER   SSN EIN ☐☐

26. PATIENT'S ACCOUNT NO.

27. ACCEPT ASSIGNMENT?
(For govt. claims, see back)
☐ YES ☐ NO

28. TOTAL CHARGE $

29. AMOUNT PAID $

30. BALANCE DUE $

31. SIGNATURE OF PHYSICIAN OR SUPPLIER INCLUDING DEGREES OR CREDENTIALS
(I certify that the statements on the reverse apply to this bill and are made a part thereof.)

SIGNED _____ DATE _____

32. SERVICE FACILITY LOCATION INFORMATION

a. NPI   b.

33. BILLING PROVIDER INFO & PH. # (   )

a. NPI   b.

NUCC Instruction Manual available at: www.nucc.org
WCMS-1500CS

APPROVED OMB 0938-0999 FORM CMS-1500 (08/05)

Vertical side labels: CARRIER | PATIENT AND INSURED INFORMATION | PHYSICIAN OR SUPPLIER INFORMATION | SECOND FOLD | FIRST FOLD WHCF-10-ENV / WHCF-10-ENV-SS

Figure 13-4

c. Using the source documents, the Capital City Medical Fee Schedule (Figure 13-5), and the blank CMS-1500 form provided (Figure 13-6), complete the following case study for patient Reba Jones (Case 13-3):

CASE 13-3

Capital City Medical—123 Unknown Boulevard, Capital City, NY 12345-2222 (555) 555-1234	Patient Information Form
Phil Wells, MD, Mannie Mends, MD, Bette R. Soone, MD	Tax ID: 75-0246810
	Group NPI: 1513171216

Patient Information:

Name: (Last, First) Jones, Reba ☐ Male ☒ Female Birth Date: 06/04/1953

Address: 414 Scotland Ln, Capital City, NY 12345 Phone: (555) 555-3777

Social Security Number: 741-10-3685 Full-Time Student: ☐ Yes ☒ No

Marital Status: ☐ Single ☒ Married ☐ Divorced ☐ Other

Employment:

Employer: _____ Phone: ( ) _____

Address: _____

Condition Related to: ☐ Auto Accident ☐ Employment ☐ Other Accident

Date of Accident: _____ State: _____

Emergency Contact: _____ **Phone: ( )** _____

Primary Insurance: Medicare Phone: ( ) _____

Address: P.O. Box , 9834, Capital City, NY 12345

Insurance Policyholder's Name: Warren Jones ☒ M ☐ F DOB: 11/21/1953

Address: _____

Phone: _____ Relationship to Insured: ☐ Self ☒ Spouse ☐ Child ☐ Other

Employer: _____ Phone: ( ) _____

Employer's Address: _____

Policy/ID No: 658303300A Group No: _____ Percent Covered: 80 % Copay Amt: $_____

Secondary Insurance: Aetna Phone: ( ) _____

Address: 1625 Healthcare Bldg, Capital City, NY 12345

Insurance Policyholder's Name: Warren Jones ☒ M ☐ F DOB: 11/21/1953

Address: Same

Phone: _____ Relationship to Insured: ☐ Self ☒ Spouse ☐ Child ☐ Other

Employer: Capital Hardware Phone: ( ) _____

Employer's Address: _____

Policy/ID No: 6758562 Group No: 5832 Percent Covered: _____ % Copay Amt: $ 30.00

Reason for Visit: I am here to have my sarcoidosis checked.

Known Allergies: _____

Referred by: _____

CASE 13-3
SOAP

04/24/20XX
Assignment of Benefits: Y
Signature on File: Y
Referring Physician: N

S: Reba Jones is here for a follow-up on her sarcoidosis. Pt. has no complaints at this time. She states that she is feeling "wonderful."

O: On exam, vitals are good. She denies any SOB, hemoptysis, or cough. Heart is regular rate and rhythm, with no gallop or murmur.

A: 1. Sarcoidosis—135, 517.8

P: 1. Continue current therapy.
 2. Keep appointment with pulmonologist.
 3. Return in 6 months.

_____

Phil Wells, MD
Family Practice
NPI: 1234567890

CASE 13-3

Patient Name Reba Jones

Capital City Medical
123 Unknown Boulevard, Capital City, NY 12345-2222

Date of Service
04-24-20XX

New Patient			Arthrocentesis/Aspiration/Injection		Laboratory		
Problem Focused	99201		Arthrocentesis/Aspiration/Injection		Amylase	82150
Expanded Problem, Focused	99202		Small Joint	20600	B12	82607
Detailed	99203		Interm Joint	20605	CBC & Diff	85025
Comprehensive	99204		Major Joint	20610	Comp Metabolic Panel	80053
Comprehensive/High Complex	99205		**Other Invasive/Noninvasive**		Chlamydia Screen	87110
Well Exam Infant (up to 12 mos.)	99381		Audiometry	92552	Cholesterol	82465
Well Exam 1–4 yrs.	99382		Cast Application		Digoxin	80162
Well Exam 5–11 yrs.	99383		Location Long Short		Electrolytes	80051
Well Exam 12–17 yrs.	99384		Catheterization	51701	Ferritin	82728
Well Exam 18–39 yrs.	99385		Circumcision	54150	Folate	82746
Well Exam 40–64 yrs.	99386		Colposcopy	57452	GC Screen	87070
			Colposcopy w/Biopsy	57454	Glucose	82947
			Cryosurgery Premalignant Lesion		Glucose 1 HR	82950
			Location (s):		Glycosylated HGB A1C	83036
Established Patient			Cryosurgery Warts		HCT	85014
Post-Op Follow Up Visit	99024		Location (s):		HDL	83718
Minimum	99211		Curettement Lesion		Hep BSAG	87340
Problem Focused	99212	X	Single	11055	Hepatitis panel, acute	80074
Expanded Problem Focused	99213		2–4	11056	HGB	85018
Detailed	99214		>4	11057	HIV	86703
Comprehensive/High Complex	99215		Diaphragm Fitting	57170	Iron & TIBC	83550
Well Exam Infant (up to 12 mos.)	99391		Ear Irrigation	69210	Kidney Profile	80069
Well exam 1–4 yrs.	99392		ECG	93000	Lead	83655
Well Exam 5–11 yrs.	99393		Endometrial Biopsy	58100	Liver Profile	80076
Well Exam 12–17 yrs.	99394		Exc. Lesion Malignant		Mono Test	86308
Well Exam 18–39 yrs.	99395		Benign		Pap Smear	88155
Well Exam 40–64 yrs.	99396		Location		Pregnancy Test	84703
Obstetrics			Exc. Skin Tags (1–15)	11200	Obstetric Panel	80055
Total OB Care	59400		Each Additional 10	11201	Pro Time	85610
Injections			Fracture Treatment		PSA	84153
Administration Sub. / IM	90772		Loc		RPR	86592
Drug			w/Reduc w/o Reduc		Sed. Rate	85651
Dosage			I & D Abscess Single/Simple	10060	Stool Culture	87045
Allergy	95115		Multiple or Comp	10061	Stool O & P	87177
Cocci Skin Test	86490		I & D Pilonidal Cyst Simple	10080	Strep Screen	87880
DPT	90701		Pilonidal Cyst Complex	10081	Theophylline	80198
Hemophilus	90646		IV Therapy—To One Hour	90760	Thyroid Uptake	84479
Influenza	90658		Each Additional Hour	90761	TSH	84443
MMR	90707		Laceration Repair		Urinalysis	81000
OPV	90712		Location Size Simp/Comp		Urine Culture	87088
Pneumovax	90732		Laryngoscopy	31505	Drawing Fee	36415
TB Skin Test	86580		Oximetry	94760	Specimen Collection	99000
TD	90718		Punch Biopsy		**Other:**	
Unlisted Immun	90749		Rhythm Strip	93040		
Tetanus Toxoid	90703		Treadmill	93015		
Vaccine/Toxoid Admin <8 Yr Old w/ Counseling	90465		Trigger Point or Tendon Sheath Inj.	20550		
Vaccine/Toxoid Administration for Adult	90471		Tympanometry	92567		

Diagnosis/ICD-9: **135, 517.8**

I acknowledge receipt of medical services and authorize the release of any medical information necessary to process this claim for healthcare payment only. I do authorize payment to the provider.

Patient Signature Reba Jones

Total Estimated Charges: _____ _____

Payment Amount: _____

Next Appointment: _____

Figure 13-5

Capital City Medical
Fee Schedule

New Patient OV		Punch Biopsy various codes		$80
Problem Focused 99201	$45	Nebulizer various codes		$45
Expanded Problem Focused 99202	$65	Cast Application various codes		$85
Detailed 99203	$85	Laryngoscopy 31505		$255
Comprehensive 99204	$105	Audiometry 92552		$85
Comprehensive/High Complex 99205	$115	Tympanometry 92567		$85
Well Exam infant (less than 1 year) 99381	$45	Ear Irrigation 69210		$25
Well Exam 1–4 yrs. 99382	$50	Diaphragm Fitting 57170		$30
Well Exam 5–11 yrs. 99383	$55	IV Therapy (up to one hour) 90760		$65
Well Exam 12–17 yrs. 99384	$65	Each additional hour 90761		$50
Well Exam 18–39 yrs. 99385	$85	Oximetry 94760		$10
Well Exam 40–64 yrs. 99386	$105	ECG 93000		$75
Established Patient OV		Holter Monitor various codes		$170
Post Op Follow Up Visit 99024	$0	Rhythm Strip 93040		$60
Minimum 99211	$35	Treadmill 93015		$375
Problem Focused 99212	$45	Cocci Skin Test 86490		$20
Expanded Problem Focused 99213	$55	X-ray, spine, chest, bone—any area various codes		$275
Detailed 99214	$65	Avulsion Nail 11730		$200
Comprehensive/High Complex 99215	$75	**Laboratory**		
Well exam infant (less than 1 year) 99391	$35	Amylase 82150		$40
Well Exam 1–4 yrs. 99392	$40	B12 82607		$30
Well Exam 5–11 yrs. 99393	$45	CBC & Diff 85025		$95
Well Exam 12–17 yrs. 99394	$55	Comp Metabolic Panel 80053		$75
Well Exam 18–39 yrs. 99395	$65	Chlamydia Screen 87110		$70
Well Exam 40–64 yrs. 99396	$75	Cholestrerol 82465		$75
Obstetrics		Digoxin 80162		$40
Total OB Care 59400	$1700	Electrolytes 80051		$70
Injections		Estrogen, Total 82672		$50
Administration 90772	$10	Ferritin 82728		$40
Allergy 95115	$35	Folate 82746		$30
DPT 90701	$50	GC Screen 87070		$60
Drug various codes	$35	Glucose 82947		$35
Influenza 90658	$25	Glycosylated HGB A1C 83036		$45
MMR 90707	$50	HCT 85014		$30
OPV 90712	$40	HDL 83718		$35
Pneumovax 90732	$35	HGB 85018		$30
TB Skin Test 86580	$15	Hep BSAG 83740		$40
TD 90718	$40	Hepatitis panel, acute 80074		$95
Tetanus Toxoid 90703	$40	HIV 86703		$100
Vaccine/Toxoid Administration for Younger		Iron & TIBC 83550		$45
Than 8 Years Old w/ counseling 90465	$10	Kidney Profile 80069		$95
Vaccine/Toxoid Administration for Adult 90471	$10	Lead 83665		$55
Arthrocentesis/Aspiration/Injection		Lipase 83690		$40
Small Joint 20600	$50	Lipid Panel 80061		$95
Interm Joint 20605	$60	Liver Profile 80076		$95
Major Joint 20610	$70	Mono Test 86308		$30
Trigger Point/Tendon Sheath Inj. 20550	$90	Pap Smear 88155		$90
Other Invasive/Noninvasive Procedures		Pap Collection/Supervision 88142		$95
Catheterization 51701	$55	Pregnancy Test 84703		$90
Circumcision 54150	$150	Obstetric Panel 80055		$85
Colposcopy 57452	$225	Pro Time 85610		$50
Colposcopy w/Biopsy 57454	$250	PSA 84153		$50
Cryosurgery Premalignant Lesion various codes	$160	RPR 86592		$55
Endometrial Biopsy 58100	$190	Sed. Rate 85651		$50
Excision Lesion Malignant various codes	$145	Stool Culture 87045		$80
Excision Lesion Benign various codes	$125	Stool O & P 87177		$105
Curettement Lesion		Strep Screen 87880		$35
Single 11055	$70	Theophylline 80198		$40
2–4 11056	$80	Thyroid Uptake 84479		$75
>4 11057	$90	TSH 84443		$50
Excision Skin Tags (1–15) 11200	$55	Urinalysis 81000		$35
Each Additional 10 11201	$30	Urine Culture 87088		$80
I & D Abscess Single/Simple 10060	$75	Drawing Fee 36415		$15
Multiple/Complex 10061	$95	Specimen Collection 99000		$10
I & D Pilonidal Cyst Simple 10080	$105			
I & D Pilonidal Cyst Complex 10081	$130			
Laceration Repair various codes	$60			

HEALTH INSURANCE CLAIM FORM

APPROVED BY NATIONAL UNIFORM CLAIM COMMITTEE 08/05

☐☐☐ PICA

1. MEDICARE ☐(Medicare #) MEDICAID ☐(Medicaid #) TRICARE CHAMPUS ☐(Sponsor's SSN) CHAMPVA ☐(Member ID#) GROUP HEALTH PLAN ☐(SSN or ID) FECA BLK LUNG ☐(SSN) OTHER ☐(ID)	1a. INSURED'S I.D. NUMBER (For Program in Item 1) PICA ☐☐☐

2. PATIENT'S NAME (Last Name, First Name, Middle Initial)	3. PATIENT'S BIRTH DATE MM DD YY SEX M☐ F☐	4. INSURED'S NAME (Last Name, First Name, Middle Initial)

5. PATIENT'S ADDRESS (No., Street)	6. PATIENT RELATIONSHIP TO INSURED Self☐ Spouse☐ Child☐ Other☐	7. INSURED'S ADDRESS (No, Street)
CITY STATE	8. PATIENT STATUS Single☐ Married☐ Other☐	CITY STATE
ZIP CODE TELEPHONE (Include Area Code) ( )	Full-Time Part-Time Employed☐ Student☐ Student☐	ZIP CODE TELEPHONE (Include Area Code) ( )

9. OTHER INSURED'S NAME (Last Name, First Name, Middle Initial)	10. IS PATIENT'S CONDITION RELATED TO:	11. INSURED'S POLICY GROUP OR FECA NUMBER
a. OTHER INSURED'S POLICY OR GROUP NUMBER	a. EMPLOYMENT? (Current or Previous) ☐YES ☐NO	a. INSURED'S DATE OF BIRTH MM DD YY SEX M☐ F☐
b. OTHER INSURED'S DATE OF BIRTH MM DD YY SEX M☐ F☐	b. AUTO ACCIDENT? PLACE (State) ☐YES ☐NO	b. EMPLOYER'S NAME OR SCHOOL NAME
c. EMPLOYER'S NAME OR SCHOOL NAME	c. OTHER ACCIDENT? ☐YES ☐NO	c. INSURANCE PLAN NAME OR PROGRAM NAME
d. INSURANCE PLAN NAME OR PROGRAM NAME	10d. RESERVED FOR LOCAL USE	d. IS THERE ANOTHER HEALTH BENEFIT PLAN? ☐YES ☐NO If yes, return to and complete item 9 a-d.

READ BACK OF FORM BEFORE COMPLETING & SIGNING THIS FORM.

12. PATIENT'S OR AUTHORIZED PERSON'S SIGNATURE I authorize the release of any medical or other information necessary to process this claim. I also request payment of government benefits either to myself or to the party who accepts assignment below. SIGNED _____ DATE _____	13. INSURED'S OR AUTHORIZED PERSON'S SIGNATURE I authorize payment of medical benefits to the undersigned physician or supplier for services described below. SIGNED _____

14. DATE OF CURRENT: ILLNESS (First symptom) OR MM DD YY INJURY (Accident) OR PREGNANCY (LMP)	15. IF PATIENT HAS HAD SAME OR SIMILAR ILLNESS, GIVE FIRST DATE MM DD YY	16. DATES PATIENT UNABLE TO WORK IN CURRENT OCCUPATION MM DD YY MM DD YY FROM TO
17. NAME OF REFERRING PHYSICIAN OR OTHER SOURCE	17a. 17b. NPI	18. HOSPITALIZATION DATES RELATED TO CURRENT SERVICES MM DD YY MM DD YY FROM TO
19. RESERVED FOR LOCAL USE		20. OUTSIDE LAB? ☐YES ☐NO $ CHARGES

21. DIAGNOSIS OR NATURE OF ILLNESS OR INJURY (Relate Items 1,2,3 or 4 to Item 24E by Line) 1.|___.___ 3.|___.___ 2.|___.___ 4.|___.___	22. MEDICAID RESUBMISSION CODE ORIGINAL REF. NO.
	23. PRIOR AUTHORIZATION NUMBER

24. A. DATE(S) OF SERVICE From To MM DD YY MM DD YY	B. PLACE OF SERVICE	C. EMG	D. PROCEDURES, SERVICES, OR SUPPLIES (Explain Unusual Circumstances) CPT/HCPCS MODIFIER	E. DIAGNOSIS POINTER	F. $ CHARGES	G. DAYS OR UNITS	H. EPSDT Family Plan	I. ID. QUAL.	J. RENDERING PROVIDER ID. #
1									NPI
2									NPI
3									NPI
4									NPI
5									NPI
6									NPI

25. FEDERAL TAX I.D. NUMBER SSN EIN ☐☐	26. PATIENT'S ACCOUNT NO.	27. ACCEPT ASSIGNMENT? (For govt. claims, see back) ☐YES ☐NO	28. TOTAL CHARGE $	29. AMOUNT PAID $	30. BALANCE DUE $
31. SIGNATURE OF PHYSICIAN OR SUPPLIER INCLUDING DEGREES OR CREDENTIALS (I certify that the statements on the reverse apply to this bill and are made a part thereof.) SIGNED DATE	32. SERVICE FACILITY LOCATION INFORMATION a. NPI b.	33. BILLING PROVIDER INFO & PH. # ( ) a. NPI b.

NUCC Instruction Manual available at: www.nucc.org
WCMS-1500CS

APPROVED OMB 0938-0999 FORM CMS-1500 (08/05)

CARRIER — *PATIENT AND INSURED INFORMATION* — *PHYSICIAN OR SUPPLIER INFORMATION*

SECOND FOLD — FIRST FOLD — WHCF-10-ENV / WHCF-10-ENV-SS

Figure 13-6

d. Using the source documents, the Capital City Medical Fee Schedule (Figure 13-7), and the blank CMS-1500 form provided (Figure 13-8), complete the following case study for patient Scott Reeves (Case 13-4):

CASE 13-4

Capital City Medical—123 Unknown Boulevard, Capital City, NY 12345-2222 (555)555-1234	Patient Information Form
Phil Wells, MD, Mannie Mends, MD, Bette R. Soone, MD	Tax ID: 75-0246810 Group NPI: 1513171216

Patient Information:

Name: (Last, First) Reeves, Scott ☒ Male ☐ Female Birth Date: 08/13/1955

Address: 35 Park Ave, Township, NY 12345 Phone: (555) 555-1700

Social Security Number: 393-55-9020 Full-Time Student: ☐ Yes ☒ No

Marital Status: ☐ Single ☒ Married ☐ Divorced ☐ Other

Employment:

Employer: Retired Phone: ( )

Address:

Condition Related to: ☐ Auto Accident ☐ Employment ☐ Other Accident

Date of Accident: State:

Emergency Contact: Phone: ( )

Primary Insurance: Medicare Phone: ( )

Address: P.O. Box, 9834, Capital City, NY 12345

Insurance Policyholder's Name: Same ☐ M ☐ F DOB: 11/21/1953

Address:

Phone: Relationship to Insured: ☒ Self ☐ Spouse ☐ Child ☐ Other

Employer: Phone: ( )

Employer's Address:

Policy/ID No: 201048952A Group No: Percent Covered: 80 % Copay Amt: $

Secondary Insurance: Phone: ( )

Address:

Insurance Policyholder's Name: ☐ M ☐ F DOB:

Address:

Phone: Relationship to Insured: ☐ Self ☐ Spouse ☐ Child ☐ Other

Employer: Phone: ( )

Employer's Address:

Policy/ID No: 6758562 Group No: 5832 Percent Covered: % Copay Amt: $

Reason for Visit: I am having an episode of gout.

Known Allergies:

Referred by:

CASE 13-4
SOAP

07/10/20XX
Assignment of Benefits: Y
Signature on File: Y
Referring Physician: N

S: Scott Reeves complains of gout in his left big toe. He says that it is very painful.

O: His left great toe presents as swollen. There is pain with and without movement. His BP in office is 152/78. He denies increased salt intake.

A: 1. Gout, great toe—274.0
    2. HTN—401.9

P: 1. Start cholchicine.
    2. Watch salt intake.
    3. Drink plenty of clear fluids.

_____

Phil Wells, MD
Family Practice
NPI: 1234567890

CASE 13-4

Capital City Medical
123 Unknown Boulevard, Capital City, NY 12345-2222

Date of Service
<u>07-10-20XX</u>

New Patient			Arthrocentesis/Aspiration/Injection			Laboratory		
Problem Focused	99201		Arthrocentesis/Aspiration/Injection			Amylase	82150	
Expanded Problem, Focused	99202		Small Joint	20600		B12	82607	
Detailed	99203		Interm Joint	20605		CBC & Diff	85025	
Comprehensive	99204		Major Joint	20610		Comp Metabolic Panel	80053	
Comprehensive/High Complex	99205		**Other Invasive/Noninvasive**			Chlamydia Screen	87110	
Well Exam Infant (up to 12 mos.)	99381		Audiometry	92552		Cholesterol	82465	
Well Exam 1–4 yrs.	99382		Cast Application			Digoxin	80162	
Well Exam 5–11 yrs.	99383		Location Long Short			Electrolytes	80051	
Well Exam 12–17 yrs.	99384		Catheterization	51701		Ferritin	82728	
Well Exam 18–39 yrs.	99385		Circumcision	54150		Folate	82746	
Well Exam 40–64 yrs.	99386		Colposcopy	57452		GC Screen	87070	
			Colposcopy w/Biopsy	57454		Glucose	82947	
			Cryosurgery Premalignant Lesion			Glucose 1 HR	82950	
			Location (s):			Glycosylated HGB A1C	83036	
Established Patient			Cryosurgery Warts			HCT	85014	
Post-Op Follow Up Visit	99024		Location (s):			HDL	83718	
Minimum	99211		Curettement Lesion			Hep BSAG	87340	
Problem Focused	99212		Single	11055		Hepatitis panel, acute	80074	
Expanded Problem Focused	99213	X	2–4	11056		HGB	85018	
Detailed	99214		>4	11057		HIV	86703	
Comprehensive/High Complex	99215		Diaphragm Fitting	57170		Iron & TIBC	83550	
Well Exam Infant (up to 12 mos.)	99391		Ear Irrigation	69210		Kidney Profile	80069	
Well exam 1–4 yrs.	99392		ECG	93000		Lead	83655	
Well Exam 5–11 yrs.	99393		Endometrial Biopsy	58100		Liver Profile	80076	
Well Exam 12–17 yrs.	99394		Exc. Lesion Malignant			Mono Test	86308	
Well Exam 18–39 yrs.	99395		Benign			Pap Smear	88155	
Well Exam 40–64 yrs.	99396		Location			Pregnancy Test	84703	
Obstetrics			Exc. Skin Taqs (1–15)	11200		Obstetric Panel	80055	
Total OB Care	59400		Each Additional 10	11201		Pro Time	85610	
Injections			Fracture Treatment			PSA	84153	
Administration Sub. / IM	90772		Loc			RPR	86592	
Drug			w/Reduc		w/o Reduc	Sed. Rate	85651	
Dosage			I & D Abscess Single/Simple	10060		Stool Culture	87045	
Allergy	95115		Multiple or Comp	10061		Stool O & P	87177	
Cocci Skin Test	86490		I & D Pilonidal Cyst Simple	10080		Strep Screen	87880	
DPT	90701		Pilonidal Cyst Complex	10081		Theophylline	80198	
Hemophilus	90646		IV Therapy—To One Hour	90760		Thyroid Uptake	84479	
Influenza	90658		Each Additional Hour	90761		TSH	84443	
MMR	90707		Laceration Repair			Urinalysis	81000	
OPV	90712		Location Size Simp/Comp			Urine Culture	87088	
Pneumovax	90732		Laryngoscopy	31505		Drawing Fee	36415	
TB Skin Test	86580		Oximetry	94760		Specimen Collection	99000	
TD	90718		Punch Biopsy			**Other:**		
Unlisted Immun	90749		Rhythm Strip	93040				
Tetanus Toxoid	90703		Treadmill	93015				
Vaccine/Toxoid Admin <8 Yr Old w/ Counseling	90465		Trigger Point or Tendon Sheath Inj.	20550				
Vaccine/Toxoid Administration for Adult	90471		Tympanometry	92567				

Diagnosis/ICD-9: **274.0, 401.9**

I acknowledge receipt of medical services and authorize the release of any medical information necessary to process this claim for healthcare payment only. I do authorize payment to the provider.

Total Estimated Charges: _____

Payment Amount: _____

Patient Signature <u>Scott Reeves</u>

Next Appointment: _____

Figure 13-7

Capital City Medical
Fee Schedule

New Patient OV			Punch Biopsy various codes	$80
Problem Focused 99201	$45		Nebulizer various codes	$45
Expanded Problem Focused 99202	$65		Cast Application various codes	$85
Detailed 99203	$85		Laryngoscopy 31505	$255
Comprehensive 99204	$105		Audiometry 92552	$85
Comprehensive/High Complex 99205	$115		Tympanometry 92567	$85
Well Exam infant (less than 1 year) 99381	$45		Ear Irrigation 69210	$25
Well Exam 1–4 yrs. 99382	$50		Diaphragm Fitting 57170	$30
Well Exam 5–11 yrs. 99383	$55		IV Therapy (up to one hour) 90760	$65
Well Exam 12–17 yrs. 99384	$65		Each additional hour 90761	$50
Well Exam 18–39 yrs. 99385	$85		Oximetry 94760	$10
Well Exam 40–64 yrs. 99386	$105		ECG 93000	$75
Established Patient OV			Holter Monitor various codes	$170
Post Op Follow Up Visit 99024	$0		Rhythm Strip 93040	$60
Minimum 99211	$35		Treadmill 93015	$375
Problem Focused 99212	$45		Cocci Skin Test 86490	$20
Expanded Problem Focused 99213	$55		X-ray, spine, chest, bone—any area various codes	$275
Detailed 99214	$65		Avulsion Nail 11730	$200
Comprehensive/High Complex 99215	$75		**Laboratory**	
Well exam infant (less than 1 year) 99391	$35		Amylase 82150	$40
Well Exam 1–4 yrs. 99392	$40		B12 82607	$30
Well Exam 5–11 yrs. 99393	$45		CBC & Diff 85025	$95
Well Exam 12–17 yrs. 99394	$55		Comp Metabolic Panel 80053	$75
Well Exam 18–39 yrs. 99395	$65		Chlamydia Screen 87110	$70
Well Exam 40–64 yrs. 99396	$75		Cholestrerol 82465	$75
Obstetrics			Digoxin 80162	$40
Total OB Care 59400	$1700		Electrolytes 80051	$70
Injections			Estrogen, Total 82672	$50
Administration 90772	$10		Ferritin 82728	$40
Allergy 95115	$35		Folate 82746	$30
DPT 90701	$50		GC Screen 87070	$60
Drug various codes	$35		Glucose 82947	$35
Influenza 90658	$25		Glycosylated HGB A1C 83036	$45
MMR 90707	$50		HCT 85014	$30
OPV 90712	$40		HDL 83718	$35
Pneumovax 90732	$35		HGB 85018	$30
TB Skin Test 86580	$15		Hep BSAG 83740	$40
TD 90718	$40		Hepatitis panel, acute 80074	$95
Tetanus Toxoid 90703	$40		HIV 86703	$100
Vaccine/Toxoid Administration for Younger			Iron & TIBC 83550	$45
Than 8 Years Old w/ counseling 90465	$10		Kidney Profile 80069	$95
Vaccine/Toxoid Administration for Adult 90471	$10		Lead 83665	$55
Arthrocentesis/Aspiration/Injection			Lipase 83690	$40
Small Joint 20600	$50		Lipid Panel 80061	$95
Interm Joint 20605	$60		Liver Profile 80076	$95
Major Joint 20610	$70		Mono Test 86308	$30
Trigger Point/Tendon Sheath Inj. 20550	$90		Pap Smear 88155	$90
Other Invasive/Noninvasive Procedures			Pap Collection/Supervision 88142	$95
Catheterization 51701	$55		Pregnancy Test 84703	$90
Circumcision 54150	$150		Obstetric Panel 80055	$85
Colposcopy 57452	$225		Pro Time 85610	$50
Colposcopy w/Biopsy 57454	$250		PSA 84153	$50
Cryosurgery Premalignant Lesion various codes	$160		RPR 86592	$55
Endometrial Biopsy 58100	$190		Sed. Rate 85651	$50
Excision Lesion Malignant various codes	$145		Stool Culture 87045	$80
Excision Lesion Benign various codes	$125		Stool O & P 87177	$105
Curettement Lesion			Strep Screen 87880	$35
Single 11055	$70		Theophylline 80198	$40
2–4 11056	$80		Thyroid Uptake 84479	$75
>4 11057	$90		TSH 84443	$50
Excision Skin Tags (1–15) 11200	$55		Urinalysis 81000	$35
Each Additional 10 11201	$30		Urine Culture 87088	$80
I & D Abscess Single/Simple 10060	$75		Drawing Fee 36415	$15
Multiple/Complex 10061	$95		Specimen Collection 99000	$10
I & D Pilonidal Cyst Simple 10080	$105			
I & D Pilonidal Cyst Complex 10081	$130			
Laceration Repair various codes	$60			

HEALTH INSURANCE CLAIM FORM

APPROVED BY NATIONAL UNIFORM CLAIM COMMITTEE 08/05

☐☐☐PICA   PICA☐☐☐

| 1. MEDICARE   MEDICAID   TRICARE   CHAMPVA   GROUP   FECA   OTHER   ☐(Medicare #) ☐(Medicaid #) ☐(Sponsor's SSN) ☐(Member ID#) HEALTH PLAN ☐(SSN or ID) BLK LUNG ☐(SSN) ☐(ID) | 1a. INSURED'S I.D. NUMBER   (For Program in Item 1) |

2. PATIENT'S NAME (Last Name, First Name, Middle Initial)
3. PATIENT'S BIRTH DATE   SEX   MM | DD | YY   M☐   F☐
4. INSURED'S NAME (Last Name, First Name, Middle Initial)

5. PATIENT'S ADDRESS (No., Street)
6. PATIENT RELATIONSHIP TO INSURED   Self☐ Spouse☐ Child☐ Other☐
7. INSURED'S ADDRESS (No, Street)

CITY   STATE
8. PATIENT STATUS   Single☐ Married☐ Other☐   Employed☐ Full-Time Student☐ Part-Time Student☐
CITY   STATE

ZIP CODE   TELEPHONE (Include Area Code) ( )
ZIP CODE   TELEPHONE (Include Area Code) ( )

9. OTHER INSURED'S NAME (Last Name, First Name, Middle Initial)
10. IS PATIENT'S CONDITION RELATED TO:
11. INSURED'S POLICY GROUP OR FECA NUMBER

a. OTHER INSURED'S POLICY OR GROUP NUMBER
a. EMPLOYMENT? (Current or Previous)   ☐YES ☐NO
a. INSURED'S DATE OF BIRTH   SEX   MM | DD | YY   M☐   F☐

b. OTHER INSURED'S DATE OF BIRTH   SEX   MM | DD | YY   M☐ F☐
b. AUTO ACCIDENT?   PLACE (State)   ☐YES ☐NO
b. EMPLOYER'S NAME OR SCHOOL NAME

c. EMPLOYER'S NAME OR SCHOOL NAME
c. OTHER ACCIDENT?   ☐YES ☐NO
c. INSURANCE PLAN NAME OR PROGRAM NAME

d. INSURANCE PLAN NAME OR PROGRAM NAME
10d. RESERVED FOR LOCAL USE
d. IS THERE ANOTHER HEALTH BENEFIT PLAN?   ☐YES ☐NO   If yes, return to and complete item 9 a-d.

READ BACK OF FORM BEFORE COMPLETING & SIGNING THIS FORM.
12. PATIENT'S OR AUTHORIZED PERSON'S SIGNATURE I authorize the release of any medical or other information necessary to process this claim. I also request payment of government benefits either to myself or to the party who accepts assignment below.

SIGNED _____   DATE_____

13. INSURED'S OR AUTHORIZED PERSON'S SIGNATURE I authorize payment of medical benefits to the undersigned physician or supplier for services described below.

SIGNED _____

14. DATE OF CURRENT: MM | DD | YY   ◀ ILLNESS (First symptom) OR INJURY (Accident) OR PREGNANCY (LMP)
15. IF PATIENT HAS HAD SAME OR SIMILAR ILLNESS, GIVE FIRST DATE   MM | DD | YY
16. DATES PATIENT UNABLE TO WORK IN CURRENT OCCUPATION   FROM MM | DD | YY   TO MM | DD | YY

17. NAME OF REFERRING PHYSICIAN OR OTHER SOURCE
17a.
17b. NPI
18. HOSPITALIZATION DATES RELATED TO CURRENT SERVICES   FROM MM | DD | YY   TO MM | DD | YY

19. RESERVED FOR LOCAL USE
20. OUTSIDE LAB?   ☐YES ☐NO $ CHARGES

21. DIAGNOSIS OR NATURE OF ILLNESS OR INJURY (Relate Items 1,2,3 or 4 to Item 24E by Line)
1. |___.___   3. |___.___
2. |___.___   4. |___.___
22. MEDICAID RESUBMISSION   CODE   ORIGINAL REF. NO.

23. PRIOR AUTHORIZATION NUMBER

24. A. DATE(S) OF SERVICE						B. PLACE OF SERVICE	C. EMG	D. PROCEDURES, SERVICES, OR SUPPLIES (Explain Unusual Circumstances)		E. DIAGNOSIS POINTER	F. $ CHARGES	G. DAYS OR UNITS	H. EPSDT Family Plan	I. ID. QUAL.	J. RENDERING PROVIDER ID. #
From			To					CPT/HCPCS	MODIFIER						
MM	DD	YY	MM	DD	YY										
1														NPI	
2														NPI	
3														NPI	
4														NPI	
5														NPI	
6														NPI	

25. FEDERAL TAX I.D. NUMBER   SSN EIN ☐☐
26. PATIENT'S ACCOUNT NO.
27. ACCEPT ASSIGNMENT? (For govt. claims, see back)   ☐YES ☐NO
28. TOTAL CHARGE $
29. AMOUNT PAID $
30. BALANCE DUE $

31. SIGNATURE OF PHYSICIAN OR SUPPLIER INCLUDING DEGREES OR CREDENTIALS (I certify that the statements on the reverse apply to this bill and are made a part thereof.)

SIGNED _____   DATE _____

32. SERVICE FACILITY LOCATION INFORMATION
a. NPI   b.
33. BILLING PROVIDER INFO & PH. # ( )
a. NPI   b.

WHCF-10-ENV / WHCF-10-ENV-SS
SECOND FOLD   FIRST FOLD
PATIENT AND INSURED INFORMATION
PHYSICIAN OR SUPPLIER INFORMATION

Figure 13-8

e. Using the source documents, the Capital City Medical Fee Schedule (Figure 13-9), and the blank CMS-1500 form provided (Figure 13-10), complete the following case study for patient Von Vandusen (Case 13-5):

CASE 13-5

Capital City Medical—123 Unknown Boulevard, Capital City, NY 12345-2222 (555) 555-1234	Patient Information Form
Phil Wells, MD, Mannie Mends, MD, Bette R. Soone, MD	Tax ID: 75-0246810
	Group NPI: 1513171216

Patient Information:

Name: (Last, First) Vandusen, Von   ☒ Male ☐ Female   Birth Date: 07/11/1947

Address: 67 Field Dr., Township, NY 12345   Phone: (555) 555-8204

Social Security Number: 172-43-1817   Full-Time Student: ☐ Yes ☒ No

Marital Status: ☐ Single ☒ Married ☐ Divorced ☐ Other

Employment:

Employer: Retired   Phone: ( )

Address:

Condition Related to: ☐ Auto Accident   ☐ Employment   ☐ Other Accident

Date of Accident: _____ State: _____

Emergency Contact: _____ **Phone: ( )** _____

Primary Insurance: Medicare   Phone: ( )

Address: P O. Box , 9834, Capital City, NY 12345

Insurance Policyholder's Name: Same   ☐ M ☐ F DOB: 11/21/1953

Address:

Phone: _____ Relationship to Insured: ☒ Self ☐ Spouse ☐ Child ☐ Other

Employer: _____ Phone: ( ) _____

Employer's Address:

Policy/ID No: 476881270A   Group No: _____ Percent Covered: 80 % Copay Amt: $_____

Secondary Insurance: _____ Phone: ( ) _____

Address:

Insurance Policyholder's Name: _____ ☐ M ☐ F DOB: _____

Address: Same

Phone: _____ Relationship to Insured: ☐ Self ☐ Spouse ☐ Child ☐ Other

Employer: _____ Phone: ( ) _____

Employer's Address:

Policy/ID No: 6758562   Group No: 5832 Percent Covered: ___% Copay Amt: $_____

Reason for Visit: Checkup on my heart condition and blood pressure

Known Allergies:

Referred by:

CASE 13-5
SOAP

10/27/20XX
Assignment of Benefits: Y
Signature on File: Y
Referring Physician: N

S: Von Vandusen is being seen today for HTN. He says that his BP is always running high, but otherwise, he feels fine.

O: BP on exam is 178/88. P: 86 and regular. Wt. 252 lbs. EKG shows old MI. Chest is clear to A&P. Pt. has mild ankle edema bilaterally.

A: 1. Essential HTN benign Lytes are normal values—401.0
2. Old MI—412

P: 1. Add Norvasc q. a.m.
2. Pt. advised to lose weight.
3. Return in 1 week to evaluate the addition of new BP med.

_____

Phil Wells, MD
Family Practice
NPI: 1234567890

CASE 13-5

Patient Name Von Vandusen

Capital City Medical
123 Unknown Boulevard, Capital City, NY 12345-2222

Date of Service
10-27-20XX

New Patient			Other Invasive/Noninvasive			Laboratory		
Problem Focused	99201		Arthrocentesis/Aspiration/Injection			Amylase	82150	
Expanded Problem, Focused	99202		Small Joint	20600		B12	82607	
Detailed	99203		Interm Joint	20605		CBC & Diff	85025	
Comprehensive	99204		Major Joint	20610		Comp Metabolic Panel	80053	
Comprehensive/High Complex	99205		**Other Invasive/Noninvasive**			Chlamydia Screen	87110	
Well Exam Infant (up to 12 mos.)	99381		Audiometry	92552		Cholesterol	82465	
Well Exam 1–4 yrs.	99382		Cast Application			Digoxin	80162	
Well Exam 5–11 yrs.	99383		Location Long Short			Electrolytes	80051	X
Well Exam 12–17 yrs.	99384		Catheterization	51701		Ferritin	82728	
Well Exam 18–39 yrs.	99385		Circumcision	54150		Folate	82746	
Well Exam 40–64 yrs.	99386		Colposcopy	57452		GC Screen	87070	
			Colposcopy w/Biopsy	57454		Glucose	82947	
			Cryosurgery Premalignant Lesion			Glucose 1 HR	82950	
			Location (s):			Glycosylated HGB A1C	83036	
Established Patient			Cryosurgery Warts			HCT	85014	
Post-Op Follow Up Visit	99024		Location (s):			HDL	83718	
Minimum	99211		Curettement Lesion			Hep BSAG	87340	
Problem Focused	99212		Single	11055		Hepatitis panel, acute	80074	
Expanded Problem Focused	99213	X	2–4	11056		HGB	85018	
Detailed	99214		>4	11057		HIV	86703	
Comprehensive/High Complex	99215		Diaphragm Fitting	57170		Iron & TIBC	83550	
Well Exam Infant (up to 12 mos.)	99391		Ear Irrigation	69210		Kidney Profile	80069	
Well exam 1–4 yrs.	99392		ECG	93000	X	Lead	83655	
Well Exam 5–11 yrs.	99393		Endometrial Biopsy	58100		Liver Profile	80076	
Well Exam 12–17 yrs.	99394		Exc. Lesion Malignant			Mono Test	86308	
Well Exam 18–39 yrs.	99395		Benign			Pap Smear	88155	
Well Exam 40–64 yrs.	99396		Location			Pregnancy Test	84703	
Obstetrics			Exc. Skin Tags (1–15)	11200		Obstetric Panel	80055	
Total OB Care	59400		Each Additional 10	11201		Pro Time	85610	
Injections			Fracture Treatment			PSA	84153	
Administration Sub. / IM	90772		Loc			RPR	86592	
Drug			w/Reduc w/o Reduc			Sed. Rate	85651	
Dosage			I & D Abscess Single/Simple	10060		Stool Culture	87045	
Allergy	95115		Multiple or Comp	10061		Stool O & P	87177	
Cocci Skin Test	86490		I & D Pilonidal Cyst Simple	10080		Strep Screen	87880	
DPT	90701		Pilonidal Cyst Complex	10081		Theophylline	80198	
Hemophilus	90646		IV Therapy—To One Hour	90760		Thyroid Uptake	84479	
Influenza	90658		Each Additional Hour	90761		TSH	84443	
MMR	90707		Laceration Repair			Urinalysis	81000	
OPV	90712		Location Size Simp/Comp			Urine Culture	87088	
Pneumovax	90732		Laryngoscopy	31505		Drawing Fee	36415	X
TB Skin Test	86580		Oximetry	94760		Specimen Collection	99000	
TD	90718		Punch Biopsy			**Other:**		
Unlisted Immun	90749		Rhythm Strip	93040				
Tetanus Toxoid	90703		Treadmill	93015				
Vaccine/Toxoid Admin <8 Yr Old w/ Counseling	90465		Trigger Point or Tendon Sheath Inj.	20550				
Vaccine/Toxoid Administration for Adult	90471		Tympanometry	92567				

Diagnosis/ICD-9: **401.0, 412**

I acknowledge receipt of medical services and authorize the release of any medical information necessary to process this claim for healthcare payment only. I do authorize payment to the provider.

Total Estimated Charges: _____

Payment Amount: _____

Patient Signature *Von Vandusen* _____

Next Appointment: _____

Figure 13-9

Capital City Medical
Fee Schedule

New Patient OV		Punch Biopsy various codes	$80
Problem Focused 99201	$45	Nebulizer various codes	$45
Expanded Problem Focused 99202	$65	Cast Application various codes	$85
Detailed 99203	$85	Laryngoscopy 31505	$255
Comprehensive 99204	$105	Audiometry 92552	$85
Comprehensive/High Complex 99205	$115	Tympanometry 92567	$85
Well Exam infant (less than 1 year) 99381	$45	Ear Irrigation 69210	$25
Well Exam 1–4 yrs. 99382	$50	Diaphragm Fitting 57170	$30
Well Exam 5–11 yrs. 99383	$55	IV Therapy (up to one hour) 90760	$65
Well Exam 12–17 yrs. 99384	$65	Each additional hour 90761	$50
Well Exam 18–39 yrs. 99385	$85	Oximetry 94760	$10
Well Exam 40–64 yrs. 99386	$105	ECG 93000	$75
Established Patient OV		Holter Monitor various codes	$170
Post Op Follow Up Visit 99024	$0	Rhythm Strip 93040	$60
Minimum 99211	$35	Treadmill 93015	$375
Problem Focused 99212	$45	Cocci Skin Test 86490	$20
Expanded Problem Focused 99213	$55	X-ray, spine, chest, bone—any area various codes	$275
Detailed 99214	$65	Avulsion Nail 11730	$200
Comprehensive/High Complex 99215	$75	**Laboratory**	
Well exam infant (less than 1 year) 99391	$35	Amylase 82150	$40
Well Exam 1–4 yrs. 99392	$40	B12 82607	$30
Well Exam 5–11 yrs. 99393	$45	CBC & Diff 85025	$95
Well Exam 12–17 yrs. 99394	$55	Comp Metabolic Panel 80053	$75
Well Exam 18–39 yrs. 99395	$65	Chlamydia Screen 87110	$70
Well Exam 40–64 yrs. 99396	$75	Cholestrerol 82465	$75
Obstetrics		Digoxin 80162	$40
Total OB Care 59400	$1700	Electrolytes 80051	$70
Injections		Estrogen, Total 82672	$50
Administration 90772	$10	Ferritin 82728	$40
Allergy 95115	$35	Folate 82746	$30
DPT 90701	$50	GC Screen 87070	$60
Drug various codes	$35	Glucose 82947	$35
Influenza 90658	$25	Glycosylated HGB A1C 83036	$45
MMR 90707	$50	HCT 85014	$30
OPV 90712	$40	HDL 83718	$35
Pneumovax 90732	$35	HGB 85018	$30
TB Skin Test 86580	$15	Hep BSAG 83740	$40
TD 90718	$40	Hepatitis panel, acute 80074	$95
Tetanus Toxoid 90703	$40	HIV 86703	$100
Vaccine/Toxoid Administration for Younger		Iron & TIBC 83550	$45
Than 8 Years Old w/ counseling 90465	$10	Kidney Profile 80069	$95
Vaccine/Toxoid Administration for Adult 90471	$10	Lead 83665	$55
Arthrocentesis/Aspiration/Injection		Lipase 83690	$40
Small Joint 20600	$50	Lipid Panel 80061	$95
Interm Joint 20605	$60	Liver Profile 80076	$95
Major Joint 20610	$70	Mono Test 86308	$30
Trigger Point/Tendon Sheath Inj. 20550	$90	Pap Smear 88155	$90
Other Invasive/Noninvasive Procedures		Pap Collection/Supervision 88142	$95
Catheterization 51701	$55	Pregnancy Test 84703	$90
Circumcision 54150	$150	Obstetric Panel 80055	$85
Colposcopy 57452	$225	Pro Time 85610	$50
Colposcopy w/Biopsy 57454	$250	PSA 84153	$50
Cryosurgery Premalignant Lesion various codes	$160	RPR 86592	$55
Endometrial Biopsy 58100	$190	Sed. Rate 85651	$50
Excision Lesion Malignant various codes	$145	Stool Culture 87045	$80
Excision Lesion Benign various codes	$125	Stool O & P 87177	$105
Curettement Lesion		Strep Screen 87880	$35
Single 11055	$70	Theophylline 80198	$40
2–4 11056	$80	Thyroid Uptake 84479	$75
>4 11057	$90	TSH 84443	$50
Excision Skin Tags (1–15) 11200	$55	Urinalysis 81000	$35
Each Additional 10 11201	$30	Urine Culture 87088	$80
I & D Abscess Single/Simple 10060	$75	Drawing Fee 36415	$15
Multiple/Complex 10061	$95	Specimen Collection 99000	$10
I & D Pilonidal Cyst Simple 10080	$105		
I & D Pilonidal Cyst Complex 10081	$130		
Laceration Repair various codes	$60		

HEALTH INSURANCE CLAIM FORM
APPROVED BY NATIONAL UNIFORM CLAIM COMMITTEE 08/05

PICA

1. MEDICARE	MEDICAID	TRICARE CHAMPUS	CHAMPVA	GROUP HEALTH PLAN	FECA BLK LUNG	OTHER	1a. INSURED'S I.D. NUMBER (For Program in Item 1)
☐ (Medicare #)	☐ (Medicaid #)	☐ (Sponsor's SSN)	☐ (Member ID#)	☐ (SSN or ID)	☐ (SSN)	☐ (ID)	

2. PATIENT'S NAME (Last Name, First Name, Middle Initial)	3. PATIENT'S BIRTH DATE SEX MM DD YY M☐ F☐	4. INSURED'S NAME (Last Name, First Name, Middle Initial)

5. PATIENT'S ADDRESS (No., Street)	6. PATIENT RELATIONSHIP TO INSURED Self☐ Spouse☐ Child☐ Other☐	7. INSURED'S ADDRESS (No., Street)

CITY	STATE	8. PATIENT STATUS Single☐ Married☐ Other☐	CITY	STATE

ZIP CODE	TELEPHONE (Include Area Code) ( )	Full-Time Part-Time Employed☐ Student☐ Student☐	ZIP CODE	TELEPHONE (Include Area Code) ( )

9. OTHER INSURED'S NAME (Last Name, First Name, Middle Initial)	10. IS PATIENT'S CONDITION RELATED TO:	11. INSURED'S POLICY GROUP OR FECA NUMBER

a. OTHER INSURED'S POLICY OR GROUP NUMBER	a. EMPLOYMENT? (Current or Previous) ☐YES ☐NO	a. INSURED'S DATE OF BIRTH SEX MM DD YY M☐ F☐

b. OTHER INSURED'S DATE OF BIRTH SEX MM DD YY M☐ F☐	b. AUTO ACCIDENT? PLACE (State) ☐YES ☐NO	b. EMPLOYER'S NAME OR SCHOOL NAME

c. EMPLOYER'S NAME OR SCHOOL NAME	c. OTHER ACCIDENT? ☐YES ☐NO	c. INSURANCE PLAN NAME OR PROGRAM NAME

d. INSURANCE PLAN NAME OR PROGRAM NAME	10d. RESERVED FOR LOCAL USE	d. IS THERE ANOTHER HEALTH BENEFIT PLAN? ☐YES ☐NO If yes, return to and complete item 9 a-d.

READ BACK OF FORM BEFORE COMPLETING & SIGNING THIS FORM.

12. PATIENT'S OR AUTHORIZED PERSON'S SIGNATURE I authorize the release of any medical or other information necessary to process this claim. I also request payment of government benefits either to myself or to the party who accepts assignment below.

SIGNED _____ DATE _____

13. INSURED'S OR AUTHORIZED PERSON'S SIGNATURE I authorize payment of medical benefits to the undersigned physician or supplier for services described below.

SIGNED _____

14. DATE OF CURRENT: ILLNESS (First symptom) OR INJURY (Accident) OR PREGNANCY (LMP) MM DD YY	15. IF PATIENT HAS HAD SAME OR SIMILAR ILLNESS, GIVE FIRST DATE MM DD YY	16. DATES PATIENT UNABLE TO WORK IN CURRENT OCCUPATION MM DD YY MM DD YY FROM TO

17. NAME OF REFERRING PHYSICIAN OR OTHER SOURCE	17a. 17b. NPI	18. HOSPITALIZATION DATES RELATED TO CURRENT SERVICES MM DD YY MM DD YY FROM TO

19. RESERVED FOR LOCAL USE		20. OUTSIDE LAB? ☐YES ☐NO $ CHARGES

21. DIAGNOSIS OR NATURE OF ILLNESS OR INJURY (Relate Items 1,2,3 or 4 to Item 24E by Line) 1. _____ 3. _____ 2. _____ 4. _____	22. MEDICAID RESUBMISSION CODE ORIGINAL REF. NO. 23. PRIOR AUTHORIZATION NUMBER

24. A. DATE(S) OF SERVICE From To MM DD YY MM DD YY	B. PLACE OF SERVICE	C. EMG	D. PROCEDURES, SERVICES, OR SUPPLIES (Explain Unusual Circumstances) CPT/HCPCS MODIFIER	E. DIAGNOSIS POINTER	F. $ CHARGES	G. DAYS OR UNITS	H. EPSDT Family Plan	I. ID. QUAL.	J. RENDERING PROVIDER ID. #
1								NPI	
2								NPI	
3								NPI	
4								NPI	
5								NPI	
6								NPI	

25. FEDERAL TAX I.D. NUMBER SSN EIN ☐☐	26. PATIENT'S ACCOUNT NO.	27. ACCEPT ASSIGNMENT? (For govt. claims, see back) ☐YES ☐NO	28. TOTAL CHARGE $	29. AMOUNT PAID $	30. BALANCE DUE $

31. SIGNATURE OF PHYSICIAN OR SUPPLIER INCLUDING DEGREES OR CREDENTIALS (I certify that the statements on the reverse apply to this bill and are made a part thereof.) SIGNED _____ DATE _____	32. SERVICE FACILITY LOCATION INFORMATION a. NPI b.	33. BILLING PROVIDER INFO & PH. # ( ) a. NPI b.

NUCC Instruction Manual available at: www.nucc.org
WCMS-1500CS

APPROVED OMB 0938-0999 FORM CMS-1500 (08/05)

CARRIER → PATIENT AND INSURED INFORMATION → PHYSICIAN OR SUPPLIER INFORMATION →

SECOND FOLD — FIRST FOLD WHCF-10-ENV / WHCF-10-ENV-SS

Figure 13-10

REVIEW QUESTIONS

MATCHING

Choose the correct answer, and write its corresponding letter in the space provided.

a. Medicare Part A
b. Respite care
c. Medicare secondary payer (MSP)
d. Crossover
e. GA

1. _____ The reassignment of the gaps in coverage that eliminates the need for filing a separate claim with Medigap
2. _____ Covers inpatient facility costs
3. _____ Care given to a hospice patient to allow the usual caregiver time to rest
4. _____ Term used when Medicare is not responsible for paying a claim first
5. _____ Modifier used on a claim form to identify that a patient has signed an ABN and that it is on file with the provider

MULTIPLE CHOICE

Circle the letter of the choice that best completes each statement or answers the question.

1. What is another name for Medicare Part C?

   a. Medigap
   b. MediCal
   c. Medicare Advantage
   d. None of the above

2. Which of the following is *not* covered by Medicare Parts A and B?

   a. Long-term care
   b. Routine dental care
   c. Routine eye care
   d. All of the above

3. Which of the following is considered medically necessary?

   a. An elective procedure
   b. An experimental or investigational procedure
   c. An essential treatment
   d. None of the above

4. Who receives a Medicare Summary Notice?

   a. Medicare beneficiaries
   b. Patients
   c. Providers
   d. Both a and b

5. What is the name of the form that Medicare will send a provider to request additional information or documentation for a claim to be processed?

   a. Advanced Beneficiary Notice
   b. Medicare Development Letter
   c. Remittance Advice Notice
   d. Explanation of Benefits Notice

SHORT ANSWER

Provide the correct response to each question that follows:

1. a. What are coinsurance days?

   _____

   _____

   _____

   b. What are the criteria for Medicare basic days?

   _____

   _____

   _____

2. What is the difference between a fee-for-service and a managed care plan?

   _____

   _____

   _____

3. Define the 72-hour rule/3-day payment window rule.

   _____

   _____

   _____

4. What should be documented in FL 20 when an independent laboratory provides an EKG or obtains a specimen from a homebound or institutionalized patient?

   _____

   _____

5. What is the result of entering a dollar amount in FL 29?

   _____

   _____

   _____

TRUE/FALSE

Identify each statement as true (T) or false (F).

1. _____ Medicare plans can be either fee-for-service or managed care.
2. _____ A nonparticipating provider can choose to accept Medicare assignment.
3. _____ An ABN does not need to be signed for every questionably covered service.
4. _____ Selling or sharing Medicare health insurance claim numbers is considered fraud.
5. _____ Routinely waiving coinsurance and/or deductibles for Medicare patients is not subject to fraud penalties.

CHAPTER 14
Medicaid Medical Billing

CHAPTER OBJECTIVES

Upon completion of this chapter in your student text, you should be able to do the following:

1. Understand the requirements for qualifying to receive Medicaid benefits.
2. Determine the schedule of benefits the Medicaid recipient will receive.
3. Discuss the method of verifying Medicaid benefits.
4. Submit a Medicaid claim and decipher claim status.

CHAPTER OUTLINE

Medicaid Guidelines

Eligibility Groups
  Categorically Needy
  Medically Needy
  Special Groups

Children's Health Insurance Program Reauthorization Act (CHIPRA)

Scope of Medicaid Services
  PACE

Amount and Duration of Medicaid Services

Payment for Medicaid Services

Medicaid Growth Trends
  Affordable Care Act Projections

The Medicaid–Medicare Relationship (Medi–Medi)

Medicaid Managed Care

Medicaid Verification

Medicaid Claims Filing
  Time Limits for Submitting Claims
  Appeal Time Limits
  Claims with Incomplete Information and Zero Paid Claims
  Newborn Claim Hints

Completing the CMS-1500 Form for Medicaid (Primary)
  Practice Exercises

KEY TERMS

◤

Using the highlighted terms and glossary in the textbook, define the following terms.

1. Aid to Families with Dependent Children (AFDC) _____
   _____

2. categorically needy _____
   _____

3. Children's Health Insurance Program (CHIP) _____
   _____

4. Children's Health Insurance Program Reauthorization Act (CHIPRA) _____
   _____

5. Early and Periodic Screening, Diagnostic and Treatment (EPSDT) _____
   _____

6. Federal Medicaid Assistant Percentages (FMAP) _____
   _____

7. medically needy _____
   _____

8. Medi–Medi _____
   _____

9. payer of last resort _____
   _____

10. restricted status _____
    _____

11. spend-down program _____
    _____

12. State Children's Health Insurance Program (SCHIP)_____
    _____

13. Supplemental Security Income (SSI) _____
    _____

14. Temporary Assistance for Needy Families (TANF) _____
    _____

15. Welfare Reform Bill _____
    _____

CRITICAL THINKING QUESTIONS

◤

Using the knowledge you have gained from reading the textbook, apply critical thinking skills to answer the following questions.

1. What is the federal government's involvement in the Medicaid program, and how does this compare with each state's involvement?
   1. _____
   2. _____

3. _____

4. _____

2. a. What are the three groups that are eligible for Medicaid, under federal law?

    1. _____

    2. _____

    3. _____

  b. What six groups are considered to be categorically needy to qualify for Medicaid?

    1. _____

    2. _____

    3. _____

    4. _____

    5. _____

    6. _____

  c. Define a medically needy person.

_____

_____

_____

3. Answer the following questions related to the Welfare Reform Bill:

  a. A patient, Christine Richards, is born to her mother, who does receive Medicaid. Her mother is a legal alien. Does Christine qualify for Medicaid? Why or why not?

_____

_____

_____

_____

_____

  b. If this patient had not been born in this country and just came here as an alien, would she qualify for Medicaid right now? Why or why not?

_____

_____

_____

_____

_____

  c. Who determines TANF eligibility?

_____

_____

_____

_____

_____

4. a. What are the 14 mandatory services that states must provide to Medicaid recipients?

1. _____
2. _____
3. _____
4. _____
5. _____
6. _____
7. _____
8. _____
9. _____
10. _____
11. _____
12. _____
13. _____
14. _____

b. What do you believe will be the future of Medicaid in 10 years? Discuss your answer with the class.

_____
_____
_____
_____
_____

5. a. You filed a Medicaid claim 60 days after the services were provided. Was this claim submitted within Medicaid's allowed time period? Why or why not?

_____
_____
_____

b. If the medical biller accidentally overlooked a Medicaid claim that had not been filed within the allowed time period, what should he do?

_____
_____
_____
_____

c. The medical biller receives a denied Medicaid claim for a patient's account and decides to appeal. What is the allowed time period to submit this appeal?

_____
_____

d. The medical biller has just received a denial for a Medicaid claim that she filed for a patient. The medical biller inspects the claim and realizes that she entered the wrong ID# for the patient. She corrects the claim and resubmits it. What is the time period allowed by Medicaid to resubmit this claim?

_____

_____

PRACTICE EXERCISES

1. Using the form locator information written out on your index cards from a prior chapter, complete the following activity. Flag those FLs that would be filled out differently for Medicaid patients.

2. Case studies are provided for additional practice in completing the CMS-1500 claim form for Medicaid physician outpatient billing. By applying what you have learned in your student text, accurately code and complete each case study. Patient demographics and a brief case history are provided. Complete the cases based on the following criteria:

    *   All patients have release of information and assignment of benefits signatures on file. Assignment of benefits is required by most states for Medicaid. SOF is not required in Item 13.

    *   All providers accept assignment for Medicaid, by law. Item 27 should not be marked.

    *   The group practice is the billing entity.

    *   The national transition to NPI numbers is complete, and legacy PINs of individual payers are no longer used. If legacy PINS are still being used by your state Medicaid program, your instructor may provide you with Medicaid PINs in addition to the NPI.

    *   2012 ICD-9-CM and CPT codes are used.

    *   Use eight-digit dates for birthdates. Use six-digit dates for all other dates.

    *   All street names should be entered with standard postal abbreviations, even if they are spelled out on the source documents.

    *   Enter the ICD-9 codes in the order they appear on the encounter form.

    *   When entering CPT codes, enter the E/M code first. Enter remaining codes in descending price order.

To complete each case study, you must determine the correct fees. Refer to the Capital City Medical Fee Schedule, which is located after each case's source documents. Use the blank CMS-1500 form provided after each case.

    a. Using the source documents, the Capital City Medical Fee Schedule (Figure 14-1), and the blank CMS-1500 form provided (Figure 14-2), complete the following case study for patient Michael Schultz (Case 14-1):

CASE 14-1

Patient Information:

Name: (Last, First) Schultz, Michael ☒ Male ☐ Female Birth Date: 10/01/1971

Address: 84 Marble St, Capital City, NY 12345 Phone: (555) 555-6918

Social Security Number: 723-44-4142 Full-Time Student: ☐ Yes ☒ No

Marital Status: ☒ Single ☐ Married ☐ Divorced ☐ Other

Employment:

Employer: Buy Now Mart Phone: (555) 555-5989

Address: 914 W. Washington St. Capital City, NY 12345

Condition Related to: ☐ Auto Accident ☐ Employment ☐ Other Accident

Date of Accident: _____ State: _____

Emergency Contact: _____ **Phone: ( )** _____

Primary Insurance: Medicaid Phone: ( ) _____

Address: 4875 Capital Blvd, Capital City, NY 12345

Insurance Policyholder's Name: Same ☐ M ☐ F DOB: _____

Address: _____

Phone: ( ) _____ Relationship to Insured: ☒ Self ☐ Spouse ☐ Child ☐ Other

Employer: _____ Phone: ( ) _____

Employer's Address: _____

Policy/ID No: 0002316983333 Group No: _____ Percent Covered: ____% Copay Amt: $5.00

Secondary Insurance: _____ Phone: ( ) _____

Address: _____

Insurance Policyholder's Name: _____ ☐ M ☐ F DOB: _____

Address: _____

Phone: ( ) _____ Relationship to Insured: ☐ Self ☐ Spouse ☐ Child ☐ Other

Employer: _____ Phone: ( ) _____

Employer's Address: _____

Policy/ID No: _____ Group No: _____ Percent Covered: ____% Copay Amt: $_____

Reason for Visit: I can't sleep and I'm stressed.

Known Allergies: _____

Referred by: _____

06/10/20XX
Assignment of Benefits: Y
Signature on File: Y
Referring Physician: N

S: Michael Schultz presents with complaints of not being able to sleep for 2 weeks. He is stressed because he has been taking care of his sick mother and working. He feels overwhelmed.

O: On exam, Pt. gets nervous and anxious. His vitals are stable. Physical findings are unremarkable. Labs are normal.

A: 1. Generalized Anxiety—300.02
2. Insomnia due to anxiety—307.42

P: 1. Start Xanax.
2. Start Levapro.
3. Return in 2 weeks.

_____
Phil Wells, MD
Family Practice
NPI: 1234567890

CASE 14-1

Patient Name Michael Schultz

Capital City Medical
123 Unknown Boulevard, Capital City, NY 12345-2222

Date of Service
06-10-20XX

New Patient			Other Invasive/Noninvasive			Laboratory		
Problem Focused	99201		Arthrocentesis/Aspiration/Injection			Amylase	82150	
Expanded Problem, Focused	99202		Small Joint		20600	B12	82607	
Detailed	99203		Interm Joint		20605	CBC & Diff	85025	X
Comprehensive	99204		Major Joint		20610	Comp Metabolic Panel	80053	
Comprehensive/High Complex	99205		Other Invasive/Noninvasive			Chlamydia Screen	87110	
Well Exam Infant (up to 12 mos.)	99381		Audiometry		92552	Cholesterol	82465	
Well Exam 1–4 yrs.	99382		Cast Application			Digoxin	80162	
Well Exam 5–11 yrs.	99383		Location Long Short			Electrolytes	80051	X
Well Exam 12–17 yrs.	99384		Catheterization		51701	Ferritin	82728	
Well Exam 18–39 yrs.	99385		Circumcision		54150	Folate	82746	
Well Exam 40–64 yrs.	99386		Colposcopy		57452	GC Screen	87070	
			Colposcopy w/Biopsy		57454	Glucose	82947	
			Cryosurgery Premalignant Lesion			Glucose 1 HR	82950	
			Location (s):			Glycosylated HGB A1C	83036	
Established Patient			Cryosurgery Warts			HCT	85014	
Post-Op Follow Up Visit	99024		Location (s):			HDL	83718	
Minimum	99211		Curettement Lesion			Hep BSAG	87340	
Problem Focused	99212		Single		11055	Hepatitis panel, acute	80074	
Expanded Problem Focused	99213	X	2–4		11056	HGB	85018	
Detailed	99214		>4		11057	HIV	86703	
Comprehensive/High Complex	99215		Diaphragm Fitting		57170	Iron & TIBC	83550	
Well Exam Infant (up to 12 mos.)	99391		Ear Irrigation		69210	Kidney Profile	80069	
Well exam 1–4 yrs.	99392		ECG		93000	Lead	83655	
Well Exam 5–11 yrs.	99393		Endometrial Biopsy		58100	Liver Profile	80076	
Well Exam 12–17 yrs.	99394		Exc. Lesion Malignant			Mono Test	86308	
Well Exam 18–39 yrs.	99395		Benign			Pap Smear	88155	
Well Exam 40–64 yrs.	99396		Location			Pregnancy Test	84703	
Obstetrics			Exc. Skin Tags (1–15)		11200	Obstetric Panel	80055	
Total OB Care	59400		Each Additional 10		11201	Pro Time	85610	
Injections			Fracture Treatment			PSA	84153	
Administration Sub. / IM	90772		Loc			RPR	86592	
Drug			w/Reduc	w/o Reduc		Sed. Rate	85651	X
Dosage			I & D Abscess Single/Simple		10060	Stool Culture	87045	
Allergy	95115		Multiple or Comp		10061	Stool O & P	87177	
Cocci Skin Test	86490		I & D Pilonidal Cyst Simple		10080	Strep Screen	87880	
DPT	90701		Pilonidal Cyst Complex		10081	Theophylline	80198	
Hemophilus	90646		IV Therapy—To One Hour		90760	Thyroid Uptake	84479	
Influenza	90658		Each Additional Hour		90761	TSH	84443	
MMR	90707		Laceration Repair			Urinalysis	81000	
OPV	90712		Location Size Simp/Comp			Urine Culture	87088	
Pneumovax	90732		Laryngoscopy		31505	Drawing Fee	36415	X
TB Skin Test	86580		Oximetry		94760	Specimen Collection	99000	
TD	90718		Punch Biopsy			**Other:**		
Unlisted Immun	90749		Rhythm Strip		93040			
Tetanus Toxoid	90703		Treadmill		93015			
Vaccine/Toxoid Admin <8 Yr Old w/ Counseling	90465		Trigger Point or Tendon Sheath Inj.		20550			
Vaccine/Toxoid Administration for Adult	90471		Tympanometry		92567			

Diagnosis/ICD-9: **300.02, 307.42**

I acknowledge receipt of medical services and authorize the release of any medical information necessary to process this claim for healthcare payment only. I do authorize payment to the provider.

Patient Signature Michael Schultz

Total Estimated Charges: _____

Payment Amount: _____

Next Appointment: _____

Figure 14-1

Capital City Medical
Fee Schedule

New Patient OV			Punch Biopsy various codes	$80
Problem Focused 99201	$45		Nebulizer various codes	$45
Expanded Problem Focused 99202	$65		Cast Application various codes	$85
Detailed 99203	$85		Laryngoscopy 31505	$255
Comprehensive 99204	$105		Audiometry 92552	$85
Comprehensive/High Complex 99205	$115		Tympanometry 92567	$85
Well Exam infant (less than 1 year) 99381	$45		Ear Irrigation 69210	$25
Well Exam 1–4 yrs. 99382	$50		Diaphragm Fitting 57170	$30
Well Exam 5–11 yrs. 99383	$55		IV Therapy (up to one hour) 90760	$65
Well Exam 12–17 yrs. 99384	$65		Each additional hour 90761	$50
Well Exam 18–39 yrs. 99385	$85		Oximetry 94760	$10
Well Exam 40–64 yrs. 99386	$105		ECG 93000	$75
Established Patient OV			Holter Monitor various codes	$170
Post Op Follow Up Visit 99024	$0		Rhythm Strip 93040	$60
Minimum 99211	$35		Treadmill 93015	$375
Problem Focused 99212	$45		Cocci Skin Test 86490	$20
Expanded Problem Focused 99213	$55		X-ray, spine, chest, bone—any area various codes	$275
Detailed 99214	$65		Avulsion Nail 11730	$200
Comprehensive/High Complex 99215	$75		**Laboratory**	
Well exam infant (less than 1 year) 99391	$35		Amylase 82150	$40
Well Exam 1–4 yrs. 99392	$40		B12 82607	$30
Well Exam 5–11 yrs. 99393	$45		CBC & Diff 85025	$95
Well Exam 12–17 yrs. 99394	$55		Comp Metabolic Panel 80053	$75
Well Exam 18–39 yrs. 99395	$65		Chlamydia Screen 87110	$70
Well Exam 40–64 yrs. 99396	$75		Cholestrerol 82465	$75
Obstetrics			Digoxin 80162	$40
Total OB Care 59400	$1700		Electrolytes 80051	$70
Injections			Estrogen, Total 82672	$50
Administration 90772	$10		Ferritin 82728	$40
Allergy 95115	$35		Folate 82746	$30
DPT 90701	$50		GC Screen 87070	$60
Drug various codes	$35		Glucose 82947	$35
Influenza 90658	$25		Glycosylated HGB A1C 83036	$45
MMR 90707	$50		HCT 85014	$30
OPV 90712	$40		HDL 83718	$35
Pneumovax 90732	$35		HGB 85018	$30
TB Skin Test 86580	$15		Hep BSAG 83740	$40
TD 90718	$40		Hepatitis panel, acute 80074	$95
Tetanus Toxoid 90703	$40		HIV 86703	$100
Vaccine/Toxoid Administration for Younger			Iron & TIBC 83550	$45
Than 8 Years Old w/ counseling 90465	$10		Kidney Profile 80069	$95
Vaccine/Toxoid Administration for Adult 90471	$10		Lead 83665	$55
Arthrocentesis/Aspiration/Injection			Lipase 83690	$40
Small Joint 20600	$50		Lipid Panel 80061	$95
Interm Joint 20605	$60		Liver Profile 80076	$95
Major Joint 20610	$70		Mono Test 86308	$30
Trigger Point/Tendon Sheath Inj. 20550	$90		Pap Smear 88155	$90
Other Invasive/Noninvasive Procedures			Pap Collection/Supervision 88142	$95
Catheterization 51701	$55		Pregnancy Test 84703	$90
Circumcision 54150	$150		Obstetric Panel 80055	$85
Colposcopy 57452	$225		Pro Time 85610	$50
Colposcopy w/Biopsy 57454	$250		PSA 84153	$50
Cryosurgery Premalignant Lesion various codes	$160		RPR 86592	$55
Endometrial Biopsy 58100	$190		Sed. Rate 85651	$50
Excision Lesion Malignant various codes	$145		Stool Culture 87045	$80
Excision Lesion Benign various codes	$125		Stool O & P 87177	$105
Curettement Lesion			Strep Screen 87880	$35
Single 11055	$70		Theophylline 80198	$40
2–4 11056	$80		Thyroid Uptake 84479	$75
>4 11057	$90		TSH 84443	$50
Excision Skin Tags (1–15) 11200	$55		Urinalysis 81000	$35
Each Additional 10 11201	$30		Urine Culture 87088	$80
I & D Abscess Single/Simple 10060	$75		Drawing Fee 36415	$15
Multiple/Complex 10061	$95		Specimen Collection 99000	$10
I & D Pilonidal Cyst Simple 10080	$105			
I & D Pilonidal Cyst Complex 10081	$130			
Laceration Repair various codes	$60			

HEALTH INSURANCE CLAIM FORM

APPROVED BY NATIONAL UNIFORM CLAIM COMMITTEE 08/05

CARRIER →

□□□PICA   PICA □□□

1. MEDICARE MEDICAID TRICARE CHAMPVA GROUP FECA OTHER	1a. INSURED'S I.D. NUMBER (For Program in Item 1)

CHAMPUS   HEALTH PLAN   BLK LUNG

□(Medicare #) □(Medicaid #) □(Sponsor's SSN) □(Member ID#) □(SSN or ID) □(SSN) □(ID)

2. PATIENT'S NAME (Last Name, First Name, Middle Initial)	3. PATIENT'S BIRTH DATE SEX	4. INSURED'S NAME (Last Name, First Name, Middle Initial)

MM DD YY   M□ F□

5. PATIENT'S ADDRESS (No., Street)	6. PATIENT RELATIONSHIP TO INSURED	7. INSURED'S ADDRESS (No., Street)

Self□ Spouse□ Child□ Other□

| CITY | STATE | 8. PATIENT STATUS | CITY | STATE |

Single□ Married□ Other□

| ZIP CODE | TELEPHONE (Include Area Code) | | ZIP CODE | TELEPHONE (Include Area Code) |

Full-Time Part-Time
Employed□ Student□ Student□

( )   ( )

| 9. OTHER INSURED'S NAME (Last Name, First Name, Middle Initial) | 10. IS PATIENT'S CONDITION RELATED TO: | 11. INSURED'S POLICY GROUP OR FECA NUMBER |

SECOND FOLD →

a. OTHER INSURED'S POLICY OR GROUP NUMBER   a. EMPLOYMENT? (Current or Previous)   a. INSURED'S DATE OF BIRTH   SEX

□YES □NO   MM DD YY   M□ F□

b. OTHER INSURED'S DATE OF BIRTH   SEX   b. AUTO ACCIDENT?   PLACE (State)   b. EMPLOYER'S NAME OR SCHOOL NAME

MM DD YY   M□ F□   □YES □NO

c. EMPLOYER'S NAME OR SCHOOL NAME   c. OTHER ACCIDENT?   c. INSURANCE PLAN NAME OR PROGRAM NAME

□YES □NO

d. INSURANCE PLAN NAME OR PROGRAM NAME   10d. RESERVED FOR LOCAL USE   d. IS THERE ANOTHER HEALTH BENEFIT PLAN?

□YES □NO   If yes, return to and complete item 9 a-d.

READ BACK OF FORM BEFORE COMPLETING & SIGNING THIS FORM.

FIRST FOLD   WHCF-10-ENV / WHCF-10-ENV-SS →

12. PATIENT'S OR AUTHORIZED PERSON'S SIGNATURE I authorize the release of any medical or other information necessary to process this claim. I also request payment of government benefits either to myself or to the party who accepts assignment below.

13. INSURED'S OR AUTHORIZED PERSON'S SIGNATURE I authorize payment of medical benefits to the undersigned physician or supplier for services described below.

SIGNED _____ DATE _____   SIGNED _____

| 14. DATE OF CURRENT: ILLNESS (First symptom) OR | 15. IF PATIENT HAS HAD SAME OR SIMILAR ILLNESS. | 16. DATES PATIENT UNABLE TO WORK IN CURRENT OCCUPATION |

MM DD YY   INJURY (Accident) OR   GIVE FIRST DATE MM DD YY   MM DD YY   MM DD YY
PREGNANCY (LMP)   FROM   TO

17. NAME OF REFERRING PHYSICIAN OR OTHER SOURCE   17a.   18. HOSPITALIZATION DATES RELATED TO CURRENT SERVICES
MM DD YY   MM DD YY
17b. NPI   FROM   TO

19. RESERVED FOR LOCAL USE   20. OUTSIDE LAB? $ CHARGES

□YES □NO

21. DIAGNOSIS OR NATURE OF ILLNESS OR INJURY (Relate Items 1,2,3 or 4 to Item 24E by Line)   22. MEDICAID RESUBMISSION
CODE   ORIGINAL REF. NO.

1. |___.___   3. |___.___

23. PRIOR AUTHORIZATION NUMBER

2. |___.___   4. |___.___

24. A. DATE(S) OF SERVICE	B.	C.	D. PROCEDURES, SERVICES, OR SUPPLIES	E.	F.	G.	H.	I.	J.
From To	PLACE OF		(Explain Unusual Circumstances)	DIAGNOSIS		DAYS OR	EPSDT Family	ID.	RENDERING
MM DD YY MM DD YY	SERVICE	EMG	CPT/HCPCS MODIFIER	POINTER	$ CHARGES	UNITS	Plan	QUAL.	PROVIDER ID. #
1								NPI	
2								NPI	
3								NPI	
4								NPI	
5								NPI	
6								NPI	

PHYSICIAN OR SUPPLIER INFORMATION →

25. FEDERAL TAX I.D. NUMBER SSN EIN	26. PATIENT'S ACCOUNT NO.	27. ACCEPT ASSIGNMENT?	28. TOTAL CHARGE	29. AMOUNT PAID	30. BALANCE DUE
□□		(For govt. claims, see back) □YES □NO	$	$	$

31. SIGNATURE OF PHYSICIAN OR SUPPLIER INCLUDING DEGREES OR CREDENTIALS (I certify that the statements on the reverse apply to this bill and are made a part thereof.)	32. SERVICE FACILITY LOCATION INFORMATION	33. BILLING PROVIDER INFO & PH. # ( )
SIGNED _____ DATE _____	a. NPI b.	a. NPI b.

APPROVED OMB 0938-0999 FORM CMS-1500 (08/05)

Figure 14-2

b. Using the source documents, the Capital City Medical Fee Schedule (Figure 14-3), and the blank CMS-1500 form provided (Figure 14-4), complete the following case study for patient Brenda Bloom (Case 14-2):

CASE 14-2

Capital City Medical—123 Unknown Boulevard, Capital City, NY 12345-2222 (555) 555-1234	Patient Information Form
	Tax ID: 75-0246810
Phil Wells, MD, Mannie Mends, MD, Bette R. Soone, MD	Group NPI: 1513171216

Patient Information:

Name: (Last, First) Bloom, Brenda   ❑ Male ☒ Female Birth Date: 12/09/1944

Address: 51 Calico St, Township, NY 12345   Phone: (555) 555-4255

Social Security Number: 133-12-0019   Full-Time Student: ❑ Yes ☒ No

Marital Status: ❑ Single ❑ Married ☒ Divorced ❑ Other

Employment:

Employer: Retired   Phone: ( )

Address:

Condition Related to: ❑ Auto Accident   ❑ Employment   ❑ Other Accident

Date of Accident: _____ State: _____

Emergency Contact: _____ **Phone: ( )** _____

Primary Insurance: Medicaid   Phone: ( )

Address: P. O. Box 9834, Capital City, NY 12345

Insurance Policyholder's Name: Same   ❑ M ❑ F DOB: _____

Address:

Phone: ( ) _____ Relationship to Insured: ☒ Self ❑ Spouse ❑ Child ❑ Other

Employer: _____ Phone: ( ) _____

Employer's Address:

Policy/ID No: 366736530A   Group No: _____ Percent Covered: 80 % Copay Amt: $ _____

Secondary Insurance: Medicaid   Phone: ( )

Address: 4875 Capital Blvd, Capital City, NY 12345

Insurance Policyholder's Name: Same   ❑ M ❑ F DOB: _____

Address:

Phone: ( ) _____ Relationship to Insured: ☒ Self ❑ Spouse ❑ Child ❑ Other

Employer: _____ Phone: ( ) _____

Employer's Address:

Policy/ID No: 0002566499883   Group No: _____ Percent Covered: ___% Copay Amt: $ 5.00

Reason for Visit: I am here for a checkup on my high blood pressure and cholesterol.

Known Allergies:

Referred by:

CASE 14-2
SOAP

09/21/20XX
Assignment of Benefits: Y
Signature on File: Y
Referring Physician: N

S: Brenda Bloom is being seen today for a regular checkup on her high blood pressure and triglycerides.

O: She presents with no new problems. Her BP in office was 132/86. Review of recent lab showed significant improvement in her triglycerides.

A: 1. HTN—401.9
2. Hypertriglyceridemia—272.1

P: 1. Continue cholesterol meds.
2. Return in 3 months.

_____

Phil Wells, MD
Family Practice
NPI: 1234567890

CASE 14-2

Patient Name <u>Brenda Bloom</u>

Capital City Medical
123 Unknown Boulevard, Capital City, NY 12345-2222

Date of Service
09-21-20XX

New Patient			Other Invasive/Noninvasive			Laboratory		
Problem Focused	99201		Arthrocentesis/Aspiration/Injection			Amylase	82150	
Expanded Problem, Focused	99202		Small Joint	20600		B12	82607	X
Detailed	99203		Interm Joint	20605		CBC & Diff	85025	
Comprehensive	99204		Major Joint	20610		Comp Metabolic Panel	80053	
Comprehensive/High Complex	99205		**Other Invasive/Noninvasive**			Chlamydia Screen	87110	
Well Exam Infant (up to 12 mos.)	99381		Audiometry	92552		Cholesterol	82465	X
Well Exam 1–4 yrs.	99382		Cast Application			Digoxin	80162	
Well Exam 5–11 yrs.	99383		Location Long Short			Electrolytes	80051	
Well Exam 12–17 yrs.	99384		Catheterization	51701		Ferritin	82728	
Well Exam 18–39 yrs.	99385		Circumcision	54150		Folate	82746	
Well Exam 40–64 yrs.	99386		Colposcopy	57452		GC Screen	87070	
			Colposcopy w/Biopsy	57454		Glucose	82947	
			Cryosurgery Premalignant Lesion			Glucose 1 HR	82950	
			Location (s):			Glycosylated HGB A1C	83036	
Established Patient			Cryosurgery Warts			HCT	85014	
Post-Op Follow Up Visit	99024		Location (s):			HDL	83718	
Minimum	99211		Curettement Lesion			Hep BSAG	87340	
Problem Focused	99212		Single	11055		Hepatitis panel, acute	80074	
Expanded Problem Focused	99213	X	2–4	11056		HGB	85018	
Detailed	99214		>4	11057		HIV	86703	
Comprehensive/High Complex	99215		Diaphragm Fitting	57170		Iron & TIBC	83550	
Well Exam Infant (up to 12 mos.)	99391		Ear Irrigation	69210		Kidney Profile	80069	
Well exam 1–4 yrs.	99392		ECG	93000		Lead	83655	
Well Exam 5–11 yrs.	99393		Endometrial Biopsy	58100		Liver Profile	80076	
Well Exam 12–17 yrs.	99394		Exc. Lesion Malignant			Mono Test	86308	
Well Exam 18–39 yrs.	99395		Benign			Pap Smear	88155	
Well Exam 40–64 yrs.	99396		Location			Pregnancy Test	84703	
Obstetrics			Exc. Skin Tags (1–15)	11200		Obstetric Panel	80055	
Total OB Care	59400		Each Additional 10	11201		Pro Time	85610	
Injections			Fracture Treatment			PSA	84153	
Administration Sub. / IM	90772		Loc			RPR	86592	
Drug			w/Reduc w/o Reduc			Sed. Rate	85651	
Dosage			I & D Abscess Single/Simple	10060		Stool Culture	87045	
Allergy	95115		Multiple or Comp	10061		Stool O & P	87177	
Cocci Skin Test	86490		I & D Pilonidal Cyst Simple	10080		Strep Screen	87880	
DPT	90701		Pilonidal Cyst Complex	10081		Theophylline	80198	
Hemophilus	90646		IV Therapy—To One Hour	90760		Thyroid Uptake	84479	
Influenza	90658		Each Additional Hour	90761		TSH	84443	
MMR	90707		Laceration Repair			Urinalysis	81000	
OPV	90712		Location Size Simp/Comp			Urine Culture	87088	
Pneumovax	90732		Laryngoscopy	31505		Drawing Fee	36415	X
TB Skin Test	86580		Oximetry	94760		Specimen Collection	99000	
TD	90718		Punch Biopsy			**Other:**		
Unlisted Immun	90749		Rhythm Strip	93040				
Tetanus Toxoid	90703		Treadmill	93015				
Vaccine/Toxoid Admin <8 Yr Old w/ Counseling	90465		Trigger Point or Tendon Sheath Inj.	20550				
Vaccine/Toxoid Administration for Adult	90471		Tympanometry	92567				

Diagnosis/ICD-9: **401.9, 272.1**

I acknowledge receipt of medical services and authorize the release of any medical information necessary to process this claim for healthcare payment only. I do authorize payment to the provider.

Patient Signature <u>Brenda Bloom</u>

Total Estimated Charges: _____

Payment Amount: _____

Next Appointment: _____

Figure 14-3

Capital City Medical
Fee Schedule

New Patient OV			Punch Biopsy various codes	$80
Problem Focused 99201	$45		Nebulizer various codes	$45
Expanded Problem Focused 99202	$65		Cast Application various codes	$85
Detailed 99203	$85		Laryngoscopy 31505	$255
Comprehensive 99204	$105		Audiometry 92552	$85
Comprehensive/High Complex 99205	$115		Tympanometry 92567	$85
Well Exam infant (less than 1 year) 99381	$45		Ear Irrigation 69210	$25
Well Exam 1–4 yrs. 99382	$50		Diaphragm Fitting 57170	$30
Well Exam 5–11 yrs. 99383	$55		IV Therapy (up to one hour) 90760	$65
Well Exam 12–17 yrs. 99384	$65		Each additional hour 90761	$50
Well Exam 18–39 yrs. 99385	$85		Oximetry 94760	$10
Well Exam 40–64 yrs. 99386	$105		ECG 93000	$75
Established Patient OV			Holter Monitor various codes	$170
Post Op Follow Up Visit 99024	$0		Rhythm Strip 93040	$60
Minimum 99211	$35		Treadmill 93015	$375
Problem Focused 99212	$45		Cocci Skin Test 86490	$20
Expanded Problem Focused 99213	$55		X-ray, spine, chest, bone—any area various codes	$275
Detailed 99214	$65		Avulsion Nail 11730	$200
Comprehensive/High Complex 99215	$75		**Laboratory**	
Well exam infant (less than 1 year) 99391	$35		Amylase 82150	$40
Well Exam 1–4 yrs. 99392	$40		B12 82607	$30
Well Exam 5–11 yrs. 99393	$45		CBC & Diff 85025	$95
Well Exam 12–17 yrs. 99394	$55		Comp Metabolic Panel 80053	$75
Well Exam 18–39 yrs. 99395	$65		Chlamydia Screen 87110	$70
Well Exam 40–64 yrs. 99396	$75		Cholestrerol 82465	$75
Obstetrics			Digoxin 80162	$40
Total OB Care 59400	$1700		Electrolytes 80051	$70
Injections			Estrogen, Total 82672	$50
Administration 90772	$10		Ferritin 82728	$40
Allergy 95115	$35		Folate 82746	$30
DPT 90701	$50		GC Screen 87070	$60
Drug various codes	$35		Glucose 82947	$35
Influenza 90658	$25		Glycosylated HGB A1C 83036	$45
MMR 90707	$50		HCT 85014	$30
OPV 90712	$40		HDL 83718	$35
Pneumovax 90732	$35		HGB 85018	$30
TB Skin Test 86580	$15		Hep BSAG 83740	$40
TD 90718	$40		Hepatitis panel, acute 80074	$95
Tetanus Toxoid 90703	$40		HIV 86703	$100
Vaccine/Toxoid Administration for Younger			Iron & TIBC 83550	$45
Than 8 Years Old w/ counseling 90465	$10		Kidney Profile 80069	$95
Vaccine/Toxoid Administration for Adult 90471	$10		Lead 83665	$55
Arthrocentesis/Aspiration/Injection			Lipase 83690	$40
Small Joint 20600	$50		Lipid Panel 80061	$95
Interm Joint 20605	$60		Liver Profile 80076	$95
Major Joint 20610	$70		Mono Test 86308	$30
Trigger Point/Tendon Sheath Inj. 20550	$90		Pap Smear 88155	$90
Other Invasive/Noninvasive Procedures			Pap Collection/Supervision 88142	$95
Catheterization 51701	$55		Pregnancy Test 84703	$90
Circumcision 54150	$150		Obstetric Panel 80055	$85
Colposcopy 57452	$225		Pro Time 85610	$50
Colposcopy w/Biopsy 57454	$250		PSA 84153	$50
Cryosurgery Premalignant Lesion various codes	$160		RPR 86592	$55
Endometrial Biopsy 58100	$190		Sed. Rate 85651	$50
Excision Lesion Malignant various codes	$145		Stool Culture 87045	$80
Excision Lesion Benign various codes	$125		Stool O & P 87177	$105
Curettement Lesion			Strep Screen 87880	$35
Single 11055	$70		Theophylline 80198	$40
2–4 11056	$80		Thyroid Uptake 84479	$75
>4 11057	$90		TSH 84443	$50
Excision Skin Tags (1–15) 11200	$55		Urinalysis 81000	$35
Each Additional 10 11201	$30		Urine Culture 87088	$80
I & D Abscess Single/Simple 10060	$75		Drawing Fee 36415	$15
Multiple/Complex 10061	$95		Specimen Collection 99000	$10
I & D Pilonidal Cyst Simple 10080	$105			
I & D Pilonidal Cyst Complex 10081	$130			
Laceration Repair various codes	$60			

Figure 14-4

c. Using the source documents, the Capital City Medical Fee Schedule (Figure 14-5), and the blank CMS-1500 form provided (Figure 14-6), complete the following case study for patient Blake McComb (Case 14-3):

CASE 14-3

Capital City Medical—123 Unknown Boulevard, Capital City, NY 12345-2222 (555) 555-1234 Phil Wells, MD, Mannie Mends, MD, Bette R. Soone, MD	Patient Information Form Tax ID: 75-0246810 Group NPI: 1513171216

Patient Information:

Name: (Last, First) McComb, Blake   ☒ Male   ☐ Female   Birth Date: 05/21/1966

Address: 6054 Spelling Rd., Capital City, NY 12345   Phone: (555) 555-9451

Social Security Number: 855-06-5872   Full-Time Student: ☐ Yes   ☒ No

Marital Status: ☐ Single   ☐ Married   ☒ Divorced   ☐ Other

Employment:

Employer: Yummy's Bakery Shop   Phone: (555) 555-6200

Address: 14 Mt. Royal Blvd., Capital City, NY 12345

Condition Related to: ☐ Auto Accident   ☐ Employment   ☐ Other Accident

Date of Accident: _____ State: _____

Emergency Contact: _____ **Phone: ( )** _____

Primary Insurance: Medicaid   Phone: ( ) _____

Address: 4875 Capital Blvd, Capital City, NY 12345

Insurance Policyholder's Name: Same   ☐ M ☐ F DOB: _____

Address: _____

Phone: ( ) _____ Relationship to Insured: ☒ Self ☐ Spouse ☐ Child ☐ Other

Employer: _____ Phone: ( ) _____

Employer's Address: _____

Policy/ID No: 03656499533 ____ Group No: ____ Percent Covered: ____% Copay Amt: $ 5.00

Secondary Insurance: _____ Phone: ( ) _____

Address: _____

Insurance Policyholder's Name: _____ ☐ M ☐ F DOB: _____

Address: _____

Phone: ( ) _____ Relationship to Insured: ☐ Self ☐ Spouse ☐ Child ☐ Other

Employer: _____ Phone: ( ) _____

Employer's Address: _____

Policy/ID No: _____ Group No: ____ Percent Covered: ____% Copay Amt: $ ____

Reason for Visit: I am here for a hearing test.

Known Allergies: _____

Referred by: _____

**CASE 14-3
SOAP**

01/29/20XX
Assignment of Benefits: Y
Signature on File: Y
Referring Physician: N

S: Blake McComb is a new patient who is here for a hearing test. He is concerned that he may be experiencing some hearing loss.

O: Pt. is generally in good health. He is alert and oriented ×3. His mood is upbeat. Audiometry shows no signs of hearing loss in either ear. He is alert to all tone levels. Nose and throat present clear. There is no impacted ceremun bilaterally.

A: 1. Hearing exam—V72.19

P: 1. Return in 1 month for PE.

_____

Phil Wells, MD
Family Practice
NPI: 1234567890

CASE 14-3

Patient Name Blake McComb

Capital City Medical
123 Unknown Boulevard, Capital City, NY 12345-2222

Date of Service
01-29-20XX

New Patient						Laboratory	
Problem Focused	99201		Arthrocentesis/Aspiration/Injection			Amylase	82150
Expanded Problem, Focused	99202	X	Small Joint	20600		B12	82607
Detailed	99203		Interm Joint	20605		CBC & Diff	85025
Comprehensive	99204		Major Joint	20610		Comp Metabolic Panel	80053
Comprehensive/High Complex	99205		**Other Invasive/Noninvasive**			Chlamydia Screen	87110
Well Exam Infant (up to 12 mos.)	99381		Audiometry	92552	X	Cholesterol	82465
Well Exam 1–4 yrs.	99382		Cast Application			Digoxin	80162
Well Exam 5–11 yrs.	99383		Location Long Short			Electrolytes	80051
Well Exam 12–17 yrs.	99384		Catheterization	51701		Ferritin	82728
Well Exam 18–39 yrs.	99385		Circumcision	54150		Folate	82746
Well Exam 40–64 yrs.	99386		Colposcopy	57452		GC Screen	87070
			Colposcopy w/Biopsy	57454		Glucose	82947
			Cryosurgery Premalignant Lesion			Glucose 1 HR	82950
			Location (s):			Glycosylated HGB A1C	83036
Established Patient			Cryosurgery Warts			HCT	85014
Post-Op Follow Up Visit	99024		Location (s):			HDL	83718
Minimum	99211		Curettement Lesion			Hep BSAG	87340
Problem Focused	99212		Single	11055		Hepatitis panel, acute	80074
Expanded Problem Focused	99213		2–4	11056		HGB	85018
Detailed	99214		>4	11057		HIV	86703
Comprehensive/High Complex	99215		Diaphragm Fitting	57170		Iron & TIBC	83550
Well Exam Infant (up to 12 mos.)	99391		Ear Irrigation	69210		Kidney Profile	80069
Well exam 1–4 yrs.	99392		ECG	93000		Lead	83655
Well Exam 5–11 yrs.	99393		Endometrial Biopsy	58100		Liver Profile	80076
Well Exam 12–17 yrs.	99394		Exc. Lesion Malignant			Mono Test	86308
Well Exam 18–39 yrs.	99395		Benign			Pap Smear	88155
Well Exam 40–64 yrs.	99396		Location			Pregnancy Test	84703
Obstetrics			Exc. Skin Tags (1–15)	11200		Obstetric Panel	80055
Total OB Care	59400		Each Additional 10	11201		Pro Time	85610
Injections			Fracture Treatment			PSA	84153
Administration Sub. / IM	90772		Loc			RPR	86592
Drug			w/Reduc w/o Reduc			Sed. Rate	85651
Dosage			I & D Abscess Single/Simple	10060		Stool Culture	87045
Allergy	95115		Multiple or Comp	10061		Stool O & P	87177
Cocci Skin Test	86490		I & D Pilonidal Cyst Simple	10080		Strep Screen	87880
DPT	90701		Pilonidal Cyst Complex	10081		Theophylline	80198
Hemophilus	90646		IV Therapy—To One Hour	90760		Thyroid Uptake	84479
Influenza	90658		Each Additional Hour	90761		TSH	84443
MMR	90707		Laceration Repair			Urinalysis	81000
OPV	90712		Location Size Simp/Comp			Urine Culture	87088
Pneumovax	90732		Laryngoscopy	31505		Drawing Fee	36415
TB Skin Test	86580		Oximetry	94760		Specimen Collection	99000
TD	90718		Punch Biopsy			**Other:**	
Unlisted Immun	90749		Rhythm Strip	93040			
Tetanus Toxoid	90703		Treadmill	93015			
Vaccine/Toxoid Admin <8 Yr Old w/ Counseling	90465		Trigger Point or Tendon Sheath Inj.	20550			
Vaccine/Toxoid Administration for Adult	90471		Tympanometry	92567			

Diagnosis/ICD-9: **V72.19**

I acknowledge receipt of medical services and authorize the release of any medical information necessary to process this claim for healthcare payment only. I do authorize payment to the provider.

Patient Signature Blake McComb

Total Estimated Charges: _____

Payment Amount: _____

Next Appointment: _____

Figure 14-5

Capital City Medical
Fee Schedule

New Patient OV			Punch Biopsy various codes	$80
Problem Focused 99201	$45		Nebulizer various codes	$45
Expanded Problem Focused 99202	$65		Cast Application various codes	$85
Detailed 99203	$85		Laryngoscopy 31505	$255
Comprehensive 99204	$105		Audiometry 92552	$85
Comprehensive/High Complex 99205	$115		Tympanometry 92567	$85
Well Exam infant (less than 1 year) 99381	$45		Ear Irrigation 69210	$25
Well Exam 1–4 yrs. 99382	$50		Diaphragm Fitting 57170	$30
Well Exam 5–11 yrs. 99383	$55		IV Therapy (up to one hour) 90760	$65
Well Exam 12–17 yrs. 99384	$65		Each additional hour 90761	$50
Well Exam 18–39 yrs. 99385	$85		Oximetry 94760	$10
Well Exam 40–64 yrs. 99386	$105		ECG 93000	$75
Established Patient OV			Holter Monitor various codes	$170
Post Op Follow Up Visit 99024	$0		Rhythm Strip 93040	$60
Minimum 99211	$35		Treadmill 93015	$375
Problem Focused 99212	$45		Cocci Skin Test 86490	$20
Expanded Problem Focused 99213	$55		X-ray, spine, chest, bone—any area various codes	$275
Detailed 99214	$65		Avulsion Nail 11730	$200
Comprehensive/High Complex 99215	$75		**Laboratory**	
Well exam infant (less than 1 year) 99391	$35		Amylase 82150	$40
Well Exam 1–4 yrs. 99392	$40		B12 82607	$30
Well Exam 5–11 yrs. 99393	$45		CBC & Diff 85025	$95
Well Exam 12–17 yrs. 99394	$55		Comp Metabolic Panel 80053	$75
Well Exam 18–39 yrs. 99395	$65		Chlamydia Screen 87110	$70
Well Exam 40–64 yrs. 99396	$75		Cholestrerol 82465	$75
Obstetrics			Digoxin 80162	$40
Total OB Care 59400	$1700		Electrolytes 80051	$70
Injections			Estrogen, Total 82672	$50
Administration 90772	$10		Ferritin 82728	$40
Allergy 95115	$35		Folate 82746	$30
DPT 90701	$50		GC Screen 87070	$60
Drug various codes	$35		Glucose 82947	$35
Influenza 90658	$25		Glycosylated HGB A1C 83036	$45
MMR 90707	$50		HCT 85014	$30
OPV 90712	$40		HDL 83718	$35
Pneumovax 90732	$35		HGB 85018	$30
TB Skin Test 86580	$15		Hep BSAG 83740	$40
TD 90718	$40		Hepatitis panel, acute 80074	$95
Tetanus Toxoid 90703	$40		HIV 86703	$100
Vaccine/Toxoid Administration for Younger Than 8 Years Old w/ counseling 90465	$10		Iron & TIBC 83550	$45
			Kidney Profile 80069	$95
Vaccine/Toxoid Administration for Adult 90471	$10		Lead 83665	$55
Arthrocentesis/Aspiration/Injection			Lipase 83690	$40
Small Joint 20600	$50		Lipid Panel 80061	$95
Interm Joint 20605	$60		Liver Profile 80076	$95
Major Joint 20610	$70		Mono Test 86308	$30
Trigger Point/Tendon Sheath Inj. 20550	$90		Pap Smear 88155	$90
Other Invasive/Noninvasive Procedures			Pap Collection/Supervision 88142	$95
Catheterization 51701	$55		Pregnancy Test 84703	$90
Circumcision 54150	$150		Obstetric Panel 80055	$85
Colposcopy 57452	$225		Pro Time 85610	$50
Colposcopy w/Biopsy 57454	$250		PSA 84153	$50
Cryosurgery Premalignant Lesion various codes	$160		RPR 86592	$55
Endometrial Biopsy 58100	$190		Sed. Rate 85651	$50
Excision Lesion Malignant various codes	$145		Stool Culture 87045	$80
Excision Lesion Benign various codes	$125		Stool O & P 87177	$105
Curettement Lesion			Strep Screen 87880	$35
Single 11055	$70		Theophylline 80198	$40
2–4 11056	$80		Thyroid Uptake 84479	$75
>4 11057	$90		TSH 84443	$50
Excision Skin Tags (1–15) 11200	$55		Urinalysis 81000	$35
Each Additional 10 11201	$30		Urine Culture 87088	$80
I & D Abscess Single/Simple 10060	$75		Drawing Fee 36415	$15
Multiple/Complex 10061	$95		Specimen Collection 99000	$10
I & D Pilonidal Cyst Simple 10080	$105			
I & D Pilonidal Cyst Complex 10081	$130			
Laceration Repair various codes	$60			

HEALTH INSURANCE CLAIM FORM

APPROVED BY NATIONAL UNIFORM CLAIM COMMITTEE 08/05

☐☐☐PICA
PICA ☐☐☐

1. MEDICARE MEDICAID TRICARE CHAMPVA GROUP FECA OTHER		1a. INSURED'S I.D. NUMBER (For Program in Item 1)

CHAMPUS HEALTH PLAN BLK LUNG

☐(Medicare #) ☐(Medicaid #) ☐(Sponsor's SSN) ☐(Member ID#) ☐(SSN or ID) ☐(SSN) ☐(ID)

2. PATIENT'S NAME (Last Name, First Name, Middle Initial)

3. PATIENT'S BIRTH DATE   SEX
MM   DD   YY
M☐   F☐

4. INSURED'S NAME (Last Name, First Name, Middle Initial)

5. PATIENT'S ADDRESS (No., Street)

6. PATIENT RELATIONSHIP TO INSURED
Self☐   Spouse☐   Child☐   Other☐

7. INSURED'S ADDRESS (No., Street)

CITY   STATE

8. PATIENT STATUS
Single☐   Married☐   Other☐

CITY   STATE

ZIP CODE   TELEPHONE (Include Area Code)
(   )

Full-Time   Part-Time
Employed☐   Student☐   Student☐

ZIP CODE   TELEPHONE (Include Area Code)
(   )

9. OTHER INSURED'S NAME (Last Name, First Name, Middle Initial)

10. IS PATIENT'S CONDITION RELATED TO:

11. INSURED'S POLICY GROUP OR FECA NUMBER

a. OTHER INSURED'S POLICY OR GROUP NUMBER

a. EMPLOYMENT? (Current or Previous)
☐YES   ☐NO

a. INSURED'S DATE OF BIRTH   SEX
MM   DD   YY
M☐   F☐

b. OTHER INSURED'S DATE OF BIRTH   SEX
MM   DD   YY
M☐   F☐

b. AUTO ACCIDENT?   PLACE (State)
☐YES   ☐NO

b. EMPLOYER'S NAME OR SCHOOL NAME

c. EMPLOYER'S NAME OR SCHOOL NAME

c. OTHER ACCIDENT?
☐YES   ☐NO

c. INSURANCE PLAN NAME OR PROGRAM NAME

d. INSURANCE PLAN NAME OR PROGRAM NAME

10d. RESERVED FOR LOCAL USE

d. IS THERE ANOTHER HEALTH BENEFIT PLAN?
☐YES   ☐NO   If yes, return to and complete item 9 a-d.

READ BACK OF FORM BEFORE COMPLETING & SIGNING THIS FORM.

12. PATIENT'S OR AUTHORIZED PERSON'S SIGNATURE I authorize the release of any medical or other information necessary to process this claim. I also request payment of government benefits either to myself or to the party who accepts assignment below.

SIGNED _____   DATE _____

13. INSURED'S OR AUTHORIZED PERSON'S SIGNATURE I authorize payment of medical benefits to the undersigned physician or supplier for services described below.

SIGNED _____

14. DATE OF CURRENT: ILLNESS (First symptom) OR
MM   DD   YY   INJURY (Accident) OR
                     PREGNANCY (LMP)

15. IF PATIENT HAS HAD SAME OR SIMILAR ILLNESS,
GIVE FIRST DATE   MM   DD   YY

16. DATES PATIENT UNABLE TO WORK IN CURRENT OCCUPATION
MM   DD   YY   MM   DD   YY
FROM   TO

17. NAME OF REFERRING PHYSICIAN OR OTHER SOURCE

17a.
17b. NPI

18. HOSPITALIZATION DATES RELATED TO CURRENT SERVICES
MM   DD   YY   MM   DD   YY
FROM   TO

19. RESERVED FOR LOCAL USE

20. OUTSIDE LAB? $ CHARGES
☐YES   ☐NO

21. DIAGNOSIS OR NATURE OF ILLNESS OR INJURY (Relate Items 1,2,3 or 4 to Item 24E by Line)

1. |____.____| 3. |____.____|
2. |____.____| 4. |____.____|

22. MEDICAID RESUBMISSION
CODE   ORIGINAL REF. NO.

23. PRIOR AUTHORIZATION NUMBER

24. A. DATE(S) OF SERVICE						B. PLACE OF SERVICE	C. EMG	D. PROCEDURES, SERVICES, OR SUPPLIES (Explain Unusual Circumstances)		E. DIAGNOSIS POINTER	F. $ CHARGES	G. DAYS OR UNITS	H. EPSDT Family Plan	I. ID. QUAL.	J. RENDERING PROVIDER ID. #
From			To					CPT/HCPCS	MODIFIER						
MM	DD	YY	MM	DD	YY										
1														NPI	
2														NPI	
3														NPI	
4														NPI	
5														NPI	
6														NPI	

25. FEDERAL TAX I.D. NUMBER   SSN EIN
☐☐

26. PATIENT'S ACCOUNT NO.

27. ACCEPT ASSIGNMENT?
(For govt. claims, see back)
☐YES   ☐NO

28. TOTAL CHARGE
$

29. AMOUNT PAID
$

30. BALANCE DUE
$

31. SIGNATURE OF PHYSICIAN OR SUPPLIER INCLUDING DEGREES OR CREDENTIALS
(I certify that the statements on the reverse apply to this bill and are made a part thereof.)

SIGNED _____ DATE _____

32. SERVICE FACILITY LOCATION INFORMATION

a. NPI   b.

33. BILLING PROVIDER INFO & PH. # (   )

a. NPI   b.

NUCC Instruction Manual available at: www.nucc.org
WCMS-1500CS

APPROVED OMB 0938-0999 FORM CMS-1500 (08/05)

CARRIER

PATIENT AND INSURED INFORMATION

PHYSICIAN OR SUPPLIER INFORMATION

SECOND FOLD

FIRST FOLD   WHCF-10-ENV / WHCF-10-ENV-SS

Figure 14-6

d. Using the source documents, the Capital City Medical Fee Schedule (Figure 14-7), and the blank CMS-1500 form provided (Figure 14-8), complete the following case study for patient Jim Hill (Case 14-4):

CASE 14-4

Capital City Medical—123 Unknown Boulevard, Capital City, NY 12345-2222 (555) 555-1234 Phil Wells, MD, Mannie Mends, MD, Bette R. Soone, MD	Patient Information Form Tax ID: 75-0246810 Group NPI: 1513171216

Patient Information:

Name: (Last, First) Hill, Jim ☒ Male ☐ Female Birth Date: 03/18/1961

Address: 736 Hillcrest St, Capital City, NY 12345 Phone: (555) 555-6176

Social Security Number: 592-70-2833 Full-Time Student: ☐ Yes ☐ No

Marital Status: ☒ Single ☐ Married ☐ Divorced ☐ Other

Employment:

Employer: Retired Phone: ( )

Address:

Condition Related to: ☐ Auto Accident ☐ Employment ☐ Other Accident

Date of Accident: State:

Emergency Contact: Phone: ( )

Primary Insurance: Medicare Phone: ( )

Address: P. O. Box 9834, Capital City, NY 12345

Insurance Policyholder's Name: Same ☐ M ☐ F DOB:

Address:

Phone: ( ) Relationship to Insured: ☒ Self ☐ Spouse ☐ Child ☐ Other

Employer: Phone: ( )

Employer's Address:

Policy/ID No: 720191114A Group No: Percent Covered: 80 % Copay Amt: $

Secondary Insurance: Medicaid Phone: ( )

Address: 4875 Capital Blvd, Capital City, NY 12345

Insurance Policyholder's Name: Same ☐ M ☐ F DOB:

Address:

Phone: ( ) Relationship to Insured: ☒ Self ☐ Spouse ☐ Child ☐ Other

Employer: Phone: ( )

Employer's Address:

Policy/ID No: 35255566874 Group No: Percent Covered: % Copay Amt: $ 5.00

Reason for Visit: Checkup for kidney disease

Known Allergies:

Referred by:

CASE 14-4
SOAP

06/11/20XX
Assignment of Benefits: Y
Signature on File: Y
Referring Physician: N

S: Jim Hill is in for his regular CRF check. He complains of feeling down. He says he hasn't been himself lately.

O: Kidney values are stable. BP: 126/72. He admits that he has lost all interest in leaving the house. He is sleeping in excess of 10 hours a day, and he is barely eating. Pt. has lost 12 lbs. in the last month. He denies any suicidal thoughts. Kidney profile is stable.

A: 1. CRF with neuropathy—585.9, 357.4
    2. Depression, mental—300.4

P: 1. Start Prozac once daily.
    2. Refill lopressor.
    3. Return in 2 weeks for evaluation of Prozac and depression.

Phil Wells, MD
Family Practice
NPI: 1234567890

CASE 14-4

Patient Name Jim Hill

Capital City Medical
123 Unknown Boulevard, Capital City, NY 12345-2222

Date of Service
06-11-20XX

New Patient			Other Invasive/Noninvasive			Laboratory		
Problem Focused	99201		Arthrocentesis/Aspiration/Injection			Amylase	82150	
Expanded Problem, Focused	99202		Small Joint	20600		B12	82607	
Detailed	99203		Interm Joint	20605		CBC & Diff	85025	
Comprehensive	99204		Major Joint	20610		Comp Metabolic Panel	80053	
Comprehensive/High Complex	99205		**Other Invasive/Noninvasive**			Chlamydia Screen	87110	
Well Exam Infant (up to 12 mos.)	99381		Audiometry	92552		Cholesterol	82465	
Well Exam 1–4 yrs.	99382		Cast Application			Digoxin	80162	
Well Exam 5–11 yrs.	99383		Location Long Short			Electrolytes	80051	
Well Exam 12–17 yrs.	99384		Catheterization	51701		Ferritin	82728	
Well Exam 18–39 yrs.	99385		Circumcision	54150		Folate	82746	
Well Exam 40–64 yrs.	99386		Colposcopy	57452		GC Screen	87070	
			Colposcopy w/Biopsy	57454		Glucose	82947	
			Cryosurgery Premalignant Lesion			Glucose 1 HR	82950	
			Location (s):			Glycosylated HGB A1C	83036	
Established Patient			Cryosurgery Warts			HCT	85014	
Post-Op Follow Up Visit	99024		Location (s):			HDL	83718	
Minimum	99211		Curettement Lesion			Hep BSAG	87340	
Problem Focused	99212		Single	11055		Hepatitis panel, acute	80074	
Expanded Problem Focused	99213	X	2–4	11056		HGB	85018	
Detailed	99214		>4	11057		HIV	86703	
Comprehensive/High Complex	99215		Diaphragm Fitting	57170		Iron & TIBC	83550	
Well Exam Infant (up to 12 mos.)	99391		Ear Irrigation	69210		Kidney Profile	80069	X
Well exam 1–4 yrs.	99392		ECG	93000		Lead	83655	
Well Exam 5–11 yrs.	99393		Endometrial Biopsy	58100		Liver Profile	80076	
Well Exam 12–17 yrs.	99394		Exc. Lesion Malignant			Mono Test	86308	
Well Exam 18–39 yrs.	99395		Benign			Pap Smear	88155	
Well Exam 40–64 yrs.	99396		Location			Pregnancy Test	84703	
Obstetrics			Exc. Skin Tags (1–15)	11200		Obstetric Panel	80055	
Total OB Care	59400		Each Additional 10	11201		Pro Time	85610	
Injections			Fracture Treatment			PSA	84153	
Administration Sub. / IM	90772		Loc			RPR	86592	
Drug			w/Reduc w/o Reduc			Sed. Rate	85651	
Dosage			I & D Abscess Single/Simple	10060		Stool Culture	87045	
Allergy	95115		Multiple or Comp	10061		Stool O & P	87177	
Cocci Skin Test	86490		I & D Pilonidal Cyst Simple	10080		Strep Screen	87880	
DPT	90701		Pilonidal Cyst Complex	10081		Theophylline	80198	
Hemophilus	90646		IV Therapy—To One Hour	90760		Thyroid Uptake	84479	
Influenza	90658		Each Additional Hour	90761		TSH	84443	
MMR	90707		Laceration Repair			Urinalysis	81000	
OPV	90712		Location Size Simp/Comp			Urine Culture	87088	
Pneumovax	90732		Laryngoscopy	31505		Drawing Fee	36415	X
TB Skin Test	86580		Oximetry	94760		Specimen Collection	99000	
TD	90718		Punch Biopsy			**Other:**		
Unlisted Immun	90749		Rhythm Strip	93040				
Tetanus Toxoid	90703		Treadmill	93015				
Vaccine/Toxoid Admin <8 Yr Old w/ Counseling	90465		Trigger Point or Tendon Sheath Inj.	20550				
Vaccine/Toxoid Administration for Adult	90471		Tympanometry	92567				

Diagnosis/ICD-9: **585.9, 357.4, 300.4**

I acknowledge receipt of medical services and authorize the release of any medical information necessary to process this claim for healthcare payment only. I do authorize payment to the provider.

Patient Signature _Jim Hill_____

Total Estimated Charges: _____

Payment Amount: _____

Next Appointment: _____

Figure 14-7

Capital City Medical
Fee Schedule

New Patient OV			Punch Biopsy various codes	$80
Problem Focused 99201	$45		Nebulizer various codes	$45
Expanded Problem Focused 99202	$65		Cast Application various codes	$85
Detailed 99203	$85		Laryngoscopy 31505	$255
Comprehensive 99204	$105		Audiometry 92552	$85
Comprehensive/High Complex 99205	$115		Tympanometry 92567	$85
Well Exam infant (less than 1 year) 99381	$45		Ear Irrigation 69210	$25
Well Exam 1–4 yrs. 99382	$50		Diaphragm Fitting 57170	$30
Well Exam 5–11 yrs. 99383	$55		IV Therapy (up to one hour) 90760	$65
Well Exam 12–17 yrs. 99384	$65		Each additional hour 90761	$50
Well Exam 18–39 yrs. 99385	$85		Oximetry 94760	$10
Well Exam 40–64 yrs. 99386	$105		ECG 93000	$75
Established Patient OV			Holter Monitor various codes	$170
Post Op Follow Up Visit 99024	$0		Rhythm Strip 93040	$60
Minimum 99211	$35		Treadmill 93015	$375
Problem Focused 99212	$45		Cocci Skin Test 86490	$20
Expanded Problem Focused 99213	$55		X-ray, spine, chest, bone—any area various codes	$275
Detailed 99214	$65		Avulsion Nail 11730	$200
Comprehensive/High Complex 99215	$75		**Laboratory**	
Well exam infant (less than 1 year) 99391	$35		Amylase 82150	$40
Well Exam 1–4 yrs. 99392	$40		B12 82607	$30
Well Exam 5–11 yrs. 99393	$45		CBC & Diff 85025	$95
Well Exam 12–17 yrs. 99394	$55		Comp Metabolic Panel 80053	$75
Well Exam 18–39 yrs. 99395	$65		Chlamydia Screen 87110	$70
Well Exam 40–64 yrs. 99396	$75		Cholestrerol 82465	$75
Obstetrics			Digoxin 80162	$40
Total OB Care 59400	$1700		Electrolytes 80051	$70
Injections			Estrogen, Total 82672	$50
Administration 90772	$10		Ferritin 82728	$40
Allergy 95115	$35		Folate 82746	$30
DPT 90701	$50		GC Screen 87070	$60
Drug various codes	$35		Glucose 82947	$35
Influenza 90658	$25		Glycosylated HGB A1C 83036	$45
MMR 90707	$50		HCT 85014	$30
OPV 90712	$40		HDL 83718	$35
Pneumovax 90732	$35		HGB 85018	$30
TB Skin Test 86580	$15		Hep BSAG 83740	$40
TD 90718	$40		Hepatitis panel, acute 80074	$95
Tetanus Toxoid 90703	$40		HIV 86703	$100
Vaccine/Toxoid Administration for Younger			Iron & TIBC 83550	$45
Than 8 Years Old w/ counseling 90465	$10		Kidney Profile 80069	$95
Vaccine/Toxoid Administration for Adult 90471	$10		Lead 83665	$55
Arthrocentesis/Aspiration/Injection			Lipase 83690	$40
Small Joint 20600	$50		Lipid Panel 80061	$95
Interm Joint 20605	$60		Liver Profile 80076	$95
Major Joint 20610	$70		Mono Test 86308	$30
Trigger Point/Tendon Sheath Inj. 20550	$90		Pap Smear 88155	$90
Other Invasive/Noninvasive Procedures			Pap Collection/Supervision 88142	$95
Catheterization 51701	$55		Pregnancy Test 84703	$90
Circumcision 54150	$150		Obstetric Panel 80055	$85
Colposcopy 57452	$225		Pro Time 85610	$50
Colposcopy w/Biopsy 57454	$250		PSA 84153	$50
Cryosurgery Premalignant Lesion various codes	$160		RPR 86592	$55
Endometrial Biopsy 58100	$190		Sed. Rate 85651	$50
Excision Lesion Malignant various codes	$145		Stool Culture 87045	$80
Excision Lesion Benign various codes	$125		Stool O & P 87177	$105
Curettement Lesion			Strep Screen 87880	$35
Single 11055	$70		Theophylline 80198	$40
2–4 11056	$80		Thyroid Uptake 84479	$75
>4 11057	$90		TSH 84443	$50
Excision Skin Tags (1–15) 11200	$55		Urinalysis 81000	$35
Each Additional 10 11201	$30		Urine Culture 87088	$80
I & D Abscess Single/Simple 10060	$75		Drawing Fee 36415	$15
Multiple/Complex 10061	$95		Specimen Collection 99000	$10
I & D Pilonidal Cyst Simple 10080	$105			
I & D Pilonidal Cyst Complex 10081	$130			
Laceration Repair various codes	$60			

(1500)

HEALTH INSURANCE CLAIM FORM

APPROVED BY NATIONAL UNIFORM CLAIM COMMITTEE 08/05

☐☐☐ PICA		PICA ☐☐☐

1. MEDICARE ☐(Medicare #) MEDICAID ☐(Medicaid #) TRICARE CHAMPUS ☐(Sponsor's SSN) CHAMPVA ☐(Member ID#) GROUP HEALTH PLAN ☐(SSN or ID) FECA BLK LUNG ☐(SSN) OTHER ☐(ID)	1a. INSURED'S I.D. NUMBER (For Program in Item 1)

2. PATIENT'S NAME (Last Name, First Name, Middle Initial)	3. PATIENT'S BIRTH DATE MM ┆ DD ┆ YY SEX M☐ F☐	4. INSURED'S NAME (Last Name, First Name, Middle Initial)

5. PATIENT'S ADDRESS (No., Street)	6. PATIENT RELATIONSHIP TO INSURED Self☐ Spouse☐ Child☐ Other☐	7. INSURED'S ADDRESS (No., Street)
CITY STATE	8. PATIENT STATUS Single☐ Married☐ Other☐	CITY STATE
ZIP CODE TELEPHONE (Include Area Code) ( )	Employed☐ Full-Time Student☐ Part-Time Student☐	ZIP CODE TELEPHONE (Include Area Code) ( )

9. OTHER INSURED'S NAME (Last Name, First Name, Middle Initial)	10. IS PATIENT'S CONDITION RELATED TO:	11. INSURED'S POLICY GROUP OR FECA NUMBER
a. OTHER INSURED'S POLICY OR GROUP NUMBER	a. EMPLOYMENT? (Current or Previous) ☐YES ☐NO	a. INSURED'S DATE OF BIRTH MM ┆ DD ┆ YY SEX M☐ F☐
b. OTHER INSURED'S DATE OF BIRTH MM ┆ DD ┆ YY SEX M☐ F☐	b. AUTO ACCIDENT? PLACE (State) ☐YES ☐NO └──┘	b. EMPLOYER'S NAME OR SCHOOL NAME
c. EMPLOYER'S NAME OR SCHOOL NAME	c. OTHER ACCIDENT? ☐YES ☐NO	c. INSURANCE PLAN NAME OR PROGRAM NAME
d. INSURANCE PLAN NAME OR PROGRAM NAME	10d. RESERVED FOR LOCAL USE	d. IS THERE ANOTHER HEALTH BENEFIT PLAN? ☐YES ☐NO If yes, return to and complete item 9 a-d.

READ BACK OF FORM BEFORE COMPLETING & SIGNING THIS FORM. 12. PATIENT'S OR AUTHORIZED PERSON'S SIGNATURE I authorize the release of any medical or other information necessary to process this claim. I also request payment of government benefits either to myself or to the party who accepts assignment below. SIGNED_____ DATE_____	13. INSURED'S OR AUTHORIZED PERSON'S SIGNATURE I authorize payment of medical benefits to the undersigned physician or supplier for services described below. SIGNED_____

14. DATE OF CURRENT: MM ┆ DD ┆ YY ◄ ILLNESS (First symptom) OR INJURY (Accident) OR PREGNANCY (LMP)	15. IF PATIENT HAS HAD SAME OR SIMILAR ILLNESS, GIVE FIRST DATE MM ┆ DD ┆ YY	16. DATES PATIENT UNABLE TO WORK IN CURRENT OCCUPATION MM ┆ DD ┆ YY MM ┆ DD ┆ YY FROM TO
17. NAME OF REFERRING PHYSICIAN OR OTHER SOURCE	17a. 17b. NPI	18. HOSPITALIZATION DATES RELATED TO CURRENT SERVICES MM ┆ DD ┆ YY MM ┆ DD ┆ YY FROM TO
19. RESERVED FOR LOCAL USE		20. OUTSIDE LAB? $ CHARGES ☐YES ☐NO
21. DIAGNOSIS OR NATURE OF ILLNESS OR INJURY (Relate Items 1,2,3 or 4 to Item 24E by Line) 1.└─┘.───── 3.└─┘.───── 2.└─┘.───── 4.└─┘.─────		22. MEDICAID RESUBMISSION CODE ORIGINAL REF. NO. 23. PRIOR AUTHORIZATION NUMBER

24. A. DATE(S) OF SERVICE From ┆ To MM DD YY MM DD YY	B. PLACE OF SERVICE	C. EMG	D. PROCEDURES, SERVICES, OR SUPPLIES (Explain Unusual Circumstances) CPT/HCPCS ┆ MODIFIER	E. DIAGNOSIS POINTER	F. $ CHARGES	G. DAYS OR UNITS	H. EPSDT Family Plan	I. ID. QUAL.	J. RENDERING PROVIDER ID. #
1								NPI	
2								NPI	
3								NPI	
4								NPI	
5								NPI	
6								NPI	

25. FEDERAL TAX I.D. NUMBER SSN EIN ☐☐	26. PATIENT'S ACCOUNT NO.	27. ACCEPT ASSIGNMENT? (For govt. claims, see back) ☐YES ☐NO	28. TOTAL CHARGE $	29. AMOUNT PAID $	30. BALANCE DUE $

31. SIGNATURE OF PHYSICIAN OR SUPPLIER INCLUDING DEGREES OR CREDENTIALS (I certify that the statements on the reverse apply to this bill and are made a part thereof.) SIGNED_____ DATE_____	32. SERVICE FACILITY LOCATION INFORMATION a. NPI b.	33. BILLING PROVIDER INFO & PH. # ( ) a. NPI b.

NUCC Instruction Manual available at: www.nucc.org
WCMS-1500CS

APPROVED OMB 0938-0999 FORM CMS-1500 (08/05)

Figure 14-8

e. Using the source documents, the Capital City Medical Fee Schedule (Figure 14-9), and the blank CMS-1500 form provided (Figure 14-10), complete the following case study for patient Jenny Powers (Case 14-5):

CASE 14-5

Capital City Medical—123 Unknown Boulevard, Capital City, NY 12345-2222 (555) 555-1234	Patient Information Form
Phil Wells, MD, Mannie Mends, MD, Bette R. Soone, MD	Tax ID: 75-0246810
	Group NPI: 1513171216

Patient Information:

Name: (Last, First) Powers, Jenny ☐ Male ☒ Female Birth Date: 06/23/1985

Address: 512 Melba St, Capital City, NY 12345 Phone: (555) 555-6008

Social Security Number: 142-19-7757 Full-Time Student: ☒ Yes ☐ No

Marital Status: ☒ Single ☐ Married ☐ Divorced ☐ Other

Employment:

Employer: _____ Phone: ( ) _____

Address: _____

Condition Related to: ☐ Auto Accident ☐ Employment ☐ Other Accident

Date of Accident: _____ State: _____

Emergency Contact: _____ **Phone: ( )** _____

Primary Insurance: Medicaid Phone: ( ) _____

Address: 4875 Capital Blvd, Capital City, NY 12345

Insurance Policyholder's Name: Same ☐ M ☐ F DOB: _____

Address: _____

Phone: ( ) _____ Relationship to Insured: ☒ Self ☐ Spouse ☐ Child ☐ Other

Employer: _____ Phone: ( ) _____

Employer's Address: _____

Policy/ID No: 6684431000 Group No: _____ Percent Covered: ____% Copay Amt: $ 5.00

Secondary Insurance: _____ Phone: ( ) _____

Address: _____

Insurance Policyholder's Name: _____ ☐ M ☐ F DOB: _____

Address: _____

Phone: ( ) _____ Relationship to Insured: ☐ Self ☐ Spouse ☐ Child ☐ Other

Employer: _____ Phone: ( ) _____

Employer's Address: _____

Policy/ID No: _____ Group No: _____ Percent Covered: ____% Copay Amt: $ _____

Reason for Visit: I am here for a follow-up on my colonoscopy.

Known Allergies: _____

Referred by: _____

CASE 14-5
SOAP

07/17/20XX
Assignment of Benefits: Y
Signature on File: Y
Referring Physician: N

S: Jenny Powers is being seen today to review the results of her recent colonoscopy. She has been having periods of diarrhea alternating with constipation.

O: The colonoscopy shows no signs of polyps or inflammation to the diverticula. There is no evidence of hemorrhoids. Pt. does present with tenderness in the right lower quadrant.

A: 1. IBS—564.1

P: 1. Start fiber supplement.
2. Pamphlets on diet and stress management given.
3. Return in 4 months.

_____

Phil Wells, MD
Family Practice
NPI: 1234567890

CASE 14-5

Capital City Medical
123 Unknown Boulevard, Capital City, NY 12345-2222

Date of Service
07-17-20XX

New Patient			Other Invasive/Noninvasive			Laboratory		
Problem Focused	99201		Arthrocentesis/Aspiration/Injection			Amylase	82150	
Expanded Problem, Focused	99202		Small Joint	20600		B12	82607	
Detailed	99203		Interm Joint	20605		CBC & Diff	85025	
Comprehensive	99204		Major Joint	20610		Comp Metabolic Panel	80053	
Comprehensive/High Complex	99205		**Other Invasive/Noninvasive**			Chlamydia Screen	87110	
Well Exam Infant (up to 12 mos.)	99381		Audiometry	92552		Cholesterol	82465	
Well Exam 1–4 yrs.	99382		Cast Application			Digoxin	80162	
Well Exam 5–11 yrs.	99383		Location Long Short			Electrolytes	80051	
Well Exam 12–17 yrs.	99384		Catheterization	51701		Ferritin	82728	
Well Exam 18–39 yrs.	99385		Circumcision	54150		Folate	82746	
Well Exam 40–64 yrs.	99386		Colposcopy	57452		GC Screen	87070	
			Colposcopy w/Biopsy	57454		Glucose	82947	
			Cryosurgery Premalignant Lesion			Glucose 1 HR	82950	
			Location (s):			Glycosylated HGB A1C	83036	
Established Patient			Cryosurgery Warts			HCT	85014	
Post-Op Follow Up Visit	99024	X	Location (s):			HDL	83718	
Minimum	99211		Curettement Lesion			Hep BSAG	87340	
Problem Focused	99212		Single	11055		Hepatitis panel, acute	80074	
Expanded Problem Focused	99213	X	2–4	11056		HGB	85018	
Detailed	99214		>4	11057		HIV	86703	
Comprehensive/High Complex	99215		Diaphragm Fitting	57170		Iron & TIBC	83550	
Well Exam Infant (up to 12 mos.)	99391		Ear Irrigation	69210		Kidney Profile	80069	
Well exam 1–4 yrs.	99392		ECG	93000		Lead	83655	
Well Exam 5–11 yrs.	99393		Endometrial Biopsy	58100		Liver Profile	80076	
Well Exam 12–17 yrs.	99394		Exc. Lesion Malignant			Mono Test	86308	
Well Exam 18–39 yrs.	99395		Benign			Pap Smear	88155	
Well Exam 40–64 yrs.	99396		Location			Pregnancy Test	84703	
Obstetrics			Exc. Skin Tags (1–15)	11200		Obstetric Panel	80055	
Total OB Care	59400		Each Additional 10	11201		Pro Time	85610	
Injections			Fracture Treatment			PSA	84153	
Administration Sub. / IM	90772		Loc			RPR	86592	
Drug			w/Reduc	w/o Reduc		Sed. Rate	85651	
Dosage			I & D Abscess Single/Simple	10060		Stool Culture	87045	
Allergy	95115		Multiple or Comp	10061		Stool O & P	87177	
Cocci Skin Test	86490		I & D Pilonidal Cyst Simple	10080		Strep Screen	87880	
DPT	90701		Pilonidal Cyst Complex	10081		Theophylline	80198	
Hemophilus	90646		IV Therapy—To One Hour	90760		Thyroid Uptake	84479	
Influenza	90658		Each Additional Hour	90761		TSH	84443	
MMR	90707		Laceration Repair			Urinalysis	81000	
OPV	90712		Location Size Simp/Comp			Urine Culture	87088	
Pneumovax	90732		Laryngoscopy	31505		Drawing Fee	36415	
TB Skin Test	86580		Oximetry	94760		Specimen Collection	99000	
TD	90718		Punch Biopsy			**Other:**		
Unlisted Immun	90749		Rhythm Strip	93040				
Tetanus Toxoid	90703		Treadmill	93015				
Vaccine/Toxoid Admin <8 Yr Old w/ Counseling	90465		Trigger Point or Tendon Sheath Inj.	20550				
Vaccine/Toxoid Administration for Adult	90471		Tympanometry	92567				

Diagnosis/ICD-9: **564.1**

I acknowledge receipt of medical services and authorize the release of any medical information necessary to process this claim for healthcare payment only. I do authorize payment to the provider.

Total Estimated Charges: _____

Payment Amount: _____

Patient Signature <u>*Jenny Powers*</u>

Next Appointment: _____

Figure 14-9

Capital City Medical
Fee Schedule

New Patient OV			Punch Biopsy various codes	$80
Problem Focused 99201	$45		Nebulizer various codes	$45
Expanded Problem Focused 99202	$65		Cast Application various codes	$85
Detailed 99203	$85		Laryngoscopy 31505	$255
Comprehensive 99204	$105		Audiometry 92552	$85
Comprehensive/High Complex 99205	$115		Tympanometry 92567	$85
Well Exam infant (less than 1 year) 99381	$45		Ear Irrigation 69210	$25
Well Exam 1–4 yrs. 99382	$50		Diaphragm Fitting 57170	$30
Well Exam 5–11 yrs. 99383	$55		IV Therapy (up to one hour) 90760	$65
Well Exam 12–17 yrs. 99384	$65		Each additional hour 90761	$50
Well Exam 18–39 yrs. 99385	$85		Oximetry 94760	$10
Well Exam 40–64 yrs. 99386	$105		ECG 93000	$75
Established Patient OV			Holter Monitor various codes	$170
Post Op Follow Up Visit 99024	$0		Rhythm Strip 93040	$60
Minimum 99211	$35		Treadmill 93015	$375
Problem Focused 99212	$45		Cocci Skin Test 86490	$20
Expanded Problem Focused 99213	$55		X-ray, spine, chest, bone—any area various codes	$275
Detailed 99214	$65		Avulsion Nail 11730	$200
Comprehensive/High Complex 99215	$75		**Laboratory**	
Well exam infant (less than 1 year) 99391	$35		Amylase 82150	$40
Well Exam 1–4 yrs. 99392	$40		B12 82607	$30
Well Exam 5–11 yrs. 99393	$45		CBC & Diff 85025	$95
Well Exam 12–17 yrs. 99394	$55		Comp Metabolic Panel 80053	$75
Well Exam 18–39 yrs. 99395	$65		Chlamydia Screen 87110	$70
Well Exam 40–64 yrs. 99396	$75		Cholestrerol 82465	$75
Obstetrics			Digoxin 80162	$40
Total OB Care 59400	$1700		Electrolytes 80051	$70
Injections			Estrogen, Total 82672	$50
Administration 90772	$10		Ferritin 82728	$40
Allergy 95115	$35		Folate 82746	$30
DPT 90701	$50		GC Screen 87070	$60
Drug various codes	$35		Glucose 82947	$35
Influenza 90658	$25		Glycosylated HGB A1C 83036	$45
MMR 90707	$50		HCT 85014	$30
OPV 90712	$40		HDL 83718	$35
Pneumovax 90732	$35		HGB 85018	$30
TB Skin Test 86580	$15		Hep BSAG 83740	$40
TD 90718	$40		Hepatitis panel, acute 80074	$95
Tetanus Toxoid 90703	$40		HIV 86703	$100
Vaccine/Toxoid Administration for Younger Than 8 Years Old w/ counseling 90465	$10		Iron & TIBC 83550	$45
			Kidney Profile 80069	$95
Vaccine/Toxoid Administration for Adult 90471	$10		Lead 83665	$55
Arthrocentesis/Aspiration/Injection			Lipase 83690	$40
Small Joint 20600	$50		Lipid Panel 80061	$95
Interm Joint 20605	$60		Liver Profile 80076	$95
Major Joint 20610	$70		Mono Test 86308	$30
Trigger Point/Tendon Sheath Inj. 20550	$90		Pap Smear 88155	$90
Other Invasive/Noninvasive Procedures			Pap Collection/Supervision 88142	$95
Catheterization 51701	$55		Pregnancy Test 84703	$90
Circumcision 54150	$150		Obstetric Panel 80055	$85
Colposcopy 57452	$225		Pro Time 85610	$50
Colposcopy w/Biopsy 57454	$250		PSA 84153	$50
Cryosurgery Premalignant Lesion various codes	$160		RPR 86592	$55
Endometrial Biopsy 58100	$190		Sed. Rate 85651	$50
Excision Lesion Malignant various codes	$145		Stool Culture 87045	$80
Excision Lesion Benign various codes	$125		Stool O & P 87177	$105
Curettement Lesion			Strep Screen 87880	$35
Single 11055	$70		Theophylline 80198	$40
2–4 11056	$80		Thyroid Uptake 84479	$75
>4 11057	$90		TSH 84443	$50
Excision Skin Tags (1–15) 11200	$55		Urinalysis 81000	$35
Each Additional 10 11201	$30		Urine Culture 87088	$80
I & D Abscess Single/Simple 10060	$75		Drawing Fee 36415	$15
Multiple/Complex 10061	$95		Specimen Collection 99000	$10
I & D Pilonidal Cyst Simple 10080	$105			
I & D Pilonidal Cyst Complex 10081	$130			
Laceration Repair various codes	$60			

Figure 14-10

224   CHAPTER 14

© 2013 Pearson Education, Inc.

REVIEW QUESTIONS

MATCHING

Choose the correct answer, and write its corresponding letter in the space provided.

a. Immigrants
b. Payer of last resort
c. Spend down
d. Cost share
e. Medi–Medi

1. _____ Incurring medical expenses that result in income being reduced to or below a state's medically needy income level
2. _____ When a person is a beneficiary of both Medicaid and Medicare
3. _____ When an insurance plan requires an enrollee to pay toward coverage
4. _____ After 1996 are ineligible for Medicaid for 5 years
5. _____ States that Medicare is always the primary plan when a patient also has Medicaid

MULTIPLE CHOICE

Circle the letter of the choice that best completes the statement or answers the question.

1. Who funds Medicaid?
   a. State government
   b. Federal government
   c. Both a and b
   d. None of the above

2. Under what condition is a provider not allowed to bill a Medicaid recipient for an uncovered service?
   a. Preauthorization was not obtained.
   b. If a service was performed and the patient knew that it may not be covered.
   c. An ABN was signed by the patient for the uncovered service.
   d. Both a and c

3. When should Medicaid coverage be verified?
   a. At each visit
   b. Once a year
   c. Every six months
   d. Every quarter

4. Which of the following would be categorically needy?
   a. Caretakers of children under 18
   b. Recipients of adoptions assistance
   c. Adults within a certain income
   d. All of the above

5. What is another name for the Welfare Reform Bill?
   a. The Personal Responsibility and Work Opportunity Reconciliation Act of 1996
   b. The Balanced Budget Act of 1997
   c. The Ticket to Work and Work Incentives Improvement Act of 1999
   d. All of the above

SHORT ANSWER

Provide the correct response to each question that follows.

1. What law allows continued Medicaid coverage for disabled persons who are still able to work?

   _____

   _____

2. What is TANF?

   _____

   _____

3. Is a PCP required for Medicaid coverage?

   _____

   _____

4. What is the function of a care coordinator?

   _____

   _____

   _____

5. What are three ways to verify Medicaid coverage for a patient?

   1. _____

   2. _____

   3. _____

TRUE/FALSE

Identify each statement as true (T) or false (F).

1. _____ Medical services under Medicaid do not have any out-of-pocket expenses for patients.
2. _____ Emergency services and family planning services covered under Medicaid do not have any out-of-pocket expenses for patients.
3. _____ The federal government has set payment caps for the SCHIP, QI, and DSH programs.
4. _____ A Medicaid recipient may have the choice of an HMO plan.
5. _____ The Affordable Care Act will begin to limit Medicaid coverage.

CHAPTER 15
TRICARE Medical Billing

CHAPTER OBJECTIVES

Upon completion of this chapter in your student text, you should be able to do the following:

1. Determine eligibility for TRICARE participants.
2. Identify different types of benefits available to veterans and their family members.
3. Submit claims to TRICARE using the CMS-1500 and the UB-04 (CMS-1450) forms.

CHAPTER OUTLINE

TRICARE
    TRICARE Eligibility
    The Patient's Financial Responsibilities
    Timely Filing
    Penalties and Interest Charges
    Authorized Providers
    Preauthorization

TRICARE Standard

TRICARE Prime

TRICARE Prime Remote

TRICARE Extra

TRICARE Senior Prime/TRICARE for Life

CHAMPVA

Submitting Claims to TRICARE

Completing the CMS-1500 Form for TRICARE (Primary)

Confidential and Sensitive Information

KEY TERMS

Using the highlighted terms and glossary in the textbook, define the following terms:

1. beneficiary _____

    _____

2. catastrophic cap _____

    _____

3. Civilian Health and Medical Program of the Uniformed Services (CHAMPUS) _____

_____

4. Civilian Health and Medical Program of the Department of Veterans Affairs (CHAMPVA) _____

_____

5. cost share _____

_____

6. Defense Enrollment Eligibility Reporting System (DEERS) _____

_____

7. military treatment facility (MTF) _____

_____

8. nonavailability statement (NAS) _____

_____

9. Palmetto Government Benefits Administrators (PGBA) _____

_____

10. primary care manager (PCM) _____

_____

11. sponsor _____

_____

12. TRICARE _____

_____

13. TRICARE Extra _____

_____

14. TRICARE for Life (TFL) _____

_____

15. TRICARE Prime _____

_____

16. TRICARE Prime Remote (TPR) _____

_____

17. TRICARE Reserve Retired (TRR) _____

_____

18. TRICARE Reserve Select (TRS) _____

_____

19. TRICARE Senior Prime _____

_____

20. TRICARE Standard _____

_____

21. TRICARE Young Adult (TYA) _____

_____

22. Wisconsin Physicians Services (WPS) _____

_____

CRITICAL THINKING QUESTIONS

Using the knowledge you have gained from reading the textbook, apply critical thinking skills to answer the following questions.

1. a. Merle Verlock is covered by TRICARE Prime. In your own words, briefly describe his plan.

   _____

   _____

   _____

   _____

   b. Explain Merle's medical access standards (wait time for appointment/care) under TRICARE Prime for the following types of care:

      1. Urgent care

      _____

      _____

      2. Routine care

      _____

      _____

      _____

      3. Referred specialty care

      _____

      _____

      _____

      4. Wellness/Preventive care

      _____

      _____

      _____

2. Jane Smith is covered by TRICARE Reserve Select. Explain how this plan works.

   _____

   _____

   _____

   _____

3. Brandon McGregory is reading over his TRICARE benefits package For TRICARE Prime, what are the consequences of not seeing a provider at an MTF, if he has one available?

   _____

   _____

   _____

4. a. Jaylynn Ramsey, who is not active duty personnel or a veteran of war, is choosing a TRICARE plan. She wants to pick the plan that allows her to access civilian medical facilities/providers as her primary health care. Which TRICARE plan is the best choice for Jaylynn?

_____

_____

   b. Jaylynn's 67-year-old uncle, Jessie Ramsey, is also choosing a TRICARE plan. He is also Medicare eligible. Which TRICARE plan is the best choice for Jessie?

_____

_____

   c. Laurel Orlando is currently an active duty marine. Which TRICARE plan is the best choice for her husband and two children?

_____

_____

5. Cedric Malcolm has CHAMPVA and needs to obtain care at the nearest VA facility. Using the Internet, locate the VA Hospital's website. Where is the closet VA Hospital in your area that Cedric can go to?

_____

_____

PRACTICE EXERCISES

1. Using the form locator information written out on your index cards from a prior chapter, complete the following activity. Flag those FLs that would be filled out differently for TRICARE patients.

2. Case studies are provided for additional practice in completing the CMS-1500 claim form for TRICARE physician outpatient billing. By applying what you have learned in your student text, accurately code and complete each case study. Patient demographics and a brief case history are provided. Complete the cases based on the following criteria:

   - All patients have release of information and assignment of benefit signatures on file.
   - All providers are participating and accept assignment.
   - The group practice is the billing entity.
   - The national transition to NPI numbers is complete, and legacy PINs of individual payers are no longer used.
   - 2012 ICD-9-CM and CPT codes are used.
   - Use eight-digit dates for birthdates. Use six digit dates for all other dates.
   - All street names should be entered using standard postal abbreviations, even if they are spelled out on the source documents.
   - Enter ICD-9 codes in the order they appear on the encounter form.
   - When entering CPT codes, enter the E/M code first. Enter remaining codes in descending price order.

In order to determine to correct fees, refer to the Capital City Medical Fee Schedule, which is located after each case's source documents. Use the blank CMS-1500 form provided after each case.

   a. Using the source documents, the Capital City Medical Fee Schedule (Figure 15-1), and the blank CMS-1500 form provided (Figure 15-2), complete the following case study for patient Staci Pratt (Case 15-1):

CASE 15-1

<table>
<tr><td>Capital City Medical—123 Unknown Boulevard, Capital City,
NY 12345-2222 (555) 555-1234
Phil Wells, MD, Mannie Mends, MD, Bette R. Soone, MD</td><td>Patient Information Form
Tax ID: 75-0246810
Group NPI: 1513171216</td></tr>
</table>

Patient Information:

Name: (Last, First) Pratt, Staci ☐ Male ☒ Female Birth Date: 05/30/1970

Address: 7 Garfield Ave, Capital City, NY 12345 Phone: (555) 555-3701

Social Security Number: 201-21-2802 Full-Time Student: ☐ Yes ☒ No

Marital Status: ☐ Single ☒ Married ☐ Divorced ☐ Other

Employment:

Employer: Township Memorial Hospital Phone: (555) 555-0700

Address: 780 Shady Street, Township, NY 12345

Condition Related to: ☐ Auto Accident ☐ Employment ☐ Other Accident

Date of Accident: _____ State: _____

Emergency Contact: _____ **Phone: ( )** _____

Primary Insurance: Tricare Phone: ( ) _____

Address: 7594 Forces-Run Rd, Militaryville, NY 12345

Insurance Policyholder's Name: Same ☐ M ☐ F DOB: _____

Address: _____

Phone: _____ Relationship to Insured: ☒ Self ☐ Spouse ☐ Child ☐ Other

Employer: _____ Phone: ( ) _____

Employer's Address: _____

Policy/ID No: 201212802 Group No: _____ Percent Covered: ___% Copay Amt: $35.00

Secondary Insurance: _____ Phone: ( ) _____

Address: _____

Insurance Policyholder's Name: _____ ☐ M ☐ F DOB: _____

Address: _____

Phone: _____ Relationship to Insured: ☐ Self ☐ Spouse ☐ Child ☐ Other

Employer: _____ Phone: ( ) _____

Employer's Address: _____

Policy/ID No: _____ Group No: _____ Percent Covered: ___% Copay Amt: $_____

Reason for Visit: Physical examination for Army Reserves.

Known Allergies: _____

Referred by: _____

CASE 15-1
SOAP

06/17/20XX
Assignment of Benefits: Y
Signature on File: Y
Referring Physician: N

S: Staci Pratt is here today for a physical examination, including a pap smear and gynecological exam. She has no complaints. This is her yearly exam for the Army Reserves.

O: Pt. denies any recent problems. Her vitals are stable. Physical exam is unremarkable. Labs are negative for any disease process. She is cleared.

A: 1. Physical/Gynecological exam for Army Reserves—V72.31

P: 1. Cleared for Army status.
2. Return p.r.n.

_____

Phil Wells, MD
Family Practice
NPI: 1234567890

CASE 15-1

Patient Name Staci Pratt

Capital City Medical
123 Unknown Boulevard, Capital City, NY 12345-2222

Date of Service
06-17-20XX

New Patient			Other Invasive/Noninvasive			Laboratory	
Problem Focused	99201		Arthrocentesis/Aspiration/Injection			Amylase	82150
Expanded Problem, Focused	99202		Small Joint	20600		B12	82607
Detailed	99203		Interm Joint	20605		CBC & Diff	85025
Comprehensive	99204		Major Joint	20610		Comp Metabolic Panel	80053
Comprehensive/High Complex	99205		**Other Invasive/Noninvasive**			Chlamydia Screen	87110
Well Exam Infant (up to 12 mos.)	99381		Audiometry	92552		Cholesterol	82465
Well Exam 1–4 yrs.	99382		Cast Application			Digoxin	80162
Well Exam 5–11 yrs.	99383		Location Long Short			Electrolytes	80051
Well Exam 12–17 yrs.	99384		Catheterization	51701		Ferritin	82728
Well Exam 18–39 yrs.	99385		Circumcision	54150		Folate	82746
Well Exam 40–64 yrs.	99386		Colposcopy	57452		GC Screen	87070
			Colposcopy w/Biopsy	57454		Glucose	82947
			Cryosurgery Premalignant Lesion			Glucose 1 HR	82950
			Location (s):			Glycosylated HGB A1C	83036
Established Patient			Cryosurgery Warts			HCT	85014
Post-Op Follow Up Visit	99024		Location (s):			HDL	83718
Minimum	99211		Curettement Lesion			Hep BSAG	87340
Problem Focused	99212		Single	11055		Hepatitis panel, acute	80074
Expanded Problem Focused	99213		2–4	11056		HGB	85018
Detailed	99214		>4	11057		HIV	86703
Comprehensive/High Complex	99215		Diaphragm Fitting	57170		Iron & TIBC	83550
Well Exam Infant (up to 12 mos.)	99391		Ear Irrigation	69210		Kidney Profile	80069
Well exam 1–4 yrs.	99392		ECG	93000		Lead	83655
Well Exam 5–11 yrs.	99393		Endometrial Biopsy	58100		Liver Profile	80076
Well Exam 12–17 yrs.	99394		Exc. Lesion Malignant			Mono Test	86308
Well Exam 18–39 yrs.	99395	X	Benign			Pap Smear	88155
Well Exam 40–64 yrs.	99396		Location			Pregnancy Test	84703
Obstetrics			Exc. Skin Tags (1–15)	11200		Obstetric Panel	80055
Total OB Care	59400		Each Additional 10	11201		Pro Time	85610
Injections			Fracture Treatment			PSA	84153
Administration Sub. / IM	90772		Loc			RPR	86592
Drug			w/Reduc w/o Reduc			Sed. Rate	85651
Dosage			I & D Abscess Single/Simple	10060		Stool Culture	87045
Allergy	95115		Multiple or Comp	10061		Stool O & P	87177
Cocci Skin Test	86490		I & D Pilonidal Cyst Simple	10080		Strep Screen	87880
DPT	90701		Pilonidal Cyst Complex	10081		Theophylline	80198
Hemophilus	90646		IV Therapy—To One Hour	90760		Thyroid Uptake	84479
Influenza	90658		Each Additional Hour	90761		TSH	84443
MMR	90707		Laceration Repair			Urinalysis	81000	X
OPV	90712		Location Size Simp/Comp			Urine Culture	87088
Pneumovax	90732		Laryngoscopy	31505		Drawing Fee	36415
TB Skin Test	86580		Oximetry	94760		Specimen Collection	99000
TD	90718		Punch Biopsy			**Other:**	
Unlisted Immun	90749		Rhythm Strip	93040			
Tetanus Toxoid	90703		Treadmill	93015			
Vaccine/Toxoid Admin <8 Yr Old w/ Counseling	90465		Trigger Point or Tendon Sheath Inj.	20550			
Vaccine/Toxoid Administration for Adult	90471		Tympanometry	92567			

Diagnosis/ICD-9: **V70.5**

I acknowledge receipt of medical services and authorize the release of any medical information necessary to process this claim for healthcare payment only. I do authorize payment to the provider.

Patient Signature _Staci Pratt_

Total Estimated Charges: _____

Payment Amount: _____

Next Appointment: _____

Figure 15-1

Capital City Medical
Fee Schedule

New Patient OV

Problem Focused 99201	$45
Expanded Problem Focused 99202	$65
Detailed 99203	$85
Comprehensive 99204	$105
Comprehensive/High Complex 99205	$115
Well Exam infant (less than 1 year) 99381	$45
Well Exam 1–4 yrs. 99382	$50
Well Exam 5–11 yrs. 99383	$55
Well Exam 12–17 yrs. 99384	$65
Well Exam 18–39 yrs. 99385	$85
Well Exam 40–64 yrs. 99386	$105

Established Patient OV

Post Op Follow Up Visit 99024	$0
Minimum 99211	$35
Problem Focused 99212	$45
Expanded Problem Focused 99213	$55
Detailed 99214	$65
Comprehensive/High Complex 99215	$75
Well exam infant (less than 1 year) 99391	$35
Well Exam 1–4 yrs. 99392	$40
Well Exam 5–11 yrs. 99393	$45
Well Exam 12–17 yrs. 99394	$55
Well Exam 18–39 yrs. 99395	$65
Well Exam 40–64 yrs. 99396	$75

Obstetrics

Total OB Care 59400	$1700

Injections

Administration 90772	$10
Allergy 95115	$35
DPT 90701	$50
Drug various codes	$35
Influenza 90658	$25
MMR 90707	$50
OPV 90712	$40
Pneumovax 90732	$35
TB Skin Test 86580	$15
TD 90718	$40
Tetanus Toxoid 90703	$40
Vaccine/Toxoid Administration for Younger Than 8 Years Old w/ counseling 90465	$10
Vaccine/Toxoid Administration for Adult 90471	$10

Arthrocentesis/Aspiration/Injection

Small Joint 20600	$50
Interm Joint 20605	$60
Major Joint 20610	$70
Trigger Point/Tendon Sheath Inj. 20550	$90

Other Invasive/Noninvasive Procedures

Catheterization 51701	$55
Circumcision 54150	$150
Colposcopy 57452	$225
Colposcopy w/Biopsy 57454	$250
Cryosurgery Premalignant Lesion various codes	$160
Endometrial Biopsy 58100	$190
Excision Lesion Malignant various codes	$145
Excision Lesion Benign various codes	$125
Curettement Lesion	
Single 11055	$70
2–4 11056	$80
>4 11057	$90
Excision Skin Tags (1–15) 11200	$55
Each Additional 10 11201	$30
I & D Abscess Single/Simple 10060	$75
Multiple/Complex 10061	$95
I & D Pilonidal Cyst Simple 10080	$105
I & D Pilonidal Cyst Complex 10081	$130
Laceration Repair various codes	$60

Punch Biopsy various codes	$80
Nebulizer various codes	$45
Cast Application various codes	$85
Laryngoscopy 31505	$255
Audiometry 92552	$85
Tympanometry 92567	$85
Ear Irrigation 69210	$25
Diaphragm Fitting 57170	$30
IV Therapy (up to one hour) 90760	$65
Each additional hour 90761	$50
Oximetry 94760	$10
ECG 93000	$75
Holter Monitor various codes	$170
Rhythm Strip 93040	$60
Treadmill 93015	$375
Cocci Skin Test 86490	$20
X-ray, spine, chest, bone—any area various codes	$275
Avulsion Nail 11730	$200

Laboratory

Amylase 82150	$40
B12 82607	$30
CBC & Diff 85025	$95
Comp Metabolic Panel 80053	$75
Chlamydia Screen 87110	$70
Cholestrerol 82465	$75
Digoxin 80162	$40
Electrolytes 80051	$70
Estrogen, Total 82672	$50
Ferritin 82728	$40
Folate 82746	$30
GC Screen 87070	$60
Glucose 82947	$35
Glycosylated HGB A1C 83036	$45
HCT 85014	$30
HDL 83718	$35
HGB 85018	$30
Hep BSAG 83740	$40
Hepatitis panel, acute 80074	$95
HIV 86703	$100
Iron & TIBC 83550	$45
Kidney Profile 80069	$95
Lead 83665	$55
Lipase 83690	$40
Lipid Panel 80061	$95
Liver Profile 80076	$95
Mono Test 86308	$30
Pap Smear 88155	$90
Pap Collection/Supervision 88142	$95
Pregnancy Test 84703	$90
Obstetric Panel 80055	$85
Pro Time 85610	$50
PSA 84153	$50
RPR 86592	$55
Sed. Rate 85651	$50
Stool Culture 87045	$80
Stool O & P 87177	$105
Strep Screen 87880	$35
Theophylline 80198	$40
Thyroid Uptake 84479	$75
TSH 84443	$50
Urinalysis 81000	$35
Urine Culture 87088	$80
Drawing Fee 36415	$15
Specimen Collection 99000	$10

HEALTH INSURANCE CLAIM FORM

APPROVED BY NATIONAL UNIFORM CLAIM COMMITTEE 08/05

☐☐☐PICA

PICA☐☐☐

1. MEDICARE	MEDICAID	TRICARE CHAMPUS	CHAMPVA	GROUP HEALTH PLAN	FECA BLK LUNG	OTHER	1a. INSURED'S I.D. NUMBER	(For Program in Item 1)
☐(Medicare #)	☐(Medicaid #)	☐(Sponsor's SSN)	☐(Member ID#)	☐(SSN or ID)	☐(SSN)	☐(ID)		

2. PATIENT'S NAME (Last Name, First Name, Middle Initial)

3. PATIENT'S BIRTH DATE MM | DD | YY   SEX   M☐ F☐

4. INSURED'S NAME (Last Name, First Name, Middle Initial)

5. PATIENT'S ADDRESS (No., Street)

6. PATIENT RELATIONSHIP TO INSURED Self☐ Spouse☐ Child☐ Other☐

7. INSURED'S ADDRESS (No., Street)

CITY   STATE

8. PATIENT STATUS Single☐ Married☐ Other☐

CITY   STATE

ZIP CODE   TELEPHONE (Include Area Code) (   )

Full-Time Part-Time Employed☐ Student☐ Student☐

ZIP CODE   TELEPHONE (Include Area Code) (   )

9. OTHER INSURED'S NAME (Last Name, First Name, Middle Initial)

10. IS PATIENT'S CONDITION RELATED TO:

11. INSURED'S POLICY GROUP OR FECA NUMBER

a. OTHER INSURED'S POLICY OR GROUP NUMBER

a. EMPLOYMENT? (Current or Previous) ☐YES ☐NO

a. INSURED'S DATE OF BIRTH MM | DD | YY   SEX   M☐ F☐

b. OTHER INSURED'S DATE OF BIRTH MM | DD | YY   SEX   M☐ F☐

b. AUTO ACCIDENT?   PLACE (State) ☐YES ☐NO

b. EMPLOYER'S NAME OR SCHOOL NAME

c. EMPLOYER'S NAME OR SCHOOL NAME

c. OTHER ACCIDENT? ☐YES ☐NO

c. INSURANCE PLAN NAME OR PROGRAM NAME

d. INSURANCE PLAN NAME OR PROGRAM NAME

10d. RESERVED FOR LOCAL USE

d. IS THERE ANOTHER HEALTH BENEFIT PLAN? ☐YES ☐NO If yes, return to and complete item 9 a-d.

READ BACK OF FORM BEFORE COMPLETING & SIGNING THIS FORM.
12. PATIENT'S OR AUTHORIZED PERSON'S SIGNATURE I authorize the release of any medical or other information necessary to process this claim. I also request payment of government benefits either to myself or to the party who accepts assignment below.

SIGNED _____ DATE _____

13. INSURED'S OR AUTHORIZED PERSON'S SIGNATURE I authorize payment of medical benefits to the undersigned physician or supplier for services described below.

SIGNED _____

14. DATE OF CURRENT: MM | DD | YY ◄ ILLNESS (First symptom) OR INJURY (Accident) OR PREGNANCY (LMP)

15. IF PATIENT HAS HAD SAME OR SIMILAR ILLNESS, GIVE FIRST DATE MM | DD | YY

16. DATES PATIENT UNABLE TO WORK IN CURRENT OCCUPATION FROM MM | DD | YY TO MM | DD | YY

17. NAME OF REFERRING PHYSICIAN OR OTHER SOURCE

17a.

17b. NPI

18. HOSPITALIZATION DATES RELATED TO CURRENT SERVICES FROM MM | DD | YY TO MM | DD | YY

19. RESERVED FOR LOCAL USE

20. OUTSIDE LAB? $ CHARGES ☐YES ☐NO

21. DIAGNOSIS OR NATURE OF ILLNESS OR INJURY (Relate Items 1,2,3 or 4 to Item 24E by Line)

1. |___.___   3. |___.___
2. |___.___   4. |___.___

22. MEDICAID RESUBMISSION CODE | ORIGINAL REF. NO.

23. PRIOR AUTHORIZATION NUMBER

24. A. DATE(S) OF SERVICE From MM DD YY To MM DD YY	B. PLACE OF SERVICE	C. EMG	D. PROCEDURES, SERVICES, OR SUPPLIES (Explain Unusual Circumstances) CPT/HCPCS	MODIFIER	E. DIAGNOSIS POINTER	F. $ CHARGES	DAYS OR UNITS	EPSDT Family Plan	I. ID. QUAL.	J. RENDERING PROVIDER ID. #
1										NPI
2										NPI
3										NPI
4										NPI
5										NPI
6										NPI

25. FEDERAL TAX I.D. NUMBER   SSN EIN ☐☐

26. PATIENT'S ACCOUNT NO.

27. ACCEPT ASSIGNMENT? (For govt. claims, see back) ☐YES ☐NO

28. TOTAL CHARGE $

29. AMOUNT PAID $

30. BALANCE DUE $

31. SIGNATURE OF PHYSICIAN OR SUPPLIER INCLUDING DEGREES OR CREDENTIALS (I certify that the statements on the reverse apply to this bill and are made a part thereof.)

SIGNED _____ DATE _____

32. SERVICE FACILITY LOCATION INFORMATION

a. NPI   b.

33. BILLING PROVIDER INFO & PH. # (   )

a. NPI   b.

NUCC Instruction Manual available at: www.nucc.org
WCMS-1500CS

APPROVED OMB 0938-0999 FORM CMS-1500 (08/05)

Sidebar text (vertical): CARRIER — PATIENT AND INSURED INFORMATION — PHYSICIAN OR SUPPLIER INFORMATION

Left margin (vertical): SECOND FOLD — WHCF-10-ENV / WHCF-10-ENV-SS — FIRST FOLD WHCF-10-ENV / WHCF-10-ENV-SS

Figure 15-2

b. Using the source documents, the Capital City Medical Fee Schedule (Figure 15-3), and the blank CMS-1500 form provided (Figure 15-4), complete the following case study for patient Jackson Trenton (Case 15-2):

CASE 15-2

Capital City Medical—123 Unknown Boulevard, Capital City, NY 12345-2222 (555) 555-1234 Phil Wells, MD, Mannie Mends, MD, Bette R. Soone, MD	Patient Information Form Tax ID: 75-0246810 Group NPI: 1513171216

Patient Information:

Name: (Last, First) Trenton, Jackson   ☒ Male   ☐ Female   Birth Date: 03/12/1942

Address: 319 W. Sun Ct, Township, NY 12345   Phone: (555) 555-7221

Social Security Number: 756-87-2918   Full-Time Student: ☐ Yes   ☒ No

Marital Status: ☐ Single   ☐ Married   ☒ Divorced   ☐ Other

Employment:

Employer: Retired   Phone: ( )

Address:

Condition Related to: ☐ Auto Accident   ☐ Employment   ☐ Other Accident

Date of Accident: _____ State: _____

Emergency Contact: _____ **Phone: ( )** _____

Primary Insurance: CHAMPVA _____ Phone: ( ) _____

Address: P. O Box 4586, Capital City, NY 12345

Insurance Policyholder's Name: Same _____ ☐ M ☐ F DOB: _____

Address:

Phone: _____ Relationship to Insured: ☒ Self ☐ Spouse ☐ Child ☐ Other

Employer: _____ Phone: ( ) _____

Employer's Address:

Policy/ID No: 756872918 _____ Group No: ____ Percent Covered: 100 % Copay Amt: $____

Secondary Insurance: _____ Phone: ( ) _____

Address:

Insurance Policyholder's Name: _____ ☐ M ☐ F DOB: _____

Address:

Phone: _____ Relationship to Insured: ☐ Self ☐ Spouse ☐ Child ☐ Other

Employer: _____ Phone: ( ) _____

Employer's Address:

Policy/ID No: _____ Group No: ____ Percent Covered: ___% Copay Amt: $____

Reason for Visit: Follow-up on post-traumatic stress disorder.

Known Allergies: _____

Referred by: _____

CASE 15-2
SOAP

01/12/20XX
Assignment of Benefits: Y
Signature on File: Y
Referring Physician: N

S: Jackson Trenton is seen today for a check on his posttraumatic stress disorder.
O: Pt. denies any problems with medication. He needs a refill on Lorazepam.
A: 1. Post-traumatic stress disorder—309.81
P: 1. Continue medications.
　　2. Return in 1 month.

_____

Phil Wells, MD
Family Practice
NPI: 1234567890

CASE 15-2

Patient Name Jackson Trenton

Capital City Medical
123 Unknown Boulevard, Capital City, NY 12345-2222

Date of Service
01-12-20XX

New Patient			Other Invasive/Noninvasive			Laboratory	
Problem Focused	99201		Arthrocentesis/Aspiration/Injection			Amylase	82150
Expanded Problem, Focused	99202		Small Joint	20600		B12	82607
Detailed	99203		Interm Joint	20605		CBC & Diff	85025
Comprehensive	99204		Major Joint	20610		Comp Metabolic Panel	80053
Comprehensive/High Complex	99205		**Other Invasive/Noninvasive**			Chlamydia Screen	87110
Well Exam Infant (up to 12 mos.)	99381		Audiometry	92552		Cholesterol	82465
Well Exam 1–4 yrs.	99382		Cast Application			Digoxin	80162
Well Exam 5–11 yrs.	99383		Location Long Short			Electrolytes	80051
Well Exam 12–17 yrs.	99384		Catheterization	51701		Ferritin	82728
Well Exam 18–39 yrs.	99385		Circumcision	54150		Folate	82746
Well Exam 40–64 yrs.	99386		Colposcopy	57452		GC Screen	87070
			Colposcopy w/Biopsy	57454		Glucose	82947
			Cryosurgery Premalignant Lesion			Glucose 1 HR	82950
			Location (s):			Glycosylated HGB A1C	83036
Established Patient			Cryosurgery Warts			HCT	85014
Post-Op Follow Up Visit	99024		Location (s):			HDL	83718
Minimum	99211		Curettement Lesion			Hep BSAG	87340
Problem Focused	99212	X	Single	11055		Hepatitis panel, acute	80074
Expanded Problem Focused	99213		2–4	11056		HGB	85018
Detailed	99214		>4	11057		HIV	86703
Comprehensive/High Complex	99215		Diaphragm Fitting	57170		Iron & TIBC	83550
Well Exam Infant (up to 12 mos.)	99391		Ear Irrigation	69210		Kidney Profile	80069
Well exam 1–4 yrs.	99392		ECG	93000		Lead	83655
Well Exam 5–11 yrs.	99393		Endometrial Biopsy	58100		Liver Profile	80076
Well Exam 12–17 yrs.	99394		Exc. Lesion Malignant			Mono Test	86308
Well Exam 18–39 yrs.	99395		Benign			Pap Smear	88155
Well Exam 40–64 yrs.	99396		Location			Pregnancy Test	84703
Obstetrics			Exc. Skin Tags (1–15)	11200		Obstetric Panel	80055
Total OB Care	59400		Each Additional 10	11201		Pro Time	85610
Injections			Fracture Treatment			PSA	84153
Administration Sub. / IM	90772		Loc			RPR	86592
Drug			w/Reduc w/o Reduc			Sed. Rate	85651
Dosage			I & D Abscess Single/Simple	10060		Stool Culture	87045
Allergy	95115		Multiple or Comp	10061		Stool O & P	87177
Cocci Skin Test	86490		I & D Pilonidal Cyst Simple	10080		Strep Screen	87880
DPT	90701		Pilonidal Cyst Complex	10081		Theophylline	80198
Hemophilus	90646		IV Therapy—To One Hour	90760		Thyroid Uptake	84479
Influenza	90658		Each Additional Hour	90761		TSH	84443
MMR	90707		Laceration Repair			Urinalysis	81000
OPV	90712		Location Size Simp/Comp			Urine Culture	87088
Pneumovax	90732		Laryngoscopy	31505		Drawing Fee	36415
TB Skin Test	86580		Oximetry	94760		Specimen Collection	99000
TD	90718		Punch Biopsy			**Other:**	
Unlisted Immun	90749		Rhythm Strip	93040			
Tetanus Toxoid	90703		Treadmill	93015			
Vaccine/Toxoid Admin <8 Yr Old w/ Counseling	90465		Trigger Point or Tendon Sheath Inj.	20550			
Vaccine/Toxoid Administration for Adult	90471		Tympanometry	92567			

Diagnosis/ICD-9: **309.81**

I acknowledge receipt of medical services and authorize the release of any
medical information necessary to process this claim for healthcare payment only. I do authorize payment to the provider.

Total Estimated Charges: _____

Payment Amount: _____

Patient Signature _Jackson Trenton_

Next Appointment: _____

Figure 15-3

Capital City Medical
Fee Schedule

New Patient OV		Punch Biopsy various codes	$80
Problem Focused 99201	$45	Nebulizer various codes	$45
Expanded Problem Focused 99202	$65	Cast Application various codes	$85
Detailed 99203	$85	Laryngoscopy 31505	$255
Comprehensive 99204	$105	Audiometry 92552	$85
Comprehensive/High Complex 99205	$115	Tympanometry 92567	$85
Well Exam infant (less than 1 year) 99381	$45	Ear Irrigation 69210	$25
Well Exam 1–4 yrs. 99382	$50	Diaphragm Fitting 57170	$30
Well Exam 5–11 yrs. 99383	$55	IV Therapy (up to one hour) 90760	$65
Well Exam 12–17 yrs. 99384	$65	Each additional hour 90761	$50
Well Exam 18–39 yrs. 99385	$85	Oximetry 94760	$10
Well Exam 40–64 yrs. 99386	$105	ECG 93000	$75
Established Patient OV		Holter Monitor various codes	$170
Post Op Follow Up Visit 99024	$0	Rhythm Strip 93040	$60
Minimum 99211	$35	Treadmill 93015	$375
Problem Focused 99212	$45	Cocci Skin Test 86490	$20
Expanded Problem Focused 99213	$55	X-ray, spine, chest, bone—any area various codes	$275
Detailed 99214	$65	Avulsion Nail 11730	$200
Comprehensive/High Complex 99215	$75	**Laboratory**	
Well exam infant (less than 1 year) 99391	$35	Amylase 82150	$40
Well Exam 1–4 yrs. 99392	$40	B12 82607	$30
Well Exam 5–11 yrs. 99393	$45	CBC & Diff 85025	$95
Well Exam 12–17 yrs. 99394	$55	Comp Metabolic Panel 80053	$75
Well Exam 18–39 yrs. 99395	$65	Chlamydia Screen 87110	$70
Well Exam 40–64 yrs. 99396	$75	Cholestrerol 82465	$75
Obstetrics		Digoxin 80162	$40
Total OB Care 59400	$1700	Electrolytes 80051	$70
Injections		Estrogen, Total 82672	$50
Administration 90772	$10	Ferritin 82728	$40
Allergy 95115	$35	Folate 82746	$30
DPT 90701	$50	GC Screen 87070	$60
Drug various codes	$35	Glucose 82947	$35
Influenza 90658	$25	Glycosylated HGB A1C 83036	$45
MMR 90707	$50	HCT 85014	$30
OPV 90712	$40	HDL 83718	$35
Pneumovax 90732	$35	HGB 85018	$30
TB Skin Test 86580	$15	Hep BSAG 83740	$40
TD 90718	$40	Hepatitis panel, acute 80074	$95
Tetanus Toxoid 90703	$40	HIV 86703	$100
Vaccine/Toxoid Administration for Younger		Iron & TIBC 83550	$45
Than 8 Years Old w/ counseling 90465	$10	Kidney Profile 80069	$95
Vaccine/Toxoid Administration for Adult 90471	$10	Lead 83665	$55
Arthrocentesis/Aspiration/Injection		Lipase 83690	$40
Small Joint 20600	$50	Lipid Panel 80061	$95
Interm Joint 20605	$60	Liver Profile 80076	$95
Major Joint 20610	$70	Mono Test 86308	$30
Trigger Point/Tendon Sheath Inj. 20550	$90	Pap Smear 88155	$90
Other Invasive/Noninvasive Procedures		Pap Collection/Supervision 88142	$95
Catheterization 51701	$55	Pregnancy Test 84703	$90
Circumcision 54150	$150	Obstetric Panel 80055	$85
Colposcopy 57452	$225	Pro Time 85610	$50
Colposcopy w/Biopsy 57454	$250	PSA 84153	$50
Cryosurgery Premalignant Lesion various codes	$160	RPR 86592	$55
Endometrial Biopsy 58100	$190	Sed. Rate 85651	$50
Excision Lesion Malignant various codes	$145	Stool Culture 87045	$80
Excision Lesion Benign various codes	$125	Stool O & P 87177	$105
Curettement Lesion		Strep Screen 87880	$35
Single 11055	$70	Theophylline 80198	$40
2–4 11056	$80	Thyroid Uptake 84479	$75
>4 11057	$90	TSH 84443	$50
Excision Skin Tags (1–15) 11200	$55	Urinalysis 81000	$35
Each Additional 10 11201	$30	Urine Culture 87088	$80
I & D Abscess Single/Simple 10060	$75	Drawing Fee 36415	$15
Multiple/Complex 10061	$95	Specimen Collection 99000	$10
I & D Pilonidal Cyst Simple 10080	$105		
I & D Pilonidal Cyst Complex 10081	$130		
Laceration Repair various codes	$60		

1500

HEALTH INSURANCE CLAIM FORM
APPROVED BY NATIONAL UNIFORM CLAIM COMMITTEE 08/05

☐☐☐ PICA   PICA ☐☐☐

1. MEDICARE   MEDICAID   TRICARE   CHAMPVA   GROUP   FECA   OTHER   1a. INSURED'S I.D. NUMBER   (For Program in Item 1)
                          CHAMPUS   HEALTH PLAN BLK LUNG
☐(Medicare #) ☐(Medicaid #) ☐(Sponsor's SSN) ☐(Member ID#) ☐(SSN or ID) ☐(SSN) ☐(ID)

2. PATIENT'S NAME (Last Name, First Name, Middle Initial)   3. PATIENT'S BIRTH DATE   SEX   4. INSURED'S NAME (Last Name, First Name, Middle Initial)
                                                    MM │ DD │ YY
                                                               M☐ F☐

5. PATIENT'S ADDRESS (No, Street)   6. PATIENT RELATIONSHIP TO INSURED   7. INSURED'S ADDRESS (No, Street)

                                     Self☐ Spouse☐ Child☐ Other☐

CITY   STATE   8. PATIENT STATUS   CITY   STATE

                                       Single☐ Married☐ Other☐

ZIP CODE   TELEPHONE (Include Area Code)   ZIP CODE   TELEPHONE (Include Area Code)
              (   )   Full-Time   Part-Time   (   )
                                 Employed☐ Student☐ Student☐

9. OTHER INSURED'S NAME (Last Name, First Name, Middle Initial)   10. IS PATIENT'S CONDITION RELATED TO: 11. INSURED'S POLICY GROUP OR FECA NUMBER

a. OTHER INSURED'S POLICY OR GROUP NUMBER   a. EMPLOYMENT? (Current or Previous)   a. INSURED'S DATE OF BIRTH   SEX
                                                                                        MM │ DD │ YY
                                             ☐YES ☐NO   M☐   F☐

b. OTHER INSURED'S DATE OF BIRTH   SEX   b. AUTO ACCIDENT?   PLACE (State)   b. EMPLOYER'S NAME OR SCHOOL NAME
   MM │ DD │ YY
                M☐ F☐   ☐YES ☐NO └___┘

c. EMPLOYER'S NAME OR SCHOOL NAME   c. OTHER ACCIDENT?   c. INSURANCE PLAN NAME OR PROGRAM NAME

                                     ☐YES ☐NO

d. INSURANCE PLAN NAME OR PROGRAM NAME   10d. RESERVED FOR LOCAL USE   d. IS THERE ANOTHER HEALTH BENEFIT PLAN?

                                                                          ☐YES ☐NO   If yes, return to and complete item 9 a-d.

READ BACK OF FORM BEFORE COMPLETING & SIGNING THIS FORM.

12. PATIENT'S OR AUTHORIZED PERSON'S SIGNATURE I authorize the release of any medical or other information   13. INSURED'S OR AUTHORIZED PERSON'S SIGNATURE I authorize payment of medical
necessary to process this claim. I also request payment of government benefits either to myself or to the party who   benefits to the undersigned physician or supplier for services described below.
accepts assignment below.

SIGNED _____   DATE _____   SIGNED _____

14. DATE OF CURRENT: ◀ ILLNESS (First symptom) OR   15. IF PATIENT HAS HAD SAME OR SIMILAR ILLNESS,   16. DATES PATIENT UNABLE TO WORK IN CURRENT OCCUPATION
   MM │ DD │ YY   INJURY (Accident) OR   GIVE FIRST DATE MM │ DD │ YY   MM │ DD │ YY   MM │ DD │ YY
                    PREGNANCY (LMP)   FROM   TO

17. NAME OF REFERRING PHYSICIAN OR OTHER SOURCE   17a.   18. HOSPITALIZATION DATES RELATED TO CURRENT SERVICES
                                                                                MM │ DD │ YY   MM │ DD │ YY
                                             17b. │ NPI   FROM   TO

19. RESERVED FOR LOCAL USE   20. OUTSIDE LAB? $ CHARGES

                              ☐YES ☐NO

21. DIAGNOSIS OR NATURE OF ILLNESS OR INJURY (Relate Items 1,2,3 or 4 to Item 24E by Line)   22. MEDICAID RESUBMISSION
                                                                                           CODE   ORIGINAL REF. NO.
1. └___·___   3. └___·___   ↓
                                                                              23. PRIOR AUTHORIZATION NUMBER
2. └___·___   4. └___·___

24. A. DATE(S) OF SERVICE						B. PLACE OF SERVICE	C. EMG	D. PROCEDURES, SERVICES, OR SUPPLIES (Explain Unusual Circumstances)		E. DIAGNOSIS POINTER	F. $ CHARGES	G. DAYS OR UNITS	H. EPSDT Family Plan	I. ID. QUAL.	J. RENDERING PROVIDER ID. #
	From			To					CPT/HCPCS	MODIFIER						
MM	DD	YY	MM	DD	YY											
1															NPI	
2															NPI	
3															NPI	
4															NPI	
5															NPI	
6															NPI	

25. FEDERAL TAX I.D. NUMBER   SSN EIN   26. PATIENT'S ACCOUNT NO.   27. ACCEPT ASSIGNMENT?   28. TOTAL CHARGE   29. AMOUNT PAID   30. BALANCE DUE
                          ☐☐   (For govt. claims, see back) $ $ $
                                                      ☐YES ☐NO

31. SIGNATURE OF PHYSICIAN OR SUPPLIER   32. SERVICE FACILITY LOCATION INFORMATION   33. BILLING PROVIDER INFO & PH. # (   )
INCLUDING DEGREES OR CREDENTIALS
(I certify that the statements on the reverse
apply to this bill and are made a part thereof.)

SIGNED _____   DATE _____   a.   NPI   b.   a.   NPI   b.

Figure 15-4

c. Using the source documents, the Capital City Medical Fee Schedule (Figure 15-5), and the blank CMS-1500 form provided (Figure 15-6), complete the following case study for patient Stephanie Reagan (Case 15-3):

CASE 15-3

Capital City Medical—123 Unknown Boulevard, Capital City, NY 12345-2222 (555) 555-1234	Patient Information Form
	Tax ID: 75-0246810
Phil Wells, MD, Mannie Mends, MD, Bette R. Soone, MD	Group NPI: 1513171216

Patient Information:

Name: (Last, First) Reagan, Stephanie ❑ Male ☒ Female Birth Date: 09/10/1984

Address: 11 Twilight Ct., Capital City, NY 12345 Phone: (555) 555-4179

Social Security Number: 877-93-1688 Full-Time Student: ❑ Yes ☒ No

Marital Status: ❑ Single ☒ Married ❑ Divorced ❑ Other

Employment:

Employer: The Bullpen Sports Bar Phone: (555) 555-2290

Address: 79 Point Plaza, Capital City, NY 12345

Condition Related to: ❑ Auto Accident ❑ Employment ❑ Other Accident

Date of Accident: _____ State: _____

Emergency Contact: _____ **Phone: ( )** _____

Primary Insurance: Tricare Phone: ( ) _____

Address: 7594 Forces-Run Rd, Militaryville, NY 12345

Insurance Policyholder's Name: Calvin Reagan ☒ M ❑ F DOB: 03/12/1983

Address: Same

Phone: _____ Relationship to Insured: ❑ Self ☒ Spouse ❑ Child ❑ Other

Employer: U. S. Air Force Phone: ( ) _____

Employer's Address: 196, Airport Rd, Capital City, NY 12345

Policy/ID No: 333-48-1076 Group No: _____ Percent Covered: ____% Copay Amt: $35.00

Secondary Insurance: _____ Phone: ( ) _____

Address: _____

Insurance Policyholder's Name: _____ ❑ M ❑ F DOB: _____

Address: _____

Phone: _____ Relationship to Insured: ❑ Self ❑ Spouse ❑ Child ❑ Other

Employer: _____ Phone: ( ) _____

Employer's Address: _____

Policy/ID No: _____ Group No: _____ Percent Covered: ____% Copay Amt: $____

Reason for Visit: I think that I have a yeast infection.

Known Allergies: _____

Referred by: _____

CASE 15-3
SOAP

10/04/20XX
Assignment of Benefits: Y
Signature on File: Y
Referring Physician: N

S: Stephanie Reagan presents in the office with complaints of burning and itching in her vaginal area. She does have a white discharge. She tried a three-day treatment of OTC yeast medicine, but it hasn't cleared up.

O: On exam, the vulva appears irritated. There is a yeast discharge present. Abdomen soft, nontender. There is no evidence of fever. She denies nausea and vomiting.

A: 1. Yeast vaginitis—112.1

P: 1. Diflucant one per day.
   2. May continue using the external vaginal itch relief cream that accompanied the OTC treatment.
   3. Return p.r.n.

_____

Phil Wells, MD
Family Practice
NPI: 1234567890

CASE 15-3

Patient Name <u>Stephanie Reagan</u>

Capital City Medical
123 Unknown Boulevard, Capital City, NY 12345-2222

Date of Service
<u>10-04-20XX</u>

New Patient			Other Invasive/Noninvasive			Laboratory	
Problem Focused	99201		Arthrocentesis/Aspiration/Injection			Amylase	82150
Expanded Problem, Focused	99202		Small Joint	20600		B12	82607
Detailed	99203		Interm Joint	20605		CBC & Diff	85025
Comprehensive	99204		Major Joint	20610		Comp Metabolic Panel	80053
Comprehensive/High Complex	99205		**Other Invasive/Noninvasive**			Chlamydia Screen	87110
Well Exam Infant (up to 12 mos.)	99381		Audiometry	92552		Cholesterol	82465
Well Exam 1–4 yrs.	99382		Cast Application			Digoxin	80162
Well Exam 5–11 yrs.	99383		Location Long Short			Electrolytes	80051
Well Exam 12–17 yrs.	99384		Catheterization	51701		Ferritin	82728
Well Exam 18–39 yrs.	99385		Circumcision	54150		Folate	82746
Well Exam 40–64 yrs.	99386		Colposcopy	57452		GC Screen	87070
			Colposcopy w/Biopsy	57454		Glucose	82947
			Cryosurgery Premalignant Lesion			Glucose 1 HR	82950
			Location (s):			Glycosylated HGB A1C	83036
Established Patient			Cryosurgery Warts			HCT	85014
Post-Op Follow Up Visit	99024		Location (s):			HDL	83718
Minimum	99211		Curettement Lesion			Hep BSAG	87340
Problem Focused	99212	X	Single	11055		Hepatitis panel, acute	80074
Expanded Problem Focused	99213		2–4	11056		HGB	85018
Detailed	99214		>4	11057		HIV	86703
Comprehensive/High Complex	99215		Diaphragm Fitting	57170		Iron & TIBC	83550
Well Exam Infant (up to 12 mos.)	99391		Ear Irrigation	69210		Kidney Profile	80069
Well exam 1–4 yrs.	99392		ECG	93000		Lead	83655
Well Exam 5–11 yrs.	99393		Endometrial Biopsy	58100		Liver Profile	80076
Well Exam 12–17 yrs.	99394		Exc. Lesion Malignant			Mono Test	86308
Well Exam 18–39 yrs.	99395		Benign			Pap Smear	88155
Well Exam 40–64 yrs.	99396		Location			Pregnancy Test	84703
Obstetrics			Exc. Skin Taqs (1–15)	11200		Obstetric Panel	80055
Total OB Care	59400		Each Additional 10	11201		Pro Time	85610
Injections			Fracture Treatment			PSA	84153
Administration Sub. / IM	90772		Loc			RPR	86592
Drug			w/Reduc w/o Reduc			Sed. Rate	85651
Dosage			I & D Abscess Single/Simple	10060		Stool Culture	87045
Allergy	95115		Multiple or Comp	10061		Stool O & P	87177
Cocci Skin Test	86490		I & D Pilonidal Cyst Simple	10080		Strep Screen	87880
DPT	90701		Pilonidal Cyst Complex	10081		Theophylline	80198
Hemophilus	90646		IV Therapy—To One Hour	90760		Thyroid Uptake	84479
Influenza	90658		Each Additional Hour	90761		TSH	84443
MMR	90707		Laceration Repair			Urinalysis	81000
OPV	90712		Location Size Simp/Comp			Urine Culture	87088
Pneumovax	90732		Laryngoscopy	31505		Drawing Fee	36415
TB Skin Test	86580		Oximetry	94760		Specimen Collection	99000
TD	90718		Punch Biopsy			**Other:**	
Unlisted Immun	90749		Rhythm Strip	93040			
Tetanus Toxoid	90703		Treadmill	93015			
Vaccine/Toxoid Admin <8 Yr Old w/ Counseling	90465		Trigger Point or Tendon Sheath Inj.	20550			
Vaccine/Toxoid Administration for Adult	90471		Tympanometry	92567			

Diagnosis/ICD-9: **112.1**

I acknowledge receipt of medical services and authorize the release of any medical information necessary to process this claim for healthcare payment only. I do authorize payment to the provider.

Patient Signature <u>Stephanie Reagan</u>

Total Estimated Charges: _____

Payment Amount: _____

Next Appointment: _____

Figure 15-5

Capital City Medical
Fee Schedule

New Patient OV		Punch Biopsy various codes	$80
Problem Focused 99201	$45	Nebulizer various codes	$45
Expanded Problem Focused 99202	$65	Cast Application various codes	$85
Detailed 99203	$85	Laryngoscopy 31505	$255
Comprehensive 99204	$105	Audiometry 92552	$85
Comprehensive/High Complex 99205	$115	Tympanometry 92567	$85
Well Exam infant (less than 1 year) 99381	$45	Ear Irrigation 69210	$25
Well Exam 1–4 yrs. 99382	$50	Diaphragm Fitting 57170	$30
Well Exam 5–11 yrs. 99383	$55	IV Therapy (up to one hour) 90760	$65
Well Exam 12–17 yrs. 99384	$65	Each additional hour 90761	$50
Well Exam 18–39 yrs. 99385	$85	Oximetry 94760	$10
Well Exam 40–64 yrs. 99386	$105	ECG 93000	$75
Established Patient OV		Holter Monitor various codes	$170
Post Op Follow Up Visit 99024	$0	Rhythm Strip 93040	$60
Minimum 99211	$35	Treadmill 93015	$375
Problem Focused 99212	$45	Cocci Skin Test 86490	$20
Expanded Problem Focused 99213	$55	X-ray, spine, chest, bone—any area various codes	$275
Detailed 99214	$65	Avulsion Nail 11730	$200
Comprehensive/High Complex 99215	$75	**Laboratory**	
Well exam infant (less than 1 year) 99391	$35	Amylase 82150	$40
Well Exam 1–4 yrs. 99392	$40	B12 82607	$30
Well Exam 5–11 yrs. 99393	$45	CBC & Diff 85025	$95
Well Exam 12–17 yrs. 99394	$55	Comp Metabolic Panel 80053	$75
Well Exam 18–39 yrs. 99395	$65	Chlamydia Screen 87110	$70
Well Exam 40–64 yrs. 99396	$75	Cholestrerol 82465	$75
Obstetrics		Digoxin 80162	$40
Total OB Care 59400	$1700	Electrolytes 80051	$70
Injections		Estrogen, Total 82672	$50
Administration 90772	$10	Ferritin 82728	$40
Allergy 95115	$35	Folate 82746	$30
DPT 90701	$50	GC Screen 87070	$60
Drug various codes	$35	Glucose 82947	$35
Influenza 90658	$25	Glycosylated HGB A1C 83036	$45
MMR 90707	$50	HCT 85014	$30
OPV 90712	$40	HDL 83718	$35
Pneumovax 90732	$35	HGB 85018	$30
TB Skin Test 86580	$15	Hep BSAG 83740	$40
TD 90718	$40	Hepatitis panel, acute 80074	$95
Tetanus Toxoid 90703	$40	HIV 86703	$100
Vaccine/Toxoid Administration for Younger		Iron & TIBC 83550	$45
Than 8 Years Old w/ counseling 90465	$10	Kidney Profile 80069	$95
Vaccine/Toxoid Administration for Adult 90471	$10	Lead 83665	$55
Arthrocentesis/Aspiration/Injection		Lipase 83690	$40
Small Joint 20600	$50	Lipid Panel 80061	$95
Interm Joint 20605	$60	Liver Profile 80076	$95
Major Joint 20610	$70	Mono Test 86308	$30
Trigger Point/Tendon Sheath Inj. 20550	$90	Pap Smear 88155	$90
Other Invasive/Noninvasive Procedures		Pap Collection/Supervision 88142	$95
Catheterization 51701	$55	Pregnancy Test 84703	$90
Circumcision 54150	$150	Obstetric Panel 80055	$85
Colposcopy 57452	$225	Pro Time 85610	$50
Colposcopy w/Biopsy 57454	$250	PSA 84153	$50
Cryosurgery Premalignant Lesion various codes	$160	RPR 86592	$55
Endometrial Biopsy 58100	$190	Sed. Rate 85651	$50
Excision Lesion Malignant various codes	$145	Stool Culture 87045	$80
Excision Lesion Benign various codes	$125	Stool O & P 87177	$105
Curettement Lesion		Strep Screen 87880	$35
Single 11055	$70	Theophylline 80198	$40
2–4 11056	$80	Thyroid Uptake 84479	$75
>4 11057	$90	TSH 84443	$50
Excision Skin Tags (1–15) 11200	$55	Urinalysis 81000	$35
Each Additional 10 11201	$30	Urine Culture 87088	$80
I & D Abscess Single/Simple 10060	$75	Drawing Fee 36415	$15
Multiple/Complex 10061	$95	Specimen Collection 99000	$10
I & D Pilonidal Cyst Simple 10080	$105		
I & D Pilonidal Cyst Complex 10081	$130		
Laceration Repair various codes	$60		

HEALTH INSURANCE CLAIM FORM

APPROVED BY NATIONAL UNIFORM CLAIM COMMITTEE 08/05

	PICA									PICA	

1. MEDICARE MEDICAID TRICARE CHAMPVA GROUP FECA OTHER
CHAMPUS HEALTH PLAN BLK LUNG
☐(Medicare #) ☐(Medicaid #) ☐(Sponsor's SSN) ☐(Member ID#) ☐(SSN or ID) ☐(SSN) ☐(ID)

1a. INSURED'S I.D. NUMBER (For Program in Item 1)

2. PATIENT'S NAME (Last Name, First Name, Middle Initial)

3. PATIENT'S BIRTH DATE SEX
MM DD YY
M☐ F☐

4. INSURED'S NAME (Last Name, First Name, Middle Initial)

5. PATIENT'S ADDRESS (No., Street)

6. PATIENT RELATIONSHIP TO INSURED
Self☐ Spouse☐ Child☐ Other☐

7. INSURED'S ADDRESS (No., Street)

CITY STATE

8. PATIENT STATUS
Single☐ Married☐ Other☐

Full-Time Part-Time
Employed☐ Student☐ Student☐

CITY STATE

ZIP CODE TELEPHONE (Include Area Code)
( )

ZIP CODE TELEPHONE (Include Area Code)
( )

9. OTHER INSURED'S NAME (Last Name, First Name, Middle Initial)

10. IS PATIENT'S CONDITION RELATED TO:

11. INSURED'S POLICY GROUP OR FECA NUMBER

a. OTHER INSURED'S POLICY OR GROUP NUMBER

a. EMPLOYMENT? (Current or Previous)
☐YES ☐NO

a. INSURED'S DATE OF BIRTH SEX
MM DD YY
M☐ F☐

b. OTHER INSURED'S DATE OF BIRTH SEX
MM DD YY
M☐ F☐

b. AUTO ACCIDENT? PLACE (State)
☐YES ☐NO

b. EMPLOYER'S NAME OR SCHOOL NAME

c. EMPLOYER'S NAME OR SCHOOL NAME

c. OTHER ACCIDENT?
☐YES ☐NO

c. INSURANCE PLAN NAME OR PROGRAM NAME

d. INSURANCE PLAN NAME OR PROGRAM NAME

10d. RESERVED FOR LOCAL USE

d. IS THERE ANOTHER HEALTH BENEFIT PLAN?
☐YES ☐NO *If yes,* return to and complete item 9 a-d.

READ BACK OF FORM BEFORE COMPLETING & SIGNING THIS FORM.

12. PATIENT'S OR AUTHORIZED PERSON'S SIGNATURE I authorize the release of any medical or other information necessary to process this claim. I also request payment of government benefits either to myself or to the party who accepts assignment below.

SIGNED_____ DATE_____

13. INSURED'S OR AUTHORIZED PERSON'S SIGNATURE I authorize payment of medical benefits to the undersigned physician or supplier for services described below.

SIGNED_____

14. DATE OF CURRENT: ILLNESS (First symptom) OR
MM DD YY INJURY (Accident) OR
PREGNANCY (LMP)

15. IF PATIENT HAS HAD SAME OR SIMILAR ILLNESS.
GIVE FIRST DATE MM DD YY

16. DATES PATIENT UNABLE TO WORK IN CURRENT OCCUPATION
FROM MM DD YY TO MM DD YY

17. NAME OF REFERRING PHYSICIAN OR OTHER SOURCE

17a.
17b. NPI

18. HOSPITALIZATION DATES RELATED TO CURRENT SERVICES
FROM MM DD YY TO MM DD YY

19. RESERVED FOR LOCAL USE

20. OUTSIDE LAB? $ CHARGES
☐YES ☐NO

21. DIAGNOSIS OR NATURE OF ILLNESS OR INJURY (Relate Items 1,2,3 or 4 to Item 24E by Line)
1. |___.___   3. |___.___
2. |___.___   4. |___.___

22. MEDICAID RESUBMISSION
CODE ORIGINAL REF. NO.

23. PRIOR AUTHORIZATION NUMBER

24. A. DATE(S) OF SERVICE						B. PLACE OF SERVICE	C. EMG	D. PROCEDURES, SERVICES, OR SUPPLIES (Explain Unusual Circumstances)		E. DIAGNOSIS POINTER	F. $ CHARGES	G. DAYS OR UNITS	H. EPSDT Family Plan	I. ID. QUAL.	J. RENDERING PROVIDER ID. #
From			To					CPT/HCPCS	MODIFIER						
MM	DD	YY	MM	DD	YY										
1														NPI	
2														NPI	
3														NPI	
4														NPI	
5														NPI	
6														NPI	

25. FEDERAL TAX I.D. NUMBER SSN EIN ☐☐

26. PATIENT'S ACCOUNT NO.

27. ACCEPT ASSIGNMENT? (For govt. claims, see back) ☐YES ☐NO

28. TOTAL CHARGE $

29. AMOUNT PAID $

30. BALANCE DUE $

31. SIGNATURE OF PHYSICIAN OR SUPPLIER INCLUDING DEGREES OR CREDENTIALS (I certify that the statements on the reverse apply to this bill and are made a part thereof.)

SIGNED_____ DATE_____

32. SERVICE FACILITY LOCATION INFORMATION
a. NPI b.

33. BILLING PROVIDER INFO & PH. # ( )
a. NPI b.

APPROVED OMB 0938-0999 FORM CMS-1500 (08/05)

CARRIER

PATIENT AND INSURED INFORMATION

PHYSICIAN OR SUPPLIER INFORMATION

SECOND FOLD

FIRST FOLD WHCF-10-ENV / WHCF-10-ENV-SS

Figure 15-6

d. Using the source documents, the Capital City Medical Fee Schedule (Figure 15-7), and the blank CMS-1500 form provided (Figure 15-8), complete the following case study for patient Allen Won (Case 15-4):

CASE 15-4

Capital City Medical—123 Unknown Boulevard, Capital City, NY 12345-2222 (555) 555-1234	Patient Information Form
	Tax ID: 75-0246810
Phil Wells, MD, Mannie Mends, MD, Bette R. Soone, MD	Group NPI: 1513171216

Patient Information:

Name: (Last, First) Won, Allen ☒ Male ☐ Female   Birth Date: 08/14/2002

Address: 448 Sunset Ln, Capital City, NY 12345   Phone: (555) 555-5312

Social Security Number: 505-72-6853   Full-Time Student: ☒ Yes ☐ No

Marital Status: ☐ Single ☐ Married ☐ Divorced ☐ Other

Employment:

Employer: _____ Phone: ( ) _____

Address: _____

Condition Related to: ☐ Auto Accident ☐ Employment ☐ Other Accident

Date of Accident: _____ State: _____

Emergency Contact: _____ **Phone: ( )** _____

Primary Insurance: Tricare   Phone: ( ) _____

Address: 7594 Forces-Run Rd, Militaryville, NY 12345

Insurance Policyholder's Name: Victor Won ☒ M ☐ F DOB: 04/24/1986

Address: Same

Phone: _____ Relationship to Insured: ☐ Self ☐ Spouse ☒ Child ☐ Other

Employer: U. S. Marine Corp.   Phone: ( ) _____

Employer's Address: 1819 Base Ave, Capital City, NY 12345

Policy/ID No: 983-50-5983   Group No: _____ Percent Covered: ____% Copay Amt: $35.00

Secondary Insurance: _____   Phone: ( ) _____

Address: _____

Insurance Policyholder's Name: _____ ☐ M ☐ F DOB: _____

Address: _____

Phone: _____ Relationship to Insured: ☐ Self ☐ Spouse ☐ Child ☐ Other

Employer: _____   Phone: ( ) _____

Employer's Address: _____

Policy/ID No: _____ Group No: _____ Percent Covered: ____% Copay Amt: $_____

Reason for Visit: My son has head lice.

Known Allergies: _____

Referred by: _____

CASE 15-4
SOAP

04/16/20XX
Assignment of Benefits: Y
Signature on File: Y
Referring Physician: N

S: Allen Won presents in the office today for head lice. He may have gotten it from a classmate who was sent home on Monday for the same problem.

O: There is evidence of lice eggs on the scalp. Skin presents unremarkable, without rash or lacerations.

A: 1. Pediculus capitas—132.0

P: 1. Lindane shampoo daily.
   2. Keep clothes and linens clean.
   3. Mother told that it may take more than one treatment to rid the head of lice. Mother was advised to shave Allen's head, for best results.

_____

Phil Wells, MD
Family Practice
NPI: 1234567890

CASE 15-4

Patient Name Allen Won

Capital City Medical
123 Unknown Boulevard, Capital City, NY 12345-2222

Date of Service
04-16-20XX

New Patient			Arthrocentesis/Aspiration/Injection			Laboratory	
Problem Focused	99201		Small Joint		20600	Amylase	82150
Expanded Problem, Focused	99202		Interm Joint		20605	B12	82607
Detailed	99203		Major Joint		20610	CBC & Diff	85025
Comprehensive	99204		**Other Invasive/Noninvasive**			Comp Metabolic Panel	80053
Comprehensive/High Complex	99205		Audiometry		92552	Chlamydia Screen	87110
Well Exam Infant (up to 12 mos.)	99381		Cast Application			Cholesterol	82465
Well Exam 1–4 yrs.	99382		Location Long Short			Digoxin	80162
Well Exam 5–11 yrs.	99383		Catheterization		51701	Electrolytes	80051
Well Exam 12–17 yrs.	99384		Circumcision		54150	Ferritin	82728
Well Exam 18–39 yrs.	99385		Colposcopy		57452	Folate	82746
Well Exam 40–64 yrs.	99386		Colposcopy w/Biopsy		57454	GC Screen	87070
			Cryosurgery Premalignant Lesion			Glucose	82947
			Location (s):			Glucose 1 HR	82950
			Cryosurgery Warts			Glycosylated HGB A1C	83036
Established Patient			Location (s):			HCT	85014
Post-Op Follow Up Visit	99024		Curettement Lesion			HDL	83718
Minimum	99211		Single		11055	Hep BSAG	87340
Problem Focused	99212	X	2–4		11056	Hepatitis panel, acute	80074
Expanded Problem Focused	99213		>4		11057	HGB	85018
Detailed	99214		Diaphragm Fitting		57170	HIV	86703
Comprehensive/High Complex	99215		Ear Irrigation		69210	Iron & TIBC	83550
Well Exam Infant (up to 12 mos.)	99391		ECG		93000	Kidney Profile	80069
Well exam 1–4 yrs.	99392		Endometrial Biopsy		58100	Lead	83655
Well Exam 5–11 yrs.	99393		Exc. Lesion Malignant			Liver Profile	80076
Well Exam 12–17 yrs.	99394		Benign			Mono Test	86308
Well Exam 18–39 yrs.	99395		Location			Pap Smear	88155
Well Exam 40–64 yrs.	99396		Exc. Skin Tags (1–15)		11200	Pregnancy Test	84703
Obstetrics			Each Additional 10		11201	Obstetric Panel	80055
Total OB Care	59400		Fracture Treatment			Pro Time	85610
Injections			Loc			PSA	84153
Administration Sub. / IM	90772		w/Reduc	w/o Reduc		RPR	86592
Drug			I & D Abscess Single/Simple		10060	Sed. Rate	85651
Dosage			Multiple or Comp		10061	Stool Culture	87045
Allergy	95115		I & D Pilonidal Cyst Simple		10080	Stool O & P	87177
Cocci Skin Test	86490		Pilonidal Cyst Complex		10081	Strep Screen	87880
DPT	90701		IV Therapy—To One Hour		90760	Theophylline	80198
Hemophilus	90646		Each Additional Hour		90761	Thyroid Uptake	84479
Influenza	90658		Laceration Repair			TSH	84443
MMR	90707		Location Size Simp/Comp			Urinalysis	81000
OPV	90712		Laryngoscopy		31505	Urine Culture	87088
Pneumovax	90732		Oximetry		94760	Drawing Fee	36415
TB Skin Test	86580		Punch Biopsy			Specimen Collection	99000
TD	90718		Rhythm Strip		93040	**Other:**	
Unlisted Immun	90749		Treadmill		93015		
Tetanus Toxoid	90703		Trigger Point or Tendon Sheath Inj.		20550		
Vaccine/Toxoid Admin <8 Yr Old w/ Counseling	90465						
Vaccine/Toxoid Administration for Adult	90471		Tympanometry		92567		

Diagnosis/ICD-9: **132.0**

I acknowledge receipt of medical services and authorize the release of any medical information necessary to process this claim for healthcare payment only. I do authorize payment to the provider.

Patient Signature _Victor Won_

Total Estimated Charges: _____

Payment Amount: _____

Next Appointment: _____

Figure 15-7

Capital City Medical
Fee Schedule

New Patient OV			Punch Biopsy various codes	$80
Problem Focused 99201	$45		Nebulizer various codes	$45
Expanded Problem Focused 99202	$65		Cast Application various codes	$85
Detailed 99203	$85		Laryngoscopy 31505	$255
Comprehensive 99204	$105		Audiometry 92552	$85
Comprehensive/High Complex 99205	$115		Tympanometry 92567	$85
Well Exam infant (less than 1 year) 99381	$45		Ear Irrigation 69210	$25
Well Exam 1–4 yrs. 99382	$50		Diaphragm Fitting 57170	$30
Well Exam 5–11 yrs. 99383	$55		IV Therapy (up to one hour) 90760	$65
Well Exam 12–17 yrs. 99384	$65		Each additional hour 90761	$50
Well Exam 18–39 yrs. 99385	$85		Oximetry 94760	$10
Well Exam 40–64 yrs. 99386	$105		ECG 93000	$75
Established Patient OV			Holter Monitor various codes	$170
Post Op Follow Up Visit 99024	$0		Rhythm Strip 93040	$60
Minimum 99211	$35		Treadmill 93015	$375
Problem Focused 99212	$45		Cocci Skin Test 86490	$20
Expanded Problem Focused 99213	$55		X-ray, spine, chest, bone—any area various codes	$275
Detailed 99214	$65		Avulsion Nail 11730	$200
Comprehensive/High Complex 99215	$75		**Laboratory**	
Well exam infant (less than 1 year) 99391	$35		Amylase 82150	$40
Well Exam 1–4 yrs. 99392	$40		B12 82607	$30
Well Exam 5–11 yrs. 99393	$45		CBC & Diff 85025	$95
Well Exam 12–17 yrs. 99394	$55		Comp Metabolic Panel 80053	$75
Well Exam 18–39 yrs. 99395	$65		Chlamydia Screen 87110	$70
Well Exam 40–64 yrs. 99396	$75		Cholestrerol 82465	$75
Obstetrics			Digoxin 80162	$40
Total OB Care 59400	$1700		Electrolytes 80051	$70
Injections			Estrogen, Total 82672	$50
Administration 90772	$10		Ferritin 82728	$40
Allergy 95115	$35		Folate 82746	$30
DPT 90701	$50		GC Screen 87070	$60
Drug various codes	$35		Glucose 82947	$35
Influenza 90658	$25		Glycosylated HGB A1C 83036	$45
MMR 90707	$50		HCT 85014	$30
OPV 90712	$40		HDL 83718	$35
Pneumovax 90732	$35		HGB 85018	$30
TB Skin Test 86580	$15		Hep BSAG 83740	$40
TD 90718	$40		Hepatitis panel, acute 80074	$95
Tetanus Toxoid 90703	$40		HIV 86703	$100
Vaccine/Toxoid Administration for Younger Than 8 Years Old w/ counseling 90465	$10		Iron & TIBC 83550	$45
			Kidney Profile 80069	$95
Vaccine/Toxoid Administration for Adult 90471	$10		Lead 83665	$55
Arthrocentesis/Aspiration/Injection			Lipase 83690	$40
Small Joint 20600	$50		Lipid Panel 80061	$95
Interm Joint 20605	$60		Liver Profile 80076	$95
Major Joint 20610	$70		Mono Test 86308	$30
Trigger Point/Tendon Sheath Inj. 20550	$90		Pap Smear 88155	$90
Other Invasive/Noninvasive Procedures			Pap Collection/Supervision 88142	$95
Catheterization 51701	$55		Pregnancy Test 84703	$90
Circumcision 54150	$150		Obstetric Panel 80055	$85
Colposcopy 57452	$225		Pro Time 85610	$50
Colposcopy w/Biopsy 57454	$250		PSA 84153	$50
Cryosurgery Premalignant Lesion various codes	$160		RPR 86592	$55
Endometrial Biopsy 58100	$190		Sed. Rate 85651	$50
Excision Lesion Malignant various codes	$145		Stool Culture 87045	$80
Excision Lesion Benign various codes	$125		Stool O & P 87177	$105
Curettement Lesion			Strep Screen 87880	$35
Single 11055	$70		Theophylline 80198	$40
2–4 11056	$80		Thyroid Uptake 84479	$75
>4 11057	$90		TSH 84443	$50
Excision Skin Tags (1–15) 11200	$55		Urinalysis 81000	$35
Each Additional 10 11201	$30		Urine Culture 87088	$80
I & D Abscess Single/Simple 10060	$75		Drawing Fee 36415	$15
Multiple/Complex 10061	$95		Specimen Collection 99000	$10
I & D Pilonidal Cyst Simple 10080	$105			
I & D Pilonidal Cyst Complex 10081	$130			
Laceration Repair various codes	$60			

HEALTH INSURANCE CLAIM FORM

APPROVED BY NATIONAL UNIFORM CLAIM COMMITTEE 08/05

☐☐☐PICA

PICA ☐☐☐

1. MEDICARE　　MEDICAID　　TRICARE　　　CHAMPVA　　GROUP　　　FECA　　　OTHER	1a. INSURED'S I.D. NUMBER　　　　　(For Program in Item 1)
CHAMPUS　　　　　　　　HEALTH PLAN　BLK LUNG	
☐(Medicare #)　☐(Medicaid #)　☐(Sponsor's SSN)　☐(Member ID#)　☐(SSN or ID)　☐(SSN)　☐(ID)	

2. PATIENT'S NAME (Last Name, First Name, Middle Initial)

3. PATIENT'S BIRTH DATE　　SEX
MM ┊ DD ┊ YY
M☐　F☐

4. INSURED'S NAME (Last Name, First Name, Middle Initial)

5. PATIENT'S ADDRESS (No., Street)

6. PATIENT RELATIONSHIP TO INSURED
Self☐　Spouse☐　Child☐　Other☐

7. INSURED'S ADDRESS (No, Street)

CITY　　　　STATE

8. PATIENT STATUS
Single☐　Married☐　Other☐
Full-Time　Part-Time
Employed☐　Student☐　Student☐

CITY　　　　STATE

ZIP CODE　　TELEPHONE (Include Area Code)
( )

ZIP CODE　　TELEPHONE (Include Area Code)
( )

9. OTHER INSURED'S NAME (Last Name, First Name, Middle Initial)

10. IS PATIENT'S CONDITION RELATED TO:

11. INSURED'S POLICY GROUP OR FECA NUMBER

a. OTHER INSURED'S POLICY OR GROUP NUMBER

a. EMPLOYMENT? (Current or Previous)
☐YES ☐NO

a. INSURED'S DATE OF BIRTH　　SEX
MM ┊ DD ┊ YY
M☐　F☐

b. OTHER INSURED'S DATE OF BIRTH　SEX
MM ┊ DD ┊ YY
M☐　F☐

b. AUTO ACCIDENT?　　PLACE (State)
☐YES ☐NO └─┘

b. EMPLOYER'S NAME OR SCHOOL NAME

c. EMPLOYER'S NAME OR SCHOOL NAME

c. OTHER ACCIDENT?
☐YES ☐NO

c. INSURANCE PLAN NAME OR PROGRAM NAME

d. INSURANCE PLAN NAME OR PROGRAM NAME

10d. RESERVED FOR LOCAL USE

d. IS THERE ANOTHER HEALTH BENEFIT PLAN?
☐YES ☐NO　If yes, return to and complete item 9 a-d.

READ BACK OF FORM BEFORE COMPLETING & SIGNING THIS FORM.
12. PATIENT'S OR AUTHORIZED PERSON'S SIGNATURE I authorize the release of any medical or other information necessary to process this claim. I also request payment of government benefits either to myself or to the party who accepts assignment below.

SIGNED _____　DATE _____

13. INSURED'S OR AUTHORIZED PERSON'S SIGNATURE I authorize payment of medical benefits to the undersigned physician or supplier for services described below.

SIGNED _____

14. DATE OF CURRENT:
MM ┊ DD ┊ YY
◄ ILLNESS (First symptom) OR INJURY (Accident) OR PREGNANCY (LMP)

15. IF PATIENT HAS HAD SAME OR SIMILAR ILLNESS, GIVE FIRST DATE　MM ┊ DD ┊ YY

16. DATES PATIENT UNABLE TO WORK IN CURRENT OCCUPATION
MM ┊ DD ┊ YY　　MM ┊ DD ┊ YY
FROM　　　TO

17. NAME OF REFERRING PHYSICIAN OR OTHER SOURCE

17a.
17b. │ NPI

18. HOSPITALIZATION DATES RELATED TO CURRENT SERVICES
MM ┊ DD ┊ YY　　MM ┊ DD ┊ YY
FROM　　　TO

19. RESERVED FOR LOCAL USE

20. OUTSIDE LAB?　　$ CHARGES
☐YES ☐NO

21. DIAGNOSIS OR NATURE OF ILLNESS OR INJURY (Relate Items 1,2,3 or 4 to Item 24E by Line)

1. └─── · ───　　　3. └─── · ───
2. └─── · ───　　　4. └─── · ───

22. MEDICAID RESUBMISSION
CODE　　　ORIGINAL REF. NO.

23. PRIOR AUTHORIZATION NUMBER

24. A. DATE(S) OF SERVICE		B.	C.	D. PROCEDURES, SERVICES, OR SUPPLIES	E.	F.	G.	H.	I.	J.
From　　　To		PLACE OF		(Explain Unusual Circumstances)	DIAGNOSIS		DAYS OR	EPSDT Family	ID.	RENDERING
MM DD YY　MM DD YY		SERVICE	EMG	CPT/HCPCS　MODIFIER	POINTER	$ CHARGES	UNITS	Plan	QUAL.	PROVIDER ID. #
1									NPI	
2									NPI	
3									NPI	
4									NPI	
5									NPI	
6									NPI	

25. FEDERAL TAX I.D. NUMBER　SSN EIN
☐☐

26. PATIENT'S ACCOUNT NO.

27. ACCEPT ASSIGNMENT?
(For govt. claims, see back)
☐YES ☐NO

28. TOTAL CHARGE
$

29. AMOUNT PAID
$

30. BALANCE DUE
$

31. SIGNATURE OF PHYSICIAN OR SUPPLIER INCLUDING DEGREES OR CREDENTIALS
(I certify that the statements on the reverse apply to this bill and are made a part thereof.)

SIGNED _____　DATE _____

32. SERVICE FACILITY LOCATION INFORMATION
a. NPI　b.

33. BILLING PROVIDER INFO & PH. # ( )
a. NPI　b.

(Side margins: CARRIER — PATIENT AND INSURED INFORMATION — PHYSICIAN OR SUPPLIER INFORMATION)

(Left margin: SECOND FOLD — FIRST FOLD WHCF-10-ENV / WHCF-10-ENV-SS)

Figure 15-8

e. Using the source documents, the Capital City Medical Fee Schedule (Figure 15-9), and the blank CMS-1500 form provided (Figure 15-10), complete the following case study for patient Gerardo Lamos (Case 15-5):

CASE 15-5

Capital City Medical—123 Unknown Boulevard, Capital City, NY 12345-2222 (555) 555-1234	Patient Information Form
Phil Wells, MD, Mannie Mends, MD, Bette R. Soone, MD	Tax ID: 75-0246810
	Group NPI: 1513171216

Patient Information:

Name: (Last, First) Lamos, Gerardo   ☒ Male ☐ Female   Birth Date: 01/21/1944

Address: 6270 Meyer Ave, Capital City, NY 12345   Phone: (555) 555-0590

Social Security Number: 431-00-8131   Full-Time Student: ☐ Yes ☐ No

Marital Status: ☐ Single ☒ Married ☐ Divorced ☐ Other

Employment:

Employer: Retired   Phone: ( )

Address:

Condition Related to: ☐ Auto Accident ☐ Employment ☐ Other Accident

Date of Accident: _____ State: _____

Emergency Contact: _____ **Phone: ( )** _____

Primary Insurance: CHAMPVA   Phone: ( )

Address: P. O Box 4586, Capital City, NY 12345

Insurance Policyholder's Name: Same   ☐ M ☐ F DOB:

Address:

Phone: _____ Relationship to Insured: ☒ Self ☐ Spouse ☐ Child ☐ Other

Employer: _____ Phone: ( ) _____

Employer's Address:

Policy/ID No: 431008131   Group No: _____ Percent Covered: 100 % Copay Amt: $_____

Secondary Insurance: _____   Phone: ( ) _____

Address:

Insurance Policyholder's Name: _____   ☐ M ☐ F DOB: _____

Address:

Phone: _____ Relationship to Insured: ☐ Self ☐ Spouse ☐ Child ☐ Other

Employer: _____ Phone: ( ) _____

Employer's Address:

Policy/ID No: _____ Group No: _____ Percent Covered: ___% Copay Amt: $_____

Reason for Visit: I think that my bronchitis is back.

Known Allergies: _____

Referred by: _____

CASE 15-5
SOAP

02/01/20XX
Assignment of Benefits: Y
Signature on File: Y
Referring Physician: N

S: Gerardo Lamos is being seen because of possible recurrence of bronchitis. He says that his chest hurts, and that he has a productive cough.

O: There is no fever present. Chest sounds congested on A&P. No wheezing, rubs, or rhonchi. Nose and oropharynx are clear. Throat does appear red due to coughing.

A: 1. Chronic bronchitis—491.9

P: 1. Avelox one daily with food.
2. Guaifenesin, one twice a day.
3. Finish all medications.

_____

Phil Well, MD
Family Practice
NPI: 1234567890

CASE 15-5

Patient Name Gerardo Lamos

Capital City Medical
123 Unknown Boulevard, Capital City, NY 12345-2222

Date of Service
02-01-20XX

New Patient			Arthrocentesis/Aspiration/Injection		Laboratory		
Problem Focused	99201		Arthrocentesis/Aspiration/Injection		Amylase	82150	
Expanded Problem, Focused	99202		Small Joint	20600	B12	82607	
Detailed	99203		Interm Joint	20605	CBC & Diff	85025	
Comprehensive	99204		Major Joint	20610	Comp Metabolic Panel	80053	
Comprehensive/High Complex	99205		**Other Invasive/Noninvasive**		Chlamydia Screen	87110	
Well Exam Infant (up to 12 mos.)	99381		Audiometry	92552	Cholesterol	82465	
Well Exam 1–4 yrs.	99382		Cast Application		Digoxin	80162	
Well Exam 5–11 yrs.	99383		Location Long Short		Electrolytes	80051	
Well Exam 12–17 yrs.	99384		Catheterization	51701	Ferritin	82728	
Well Exam 18–39 yrs.	99385		Circumcision	54150	Folate	82746	
Well Exam 40–64 yrs.	99386		Colposcopy	57452	GC Screen	87070	
			Colposcopy w/Biopsy	57454	Glucose	82947	
			Cryosurgery Premalignant Lesion		Glucose 1 HR	82950	
			Location (s):		Glycosylated HGB A1C	83036	
Established Patient			Cryosurgery Warts		HCT	85014	
Post-Op Follow Up Visit	99024		Location (s):		HDL	83718	
Minimum	99211		Curettement Lesion		Hep BSAG	87340	
Problem Focused	99212	X	Single	11055	Hepatitis panel, acute	80074	
Expanded Problem Focused	99213		2–4	11056	HGB	85018	
Detailed	99214		>4	11057	HIV	86703	
Comprehensive/High Complex	99215		Diaphragm Fitting	57170	Iron & TIBC	83550	
Well Exam Infant (up to 12 mos.)	99391		Ear Irrigation	69210	Kidney Profile	80069	
Well exam 1–4 yrs.	99392		ECG	93000	Lead	83655	
Well Exam 5–11 yrs.	99393		Endometrial Biopsy	58100	Liver Profile	80076	
Well Exam 12–17 yrs.	99394		Exc. Lesion Malignant		Mono Test	86308	
Well Exam 18–39 yrs.	99395		Benign		Pap Smear	88155	
Well Exam 40–64 yrs.	99396		Location		Pregnancy Test	84703	
Obstetrics			Exc. Skin Tags (1–15)	11200	Obstetric Panel	80055	
Total OB Care	59400		Each Additional 10	11201	Pro Time	85610	
Injections			Fracture Treatment		PSA	84153	
Administration Sub. / IM	90772		Loc		RPR	86592	
Drug			w/Reduc w/o Reduc		Sed. Rate	85651	
Dosage			I & D Abscess Single/Simple	10060	Stool Culture	87045	
Allergy	95115		Multiple or Comp	10061	Stool O & P	87177	
Cocci Skin Test	86490		I & D Pilonidal Cyst Simple	10080	Strep Screen	87880	
DPT	90701		Pilonidal Cyst Complex	10081	Theophylline	80198	
Hemophilus	90646		IV Therapy—To One Hour	90760	Thyroid Uptake	84479	
Influenza	90658		Each Additional Hour	90761	TSH	84443	
MMR	90707		Laceration Repair		Urinalysis	81000	
OPV	90712		Location Size Simp/Comp		Urine Culture	87088	
Pneumovax	90732		Laryngoscopy	31505	Drawing Fee	36415	
TB Skin Test	86580		Oximetry	94760	Specimen Collection	99000	
TD	90718		Punch Biopsy		**Other:**		
Unlisted Immun	90749		Rhythm Strip	93040			
Tetanus Toxoid	90703		Treadmill	93015			
Vaccine/Toxoid Admin <8 Yr Old w/ Counseling	90465		Trigger Point or Tendon Sheath Inj.	20550			
Vaccine/Toxoid Administration for Adult	90471		Tympanometry	92567			

Diagnosis/ICD-9: **491.9**

I acknowledge receipt of medical services and authorize the release of any medical information necessary to process this claim for healthcare payment only. I do authorize payment to the provider.

Patient Signature *Gerardo Lamos*

Total Estimated Charges: _____

Payment Amount: _____

Next Appointment: _____

Figure 15-9

Capital City Medical
Fee Schedule

New Patient OV		Punch Biopsy various codes	$80
Problem Focused 99201	$45	Nebulizer various codes	$45
Expanded Problem Focused 99202	$65	Cast Application various codes	$85
Detailed 99203	$85	Laryngoscopy 31505	$255
Comprehensive 99204	$105	Audiometry 92552	$85
Comprehensive/High Complex 99205	$115	Tympanometry 92567	$85
Well Exam infant (less than 1 year) 99381	$45	Ear Irrigation 69210	$25
Well Exam 1–4 yrs. 99382	$50	Diaphragm Fitting 57170	$30
Well Exam 5–11 yrs. 99383	$55	IV Therapy (up to one hour) 90760	$65
Well Exam 12–17 yrs. 99384	$65	Each additional hour 90761	$50
Well Exam 18–39 yrs. 99385	$85	Oximetry 94760	$10
Well Exam 40–64 yrs. 99386	$105	ECG 93000	$75
Established Patient OV		Holter Monitor various codes	$170
Post Op Follow Up Visit 99024	$0	Rhythm Strip 93040	$60
Minimum 99211	$35	Treadmill 93015	$375
Problem Focused 99212	$45	Cocci Skin Test 86490	$20
Expanded Problem Focused 99213	$55	X-ray, spine, chest, bone—any area various codes	$275
Detailed 99214	$65	Avulsion Nail 11730	$200
Comprehensive/High Complex 99215	$75	**Laboratory**	
Well exam infant (less than 1 year) 99391	$35	Amylase 82150	$40
Well Exam 1–4 yrs. 99392	$40	B12 82607	$30
Well Exam 5–11 yrs. 99393	$45	CBC & Diff 85025	$95
Well Exam 12–17 yrs. 99394	$55	Comp Metabolic Panel 80053	$75
Well Exam 18–39 yrs. 99395	$65	Chlamydia Screen 87110	$70
Well Exam 40–64 yrs. 99396	$75	Cholestrerol 82465	$75
Obstetrics		Digoxin 80162	$40
Total OB Care 59400	$1700	Electrolytes 80051	$70
Injections		Estrogen, Total 82672	$50
Administration 90772	$10	Ferritin 82728	$40
Allergy 95115	$35	Folate 82746	$30
DPT 90701	$50	GC Screen 87070	$60
Drug various codes	$35	Glucose 82947	$35
Influenza 90658	$25	Glycosylated HGB A1C 83036	$45
MMR 90707	$50	HCT 85014	$30
OPV 90712	$40	HDL 83718	$35
Pneumovax 90732	$35	HGB 85018	$30
TB Skin Test 86580	$15	Hep BSAG 83740	$40
TD 90718	$40	Hepatitis panel, acute 80074	$95
Tetanus Toxoid 90703	$40	HIV 86703	$100
Vaccine/Toxoid Administration for Younger Than 8 Years Old w/ counseling 90465	$10	Iron & TIBC 83550	$45
		Kidney Profile 80069	$95
Vaccine/Toxoid Administration for Adult 90471	$10	Lead 83665	$55
Arthrocentesis/Aspiration/Injection		Lipase 83690	$40
Small Joint 20600	$50	Lipid Panel 80061	$95
Interm Joint 20605	$60	Liver Profile 80076	$95
Major Joint 20610	$70	Mono Test 86308	$30
Trigger Point/Tendon Sheath Inj. 20550	$90	Pap Smear 88155	$90
Other Invasive/Noninvasive Procedures		Pap Collection/Supervision 88142	$95
Catheterization 51701	$55	Pregnancy Test 84703	$90
Circumcision 54150	$150	Obstetric Panel 80055	$85
Colposcopy 57452	$225	Pro Time 85610	$50
Colposcopy w/Biopsy 57454	$250	PSA 84153	$50
Cryosurgery Premalignant Lesion various codes	$160	RPR 86592	$55
Endometrial Biopsy 58100	$190	Sed. Rate 85651	$50
Excision Lesion Malignant various codes	$145	Stool Culture 87045	$80
Excision Lesion Benign various codes	$125	Stool O & P 87177	$105
Curettement Lesion		Strep Screen 87880	$35
Single 11055	$70	Theophylline 80198	$40
2–4 11056	$80	Thyroid Uptake 84479	$75
>4 11057	$90	TSH 84443	$50
Excision Skin Tags (1–15) 11200	$55	Urinalysis 81000	$35
Each Additional 10 11201	$30	Urine Culture 87088	$80
I & D Abscess Single/Simple 10060	$75	Drawing Fee 36415	$15
Multiple/Complex 10061	$95	Specimen Collection 99000	$10
I & D Pilonidal Cyst Simple 10080	$105		
I & D Pilonidal Cyst Complex 10081	$130		
Laceration Repair various codes	$60		

HEALTH INSURANCE CLAIM FORM

APPROVED BY NATIONAL UNIFORM CLAIM COMMITTEE 08/05

☐☐PICA | PICA ☐☐☐

| 1. MEDICARE ☐(Medicare #) | MEDICAID ☐(Medicaid #) | TRICARE CHAMPUS ☐(Sponsor's SSN) | CHAMPVA ☐(Member ID#) | GROUP HEALTH PLAN ☐(SSN or ID) | FECA BLK LUNG ☐(SSN) | OTHER ☐(ID) | 1a. INSURED'S I.D. NUMBER | (For Program in Item 1) |

2. PATIENT'S NAME (Last Name, First Name, Middle Initial)

3. PATIENT'S BIRTH DATE MM DD YY **SEX** M☐ F☐

4. INSURED'S NAME (Last Name, First Name, Middle Initial)

5. PATIENT'S ADDRESS (No., Street)

6. PATIENT RELATIONSHIP TO INSURED
Self☐ Spouse☐ Child☐ Other☐

7. INSURED'S ADDRESS (No., Street)

CITY | STATE

8. PATIENT STATUS
Single☐ Married☐ Other☐
Employed☐ Full-Time Student☐ Part-Time Student☐

CITY | STATE

ZIP CODE | TELEPHONE (Include Area Code) ( )

ZIP CODE | TELEPHONE (Include Area Code) ( )

9. OTHER INSURED'S NAME (Last Name, First Name, Middle Initial)

10. IS PATIENT'S CONDITION RELATED TO:

11. INSURED'S POLICY GROUP OR FECA NUMBER

a. OTHER INSURED'S POLICY OR GROUP NUMBER

a. EMPLOYMENT? (Current or Previous)
☐YES ☐NO

a. INSURED'S DATE OF BIRTH MM DD YY SEX M☐ F☐

b. OTHER INSURED'S DATE OF BIRTH MM DD YY SEX M☐ F☐

b. AUTO ACCIDENT? PLACE (State)
☐YES ☐NO ☐

b. EMPLOYER'S NAME OR SCHOOL NAME

c. EMPLOYER'S NAME OR SCHOOL NAME

c. OTHER ACCIDENT?
☐YES ☐NO

c. INSURANCE PLAN NAME OR PROGRAM NAME

d. INSURANCE PLAN NAME OR PROGRAM NAME

10d. RESERVED FOR LOCAL USE

d. IS THERE ANOTHER HEALTH BENEFIT PLAN?
☐YES ☐NO *If yes, return to and complete item 9 a-d.*

READ BACK OF FORM BEFORE COMPLETING & SIGNING THIS FORM.
12. PATIENT'S OR AUTHORIZED PERSON'S SIGNATURE I authorize the release of any medical or other information necessary to process this claim. I also request payment of government benefits either to myself or to the party who accepts assignment below.

SIGNED _____ DATE _____

13. INSURED'S OR AUTHORIZED PERSON'S SIGNATURE I authorize payment of medical benefits to the undersigned physician or supplier for services described below.

SIGNED _____

| 14. DATE OF CURRENT: MM DD YY | ◄ ILLNESS (First symptom) OR INJURY (Accident) OR PREGNANCY (LMP) | 15. IF PATIENT HAS HAD SAME OR SIMILAR ILLNESS, GIVE FIRST DATE MM DD YY | 16. DATES PATIENT UNABLE TO WORK IN CURRENT OCCUPATION FROM MM DD YY TO MM DD YY |

17. NAME OF REFERRING PHYSICIAN OR OTHER SOURCE | 17a. | 17b. NPI | 18. HOSPITALIZATION DATES RELATED TO CURRENT SERVICES FROM MM DD YY TO MM DD YY

19. RESERVED FOR LOCAL USE | 20. OUTSIDE LAB? ☐YES ☐NO | $ CHARGES

21. DIAGNOSIS OR NATURE OF ILLNESS OR INJURY (Relate Items 1,2,3 or 4 to Item 24E by Line)
1. |____.____ 3. |____.____
2. |____.____ 4. |____.____

22. MEDICAID RESUBMISSION CODE | ORIGINAL REF. NO.

23. PRIOR AUTHORIZATION NUMBER

24. A. DATE(S) OF SERVICE				B. PLACE OF SERVICE	C. EMG	D. PROCEDURES, SERVICES, OR SUPPLIES (Explain Unusual Circumstances) CPT/HCPCS MODIFIER	E. DIAGNOSIS POINTER	F. $ CHARGES	G. DAYS OR UNITS	H. EPSDT Family Plan	I. ID. QUAL.	J. RENDERING PROVIDER ID. #
From MM DD YY	To MM DD YY											
1											NPI	
2											NPI	
3											NPI	
4											NPI	
5											NPI	
6											NPI	

| 25. FEDERAL TAX I.D. NUMBER ☐☐ SSN EIN | 26. PATIENT'S ACCOUNT NO. | 27. ACCEPT ASSIGNMENT? (For govt. claims, see back) ☐YES ☐NO | 28. TOTAL CHARGE $ | 29. AMOUNT PAID $ | 30. BALANCE DUE $ |

31. SIGNATURE OF PHYSICIAN OR SUPPLIER INCLUDING DEGREES OR CREDENTIALS (I certify that the statements on the reverse apply to this bill and are made a part thereof.)

SIGNED _____ DATE _____

32. SERVICE FACILITY LOCATION INFORMATION

a. NPI | b.

33. BILLING PROVIDER INFO & PH. # ( )

a. NPI | b.

NUCC Instruction Manual available at: www.nucc.org
WCMS-1500CS

APPROVED OMB 0938-0999 FORM CMS-1500 (08/05)

Vertical margin text (right): CARRIER | PATIENT AND INSURED INFORMATION | PHYSICIAN OR SUPPLIER INFORMATION

Vertical margin text (left): SECOND FOLD | FIRST FOLD — WHCF-10-ENV / WHCF-10-ENV-SS

Figure 15-10

3. Using the information from Chapter 15 in your student text, complete the following table by comparing the TRICARE plans:

	TRICARE Standard/Extra	TRICARE Prime/Prime Remote
Type of Program		
Availability		
Enrollment		
Enrollment Fees		
Costs		
Provider choices		
MTF priority		
Primary care managers		
Referral and authorization requirements		
Clinical preventive care		

REVIEW QUESTIONS

MATCHING

Choose the correct answer, and write its corresponding letter in the space provided.

a. HCF
b. Nonavailability statement
c. Catastrophic cap
d. DEERS
e. CHAMPUS

1. _____ Database listing all eligible TRICARE recipients and their status of TRICARE coverage
2. _____ Former title of TRICARE
3. _____ An electronic document stating that a specific service required for a TRICARE patient is not provided at a nearby MTF, allowing for civilian medical services
4. _____ Assist the patient with the referral or preauthorization process.
5. _____ A limit placed on the total amount of medical expenses

MULTIPLE CHOICE

Circle the letter of the choice that best completes the statement or answers the question.

1. When does the TRICARE fiscal year begin?
   a. October 1
   b. January 1
   c. July 1
   d. January 15

2. For how many days is a NAS valid after the initial issuing date?
   a. 90 days
   b. 30 days
   c. 15 days
   d. 60 days

3. A non-par can charge how much for a visit?
   a. Up to 90% of charges.
   b. Up to 100% of charges
   c. Up to 115% of charges
   d. None of the above

4. The active duty service member under TRICARE is known as the _____.
   a. sponsor
   b. beneficiary
   c. Both a and b
   d. None of the above

5. An individual who qualifies for TRICARE under an active duty service member is known as the _____.
   a. sponsor
   b. beneficiary
   c. Both a and b
   d. None of the above

SHORT ANSWER

Provide the correct response to each question that follows:

1. What are the five TRICARE programs?

   1. _____

   2. _____

   3. _____

   4. _____

   5. _____

2. When might an NAS need to be filed?

   _____

3. What claim form is used by TRICARE and CHAMPVA for the following services?

   Inpatient_____

   Outpatient _____

4. How would the medical office specialist determine where to send a claim for the following programs?

   TRICARE

   _____

   _____

   _____

   CHAMPVA

   _____

   _____

   _____

5. a. Who is covered under CHAMPVA?

      _____

      _____

   b. To have CHAMPVA cover medical services, what type of facility must be used?

      _____

   c. What is required if a veteran wants to obtain community medical treatment?

      _____

      _____

   d. Do all medical services for veterans need approval prior to treatment?

      _____

TRUE/FALSE

Identify the statement as true (T) or false (F).

1. _____ All referrals and authorizations must be arranged by a TRICARE primary care manager (PCM) to ensure coverage of services to be provided.

2. _____ TRICARE Prime Remote is offered only in the United States and does not require enrollment in this program.

3. _____ If a patient has another type of insurance, Tricare is secondary.

4. _____ CHAMPVA is the primary payer to Medicare for services covered by both programs.

5. _____ MTF services do not vary per facility.

CHAPTER 16
Explanation of Benefits and Payment Adjudication

CHAPTER OBJECTIVES
◪

Upon completion of this chapter in your student text, you should be able to do the following:

1. Define the steps for filing a medical claim.
2. Understand the importance of the Explanation of Benefits and Electronic Remittance Advice forms.
3. Calculate accurate payment by a carrier or third-party payer.
4. Make adjustments to patient accounts.
5. Review reason codes.

CHAPTER OUTLINE
◪

Steps for Filing a Medical Claim

Claims Process

Determining the Fees
  Charge-Based Fee Structures
  Resource-Based Fee Structures

History of the Resource-Based Relative Value Scale

The RBRVS System

Determining the Medicare Fee

Allowed Charges

Payers' Policies

Capitation

Calculations of Patient Charges
  Deductible
  Copayments
  Coinsurance
  Excluded Services

Balance Billing

Processing an Explanation of Benefits
  Information on an EOB

Reviewing Claims Information

Adjustments to Patient Accounts
  Processing Reimbursement Information
  *Confirming Amount Paid, Making Adjustments, and Determining the
  Amount Due from Patient*

Methods of Receiving Funds
Check by Mail
Electronic Funds Transfer
Lockbox Services

KEY TERMS

Using the highlighted terms and glossary in the textbook, define the following terms:

1. adjudication_____

   _____

2. adjustment_____

   _____

3. allowed charge _____

   _____

4. appeal_____

   _____

5. balance billing_____

   _____

6. capitation plan _____

   _____

7. charge-based fees _____

   _____

8. conversion factor _____

   _____

9. coordination of benefits (COB) _____

   _____

10. Electronic Remittance Advice (ERA) _____

    _____

11. excluded services_____

    _____

12. Explanation of Benefits (EOB) _____

    _____

13. Geographic Practice Cost Index (GPCI) _____

    _____

14. lifetime maximum_____

    _____

15. manual review_____

    _____

16. Medicare conversion factor (MCF) _____

    _____

17. Medicare Fee Schedule (MFS)_____

    _____

18. nationally uniform relative value _____

_____

19. out-of-pocket expenses _____

_____

20. pending claim _____

_____

21. per member per month (PMPM) _____

_____

22. reason codes _____

_____

23. relative value unit (RVU) _____

_____

24. remark codes _____

_____

25. resource-based fees _____

_____

26. resource-based relative value scale (RBRVS) _____

_____

27. retention schedule _____

_____

28. turnaround time _____

_____

29. usual, customary, and reasonable (UCR)_____

_____

30. withhold_____

_____

31. write-offs _____

_____

CRITICAL THINKING QUESTIONS

Using the knowledge you have gained from reading the textbook, apply critical thinking skills to answer the following questions.

1. Before an EOB is received, what steps must be completed by the medical office specialist?

   1. _____

   2. _____

   3. _____

   4. _____

   5. _____

   6. _____

   7. _____

   8. _____

2. a. The insurance carrier has determined that a provided service is covered, but there is no reimbursement paid to the rendering provider. Will an EOB still be sent out? If so, who will receive the EOB? _____

b. Refer to the preceding question. Would an ERA be sent out? If so, who will receive the ERA?
_____

3. You are a claim examiner and have decided that a claim needs to be pulled for a manual review. What would you request from the rendering medical provider to help you to determine whether the claim should be paid or denied?

_____

_____

4. You are a medical billing specialist and have just received an EOB from an insurance carrier. What information is listed on the EOB?

_____

_____

_____

_____

_____

5. a. As the medical office specialist, you have just received an EOB on patient Irma Winslott. What steps must be taken before you post this information?

_____

_____

_____

_____

_____

b. Once you have taken the steps described in your answer to the previous question and accuracy has been established, where would you post this information?

_____

_____

_____

c. If an error has been identified on Irma's EOB, what is the first step to locating the error?

_____

_____

_____

d. Irma's claim has been sent back to the office as denied, and it is clear that this claim should have been paid. What should you do to obtain payment?

_____

_____

_____

PRACTICE EXERCISES

1. a. Using the information in Chapter 16 of your student text, determine the Medicare allowed fee for the following geographical areas by using the GPCIs and conversion factor for 2011, which is $33,974:

Locality	Work GPCI	Practice Expense GPCI	Malpractice Expense GPCI
Capital City	1.050	1.042	0.155
Township	1.020	1.106	0.080

Code	Work RVU	Practice RVU	Malpractice RVU
99203	1.25	1.16	0.20
99213	0.94	0.98	0.15

b. Use the initial 2011 conversion factor of $33.9764 to complete the following:

	Capital City	Township
99203:		
99213:		

2. Using the given information, calculate the following charges:

Mason Winston was seen in the office today for immunizations. The total charges are $100. The allowed amount is $80. His benefits pay 80 percent. His policy has a deductible of $25.

Usual Charge _____

Allowed Charge _____

Deductible _____

Policy pays _____ of the allowed charge after deductible, which is _____.

Patient responsible for the _____ of the allowed charge plus the deductible, which is _____.

Provider writes off the difference between the usual and allowed _____.

3. On the following examples of information provided in an explanation of benefits, complete the tables with the payment information given for each:

a.

Physician Charges	Allowed Amounts	Insurance Pays	Deductible
75.00	52.00	80%	150.00*
145.00	103.00		
110.00	86.00		

Charge	Adjustment	Allowed	Deductible	Co-pay	Ins. Pays	Coinsurance
$	$	$	$	$	$	$
$	$	$	$	$	$	$
$	$	$	$	$	$	$
TOTALS $	$	$	$	$	$	$

*Deductible not met.

Balance due from patient:

Patient's deductible: $_____

Patient's coinsurance: $_____

Total due: $_____

Total insurance pays: $_____

Total physician write-off: $_____

b.

Physician Charges	Allowed Amounts	Insurance Pays	Deductible
3,625.00	75%	70%	350.00*

Charge	Adjustment	Allowed	Deductible	Copay	Ins. Pays	Coinsurance
$	$	$	$	$	$	$
TOTALS $	$	$	$	$	$	$

*$50.00 of deductible has been met.

Balance due from patient:

Patient's deductible: $_____

Patient's coinsurance: $_____

Total due: $_____

Total insurance pays: $_____

Total physician write-off: $_____

4. a. Complete the following EOB:

Today's Date

Payer Name & Address

Health Insurance Co.
777 Corporate Way
Capital City, NY 12345

Provider's Name & Address

Phil Wells, M.D.
123 Unknown Boulevard
Capital City, TX 12345

This statement covers payments for the following patient(s):
Claim Detail Section (*Hint:* If there are numbers in the "SEE REMARKS" column, see the Remarks Section for an explanation.)

Patient Name: McGee, Regina	**Patient Account #:** RM0562
Patient ID#: 319-91-6257	**Insured's Name:** McGee, Regina
Group #: 55216	
Provider Name: Phil Wells, M.D.	**Inventory #:** 44597 **Claim Control #:** 28940

Service Date(s)	Procedure	Charges	Adjustment	Allowed	Co-pay	Deduct/Not Covered	Coins	Paid At.	Provider Paid/Remarks
07/09/2007	99213 OV	55.00		32.00	0.00	0.00		80%	
07/09/2007	69210 Ear Irr.	25.00		10.00	0.00	0.00		80%	
TOTALS									

BALANCE DUE FROM PATIENT: PT'S DED/NOT COV $_____

PT'S COINS. $_____

031 Met Maximum Limit

PAYMENT SUMMARY SECTION (Totals)

Charges	Adjustment	Allowed	Copay	Deduct/Not Covered	Coins	Total Paid

THIS IS NOT A BILL

b. Answer the following questions Regina has concerning her EOB:

1. What does it mean when the statement, "THIS IS NOT A BILL" appears on the EOB?

_____

_____

_____

_____

_____

2. Explain to Regina what the difference is between the copay and deductible.

_____

_____

_____

_____

_____

3. Explain to Regina what the Deduct/Not Covered column means.

_____

_____

_____

_____

_____

4. Explain to Regina why there is a difference between the allowed charge and the insurance carrier's actual payment.

_____

_____

_____

_____

_____

5. Using the EOB provided, fill in the following information:

Health Insurance Company

Health Insurance HMO

777 Corporate Way

Capital City, WI 12345

800-555-9876

Explanation of Benefits

Insured Name:	Gavin Retort
Insured ID/SS#:	505-11-3223
Policy:	
Claim Number:	LP-60042-003
Control Number:	208652144
Date:	01/31/08

Below is an Explanation of Benefits for your Medical Coveage

Patient: Gavin Retort **Patient ID/SS#:** 505-11-3223

Provider Name: Phil Wells, M.D. **Patient Account #:** GR375100

Service Code	Service Description	Service Date(s)	Provider Charge	Allowed Amount	Discount Amount	Not Covered	Deductible	Copay	Pay At	Remarks	Amount Paid
99386	Well Exam	01/16/08	$105.00	$77.60	$27.40	$0.00	$0.00	$20.00	100%	0054	$57.60
TOTALS			$105.00	$77.60	$27.40	$0.00	$0.00	$20.00			$47.60

Remarks

0054 PPO-Preferred Provider benefits applied. Your provider has agreed to the negotiated rate in accordance with the Private Healthcare Systems provider agreement. You should not be billed for this amount.

Payment Summary

Payment Sent To:	Phil Wells, M.D.
Payment Amount:	$67.60
Payment Date:	01/31/08
Patient's Portion:	$20.00

Total Payment Summary

Payment(s) Sent To:	Phil Wells, M.D.
Total Payment Amount:	$67.60
Payment Date:	01/31/08

*TOTAL PATIENT PORTION: $20.00

Insurance company name: _____

Patient's name: _____

Patient's ID: _____

Provider's name: _____

Date of service: _____

Total charge: _____

Procedure(s): _____

Copay: _____

Deductible: _____

Coinsurance due from patient: _____

Allowed amount: _____

Discount amount: _____

Noncovered items: _____

Rate of benefit (%): _____

Amount paid: _____

Remarks: _____

Outcome: ☐ Bill patient balance ☐ Call carrier

☐ Appeal ☐ Claim paid in full

REVIEW QUESTIONS

MATCHING

Choose the correct answer, and place its corresponding letter in the space provided.

a. discount amount
b. deductible
c. allowed charges
d. coinsurance
e. adjustment

1. _____ Difference between provider charges and allowed amount; amount physician must write off
2. _____ Maximum allowed amount for a covered charge that includes the amount both the insurance carrier and the patient will pay
3. _____ Amount of money owed by a patient every year that must be met before health insurance pays at 100 percent
4. _____ The percentage of money owed by a patient for provided medical services
5. _____ A positive or negative change to a patient's account balance, including corrections and write-offs

MULTIPLE CHOICE

Circle the letter of the choice that best completes the statement or answers the question.

1. Which of the following is stated on an EOB?
   a. The status of a claim
   b. The patient's demographics, including services provided
   c. Charges, adjustments, and any patient out-of-pocket expenses
   d. All of the above

2. Which of the following is a reason that a manually reviewed claim would be denied?
   a. Lack of required preauthorization
   b. Lack of medical necessity
   c. Lack of eligibility for a reported procedure
   d. All of the above

3. What is balance billing?
   a. Accepting allowed amount
   b. Billing patient for amount left after insurance payment
   c. Billing patient for discounted amount
   d. Both b and c

4. The act of billing a patient for any monetary amount left after the insurance carrier has made payment is known as _____.
   a. adjudication
   b. balance billing
   c. turn-around billing
   d. direct payment

5. EOB explanation codes often used by insurance carriers are also known as _____.
   a. reason codes
   b. direct codes
   c. remark codes
   d. Both a and c

SHORT ANSWER

Provide the correct response to each question that follows.

1. What are four examples of a patient's out-of-pocket expenses?
    1. _____
    2. _____
    3. _____
    4. _____

2. When should a patient's out-of-pocket expenses be collected? _____

3. What is an ERA? _____

4. What are the three explanations for the status of a claim?
    1. _____
    2. _____
    3. _____

5. Answer the following questions related to RBRVS calculations for reimbursement:
    a. Briefly explain the three cost elements related to the National Uniform Relative Value.
        1. Provider's work_____

        2. Practice expense _____

        3. Professional liability insurance _____

    b. Briefly explain the Geographic Practice Cost Index (GPCI). _____

    c. Briefly explain the Nationally Uniform Conversion Factor. _____

    d. How often is the Nationally Uniform Conversion Factor updated? _____

TRUE/FALSE

Identify the statement as true (T) or false (F).

1. _____ More than one patient can be listed on an EOB.

2. _____ A dated front and back copy of the patient's insurance card should be filed in the patient's medical chart.

3. _____ A lockbox service helps with faster collection of payments.

4. _____ A nonparticipating provider can bill a patient for fees not covered by the insurance carrier's allowed charge.

5. _____ A participating provider can bill a patient for fees not covered by the insurance carrier's allowed charge.

CHAPTER 17
Refunds, Follow-up, and Appeals

CHAPTER OBJECTIVES

Upon completion of this chapter in your student text, you should be able to do the following:

1. Understand reimbursement follow-up.
2. Know the common problems and solutions for denied or delayed payments.
3. Use problem-solving and communication skills to answer patients' questions about claims.
4. Format medical records with proper documentation.
5. Understand the appeals process and register a formal appeal.
6. Understand ERISA rules and regulations.
7. Write letters of appeal on denied claims.
8. Understand refund guidelines.
9. Rebill insurance claims.
10. Discuss the three levels of Medicare appeals.
11. Calculate and issue refunds.

CHAPTER OUTLINE

Claims Rejection Follow-Up

Rebilling

Denied or Delayed Payments

Answering Patients' Questions about Claims

Claim Rejection Appeal

Peer Review

State Insurance Commissioner

Carrier Audits

Documentation
   Documentation Guidelines
   SOAP Record-Keeping Format

Necessity of Appeals

Registering a Formal Appeal

The Appeals Process
   Reason Codes That Require a Formal Appeal

Employee Retirement Income Security Act of 1974
   Waiting Period for an ERISA Claim
   Appeal to ERISA

KEY TERMS

Using the highlighted terms and glossary in the textbook, define the following terms:

1. administrative law judge (ALJ) hearing _____

   _____

2. documentation _____

   _____

3. Employee Retirement Income Security Act (ERISA) of 1974 _____

   _____

4. follow-up _____

   _____

5. insurance commissioner _____

   _____

6. peer review _____

   _____

7. qualified independent contractors (QICs) _____

   _____

8. redetermination_____

   _____

9. SOAP format_____

   _____

CRITICAL THINKING QUESTIONS

Using the knowledge you have gained from reading the textbook, apply critical thinking skills to answer the following questions:

1. Answer the following questions related to responding to a patient's questions about a claim:

   a. Mr. Tim calls, and he is upset about a bill that he received from your clinic. What should you do first, and why? _____

   _____

   _____

b. When looking up Mr. Tim's information, you find the claim was denied, and the reason was stated as no coverage at the time of service. What should you do?

_____

_____

_____

_____

2. Identify a solution for each given scenario when a claim needs to be rebilled.

a. A patient was seen by a podiatrist for pain in his right heel. An X-ray was taken that showed evidence of a heel spur. The physician documented a cortisone injection in the right heel in the patient's chart, but forgot to document the injection on the superbill. A week after the claim submittal, you identify that the cortisone injection wasn't billed. What should be done to receive reimbursement for the injection?

_____

_____

_____

b. A patient had two different ultrasounds for a related problem within 2 weeks of each other. She had a pelvic ultrasound on May 13 and a transvaginal ultrasound on May 24. You discover that the transvaginal ultrasound was never billed. What should be done to receive reimbursement for the second ultrasound?

_____

_____

_____

3. a. Who is notified by an insurance carrier when a claim has been denied?

_____

b. You are sending an appeal letter to an insurance carrier for a denied claim to be reconsidered for reimbursement. What is the first step that must be taken before you begin to write the appeal letter?

_____

_____

c. You have received a denied claim letter from Max Cambridge's insurance carrier. What types of actions should be taken to assure Mr. Cambridge that you are making your best effort in seeking a resolution to this problem?

_____

_____

_____

4. Part of your job description is to ensure that an insurance audit runs smoothly. What are the three main steps to avoid problems during an insurance audit?

1. _____

2. _____

3. _____

5. Answer the following questions regarding researching the validity of a refund request by an insurance carrier or patient:

a. An insurance carrier sends a request for a refund because a patient's coverage was canceled prior to the date that services were rendered. What should you do before preparing the refund?

_____

_____

_____

b. An insurance carrier sends a request for a refund because of an overpayment. What should you do before preparing the refund?

_____

_____

_____

c. An insurance carrier sends a request for a refund because it paid as the primary payer when it should have paid as the secondary payer. What should you do before preparing the refund?

_____

_____

_____

d. A patient requests a refund for overpayment of her Medicare deductible for the year. She forgot that she had previously paid the deductible 2 weeks ago at another physician's office. After contacting Medicare, you find out that she has in fact paid the deductible previous to her appointment at your office. What should you do?

_____

_____

_____

e. A patient prepays for services that end up being covered by his insurance carrier. What should you do before preparing the refund?

_____

_____

_____

PRACTICE EXERCISES

1. a. Using the information presented in Chapter 17 of your student text, read the given items and determine what part of the SOAP format each is. Write S for subjective, O for objective, A for assessment, and P for plan, in the spaces provided.

1. Cymbalta 60 mg qday. _____

2. Patient states he has had right upper abdominal pain for 3 days. _____

3. CBC and CMP were run to check for kidney infection. _____

4. Primary complaint is regarding left knee pain for 1 month. _____

5. It was determined that the patient has atrial fibrillation. _____

b. In your own words, explain the difference between subjective and objective data.

_____

_____

_____

_____

Read the given scenarios and decide whether each query can be responded to by telephone or by written appeal. Provide your answers in the spaces shown.

a. An insurance carrier sends a letter of request to a patient for an update on the patient's address.

_____

b. An insurance carrier contacts the office for additional clinical documentation to process a claim.

_____

c. An emergency procedure was performed without preauthorization.

_____

d. A claim was denied because the procedure was not considered to be medically necessary. The physician believes that it was.

_____

2. Read the following delayed or denied claim scenarios, decide what would be the appropriate solution for each, and provide your answers in the spaces shown.

a. A patient has a surgical procedure that didn't have the required preauthorization.

_____

_____

b. A patient is seen for a preexisting condition that is not covered by the insurance carrier.

_____

_____

3. In the following space, write an appeal for patient Mary Thompson. She had an abdominal and a pelvic CT performed that the insurance carrier ruled as medically unnecessary. She recently had an abdominopelvic ultrasound, which was negative for any disease process, but she still complains of severe pain in her abdomen. Be sure to use positive reinforcement within your appeal letter.

_____

_____

_____

_____

_____

_____

_____

_____

_____

_____

_____

_____
_____
_____
_____
_____
_____
_____
_____
_____
_____
_____
_____
_____
_____
_____
_____
_____
_____
_____
_____
_____
_____
_____
_____
_____
_____
_____
_____

4. A patient requests a refund on his $200 deductible. He forgot that he paid it previously at his last appointment. You check his records, and he has, in fact, paid it twice this year. He does have an outstanding balance of $80 with your office. What is the amount that the patient will receive for a refund?

_____

REVIEW QUESTIONS

MATCHING

Choose the correct answer, and place its corresponding letter in the space provided.

a. peer review
b. insurance commissioner
c. redetermination
d. denied claim
e. claim appeal

1. _____ An unbiased group of physicians that determines adequate payment for provided medical services after an appeal has been denied by an insurance carrier

2. _____ Medicare review of a first-level appealed claim

3. _____ Written request for a review of a denied claim that asks an insurance carrier to reconsider reimbursement for rendered medical services

4. _____ Regulates insurance companies and serves as a liaison between the patient and carrier and between the physician and carrier; can aid in settling complaints related to claim reimbursement

5. _____ A claim that is not paid by the insurance carrier due to issues such as lack of coverage, preexisting conditions, or non-covered benefit

MULTIPLE CHOICE

Circle the letter of the choice that best completes the statement or answers the question.

1. Which of the following is a reason that an insurance carrier may ask a medical provider to rebill?
   a. Missing or incomplete claim information
   b. Errors on a claim
   c. A service provided was not medically necessary
   d. Both a and b

2. Overpayment can occur for all of the following reasons *except*:
   a. the patient pays too much.
   b. both payers pay as primary.
   c. both patient and payer pay at the same time.
   d. None of the above

3. Who can file a complaint with the Insurance Commissioner?
   a. The patient
   b. The physician
   c. The insurance carrier
   d. Both a and b

4. Which of the following is an acceptable signature on an appeal letter?
   a. Signature of the provider on the claim form only, but not on the appeal letter
   b. Actual signature or stamped signature of the provider or authorized employee
   c. Signature of the provider represented by the signature and initials of an authorized employee
   d. Both b and c

5. A wrongful retention of an insurance carrier's overpayment is known as _____.
   a. Conversion
   b. Contestment
   c. Reception
   d. Both a and c

SHORT ANSWER

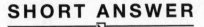

Provide the correct response to each of the following questions:

1. Why is it important to alert the payer if you are rebilling a claim?

   _____

   _____

   _____

2. List two ways that follow-up of an outstanding claim can be accomplished.
   1. _____

      _____

   2. _____

      _____

3. a. What is a disallowance?

      _____

      _____

   b. When appealing a disallowance, the medical office specialist should include what important information?

      _____

      _____

4. Name six persons to whom to redirect an appeal and why.
   1. _____

      _____

   2. _____

      _____

   3. _____

      _____

   4. _____

      _____

   5. _____

      _____

   6. _____

      _____

5. What are three reasons that an overpayment from an insurance carrier can occur?

   1. _____

   2. _____

   3. _____

TRUE/FALSE

Identify each statement as true (T) or false (F).

1. _____ An insurance claim must be monitored until payment is received.

2. _____ If a claim states that the patient's coverage has been cancelled, the medical office specialist should rebill.

3. _____ Valid court rulings and federal and state laws should be used as references in appeal letters.

4. _____ The medical office specialist should always research a refund requested by an insurance carrier before submitting the refund.

5. _____ Insurance carriers are not allowed to automatically recoup overpayments that were issued to a medical provider.

CHAPTER 18
Workers' Compensation

CHAPTER OBJECTIVES

Upon completion of this chapter in your student text, you should be able to do the following:

1. Understand the history of workers' compensation.
2. Distinguish between federal workers' compensation and state workers' compensation.
3. List the classifications of a work-related injury.
4. Know injured workers' responsibilities and rights.
5. Understand the responsibility of the treating doctor/physician of record.
6. Understand the role of an ombudsman in assisting with claims.
7. Know the four types of workers' compensation benefits.
8. Be able to discuss the different types of disability.
9. Accurately complete a CMS-1500 form for a workers' compensation claim.
10. Determine the workers' compensation fee based on the Medicare Fee Schedule.

CHAPTER OUTLINE

History of Workers' Compensation

Federal Workers' Compensation Programs

State Workers' Compensation Plans

Overview of Covered Injuries, Illnesses, and Benefits
   Occupational Diseases and Illnesses
   Work-Related Injury Classifications

Injured Worker Responsibilities and Rights

Treating Doctor's Responsibilities
   Selecting a Designated Doctor and Scheduling an Appointment
   Communicating with the Designated Doctor
   What the Designated Doctor Will Do
   Disputing the Designated Doctor's Findings

Disputing Maximum Medical Improvement or Impairment Rating

Ombudsmen

Types of Workers' Compensation Benefits
   Income Benefits
   Death and Burial Benefits

Eligible Beneficiaries
  Dependent Child, Grandchild, and Other Eligible Parties
Benefits and Compensation Termination
  Types of Government Disability Policies
Verifying Insurance Benefits
Preauthorization
  Requirements for the Preauthorization Request
Filing Insurance Claims
Completing the CMS-1500 for Workers' Compensation Claims
Independent Review Organizations
  How to Obtain an Independent Review
  The IRO Decision
Medical Records
Fraud
  Penalties
  Medical Provider Fraud
Calculating Reimbursements

KEY TERMS

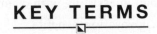

Using the highlighted terms and glossary in the textbook, define the following terms.

1. Admission of Liability _____
   _____

2. burial benefits _____
   _____

3. death benefits _____
   _____

4. designated doctor _____
   _____

5. disability _____
   _____

6. disability compensation programs _____
   _____

7. District of Columbia Workers' Compensation Act _____
   _____

8. Employer's First Report of Injury or Illness _____
   _____

9. Energy Employees' Occupational Illness Compensation Program Act (EEOICP) _____
   _____

10. Federal Coal Mine Health and Safety Act (Black Lung Benefits Reform Act) _____
    _____

11. Federal Employees' Compensation Act (FECA) _____

12. final report_____

13. fraud indicators_____

14. impairment _____

15. impairment income benefits _____

16. impairment rating_____

17. income benefits _____

18. independent review organization (IRO) _____

19. lifetime income benefits _____

20. Longshore and Harbor Workers' Compensation Act (LHWCA)_____

21. maximum medical improvement _____

22. medical benefits _____

23. Notice of Contest _____

24. occupational diseases and illnesses_____

25. Occupational Safety and Health Act _____

26. Occupational Safety and Health Administration (OSHA) _____

27. Office of Workers' Compensation Programs (OWCP) _____

28. ombudsmen_____

29. physician of record_____

30. Social Security Disability Insurance (SSDI) _____

31. supplemental income benefits _____

32. temporary income benefits _____
_____

33. treating doctor _____
_____

34. Veteran's Disability Compensation _____
_____

35. Veteran's Disability Pension Benefits _____
_____

36. vocational rehabilitation _____
_____

37. Work Status Report _____
_____

CRITICAL THINKING QUESTIONS

Using the knowledge you have gained from reading the textbook, apply critical thinking skills to answer the following questions.

1. In the following scenarios, determine what type of income benefit each patient qualifies for:

    a. Injured worker Melissa McCain was in an accident in a work vehicle, which resulted in amputation of both legs as a result of injuries sustained. What type of income benefits does she qualify for?

    _____

    b. Injured worker Joe Williams was injured at work and assigned an impairment rating of 18%. He is earning 80% less than the state wage and did not take a lump sum payment of impairment income benefits. What type of income benefits does he qualify for?

    _____

    c. Injured worker Howard White was burned on the hand and has been off for 7 days. What type of income benefit does he qualify for?

    _____

2. a. You have just made an initial appointment for Jackie Alberto for a workers' compensation appointment. How would you verify that she is covered under a workers' compensation plan?

    _____
    _____
    _____

    b. Injured worker Miles Wetherby has not filed an injury report with his employer. Can his regular health insurance plan cover his visit to your office for this injury?

    _____
    _____
    _____

3. After reading each given scenario, determine whether each injury would be either covered or not covered by workers' compensation insurance. Write C for covered and NC for not covered in the spaces provided.

    a. Rodger Ludwig injures his back while helping a patient onto the exam table.

    _____

    b. Marissa Javen trips and sprains her left ankle while getting on the elevator at work.

    _____

    c. Henry Wakeman cuts off the tip of his right index finger while using the meat slicer at work. He had stopped at the bar before his shift that day and had a few shots of whiskey.

    _____

    d. Bret Galloway is a welder. Lately, he has been experiencing moderate pain and numbness in his left arm, especially near the elbow. After examination, it is determined that he has cubital tunnel.

    _____

    e. Eddie Mann works in an automotive shop. He has been warned on many occasions that he is to wear safety glasses when performing certain procedures, yet he fails to abide by the rules because the glasses are "too uncomfortable." A piece of metal suddenly embeds in his left eye and scratches the cornea significantly.

    _____

    f. Elise Stanton is a mail carrier. Yesterday while working, a straight-end wind caused a branch to break off of a tree and strike her in the head, causing a mild contusion.

    _____

4. Read the given statements and determine the type of workers' compensation fraud being committed for each scenario presented. Write whether each indicates *employer fraud*, *employee fraud*, *attorney fraud*, or *medical provider fraud* in the spaces provided.

    a. A single procedure is unbundled when billed.

    _____

    b. A suspicious injury occurs right before punch-out time on Friday afternoon.

    _____

    c. Reporting of a smaller amount of payroll than what is true.

    _____

    d. Underutilization.

    _____

    e. A worker who is under workers' compensation has been bartending full time. His friend owns the bar, so he is being paid "off the books."

    _____

    f. A worker who has claimed a back injury was seen moving a couch into his house.

    _____

    g. An attorney charges for an unexplainable number of hours worked with the injured workers' case.

    _____

5. a. What would you do if you suspected that a patient was committing workers' compensation fraud? Would you notify anyone? If so, whom?

_____

_____

b. What would you do if you suspected that the physician you work for was committing workers' compensation fraud? Would you notify anyone? If so, whom?

_____

_____

c. An injured worker is being investigated by the local district attorney for possible workers' compensation fraud. She has been receiving both medical and income benefits. She is compensated $2500 per month by the state. If she is found guilty of workers' compensation fraud, what penalties can she encounter? What type of crime is this considered to be?

_____

_____

_____

_____

_____

PRACTICE EXERCISES

1. Using the form locator information written out on your index cards from a prior chapter, complete the following activity. Flag those FLs that would be filled out differently for workers' compensation patients.

2. Follow the directions in your student text on calculating the workers' compensation reimbursement for the CPT codes listed, and use your state to complete this exercise.

CPT Code	MFS	WC
99202		
99203		
99201		
99211		
99213		
99214		

3. The given case studies are provided for additional practice in completing the CMS-1500 claim form for workers' compensation physician outpatient billing. By applying what you have learned in your student text, accurately code and complete each case study. Patient demographics and a brief case history are provided. Complete the cases on the basis of the following assumptions:

- All patients have release of information and assignment of benefit signatures on file as a condition for workers' compensation. Items 12 and 13 should not be completed.

- All providers are participating and accept assignment by law. Item 27 should not be marked.

- The group practice is the billing entity.

- The national transition to NPI numbers is complete, and legacy PINs of individual payers are no longer used. If legacy PINS are still being used by your state's workers' compensation program, your instructor may provide legacy PINs in addition to the NPI.

- 2012 ICD-9-CM and CPT codes are used.

- Use eight-digit dates for birthdates. Use six-digit dates for all other dates.

- All street names should be entered with standard postal abbreviations, even if they are spelled out on the source documents.

- Enter ICD-9 codes in the order they appear on the encounter form.

- When entering CPT codes, enter the E/M code first. Enter remaining CPT codes in descending price order.

- Enter the workers' compensation assigned claim number in Item 1a. (Requirements will vary by state.)

Complete each case study. To determine the correct fees, refer to the Capital City Medical Fee Schedule, which is located after each case's source documents. Use the blank CMS-1500 form provided after each case.

a. Using the source documents, the Capital City Medical Fee Schedule (Figure 18-1), and the blank CMS-1500 form provided (Figure 18-2), complete the following case study for patient Zoe Rocco (Case 18-1):

CASE 18-1

Capital City Medical—123 Unknown Boulevard, Capital City, NY 12345-2222 (555) 555-1234 Phil Wells, MD, Mannie Mends, MD, Bette R. Soone, MD	Patient Information Form Tax ID: 75-0246810 Group NPI: 1513171216

Patient Information:

Name: (Last, First) Rocco, Zoe   ☒ Male ☐ Female   Birth Date: 01/04/1968

Address: 431 Mason Dr, Capital City, NY 12345   Phone: (555) 555-4334

Social Security Number: 361-71-6650   Full-Time Student: ☐ Yes ☒ No

Marital Status: ☐ Single ☒ Married ☐ Divorced ☐ Other

Employment:

Employer: Quality Steel Company   Phone: (555) 555-7835

Address: 600 Silver Rd, Capital City, NY 12345

Condition Related to: ☐ Auto Accident ☒ Employment ☐ Other Accident

Date of Accident: 09/19/20XX   State: Township

Emergency Contact: _____ **Phone: ( )** _____

Primary Insurance: Capital Workers' Compensation Insurance Co.   Phone: ( ) _____

Address: 40 Hurt Rd, Capital City, NY 12345

Insurance Policyholder's Name: _____ ☐ M ☐ F DOB: _____

Address: _____

Phone: _____ Relationship to Insured: ☒ Self ☐ Spouse ☐ Child ☐ Other

Employer: _____ Phone: ( ) _____

Employer's Address: _____

Policy/ID No: WCZR5742   Group No: _____ Percent Covered: ____% Copay Amt: $_____

Secondary Insurance: _____ Phone: ( ) _____

Address: _____

Insurance Policyholder's Name: _____ ☐ M ☐ F DOB: _____

Address: _____

Phone: _____ Relationship to Insured: ☐ Self ☐ Spouse ☐ Child ☐ Other

Employer: _____ Phone: ( ) _____

Employer's Address: _____

Policy/ID No: _____ Group No: _____ Percent Covered: ____% Copay Amt: $_____

Reason for Visit: I have been having extreme pain in my right elbow.

Known Allergies: _____

Referred by: _____

09/20/20XX
Assignment of Benefits: Y
Signature on File: Y
Referring Physician: N

S: New patient Zoe Rocco is complaining of severe pain in his right elbow, which began a week ago.

O: Pt. has limited ROM in the right elbow. It is sensitive to touch. No redness, ulcerations, or rash is present. Pt. does have numbness and tingling. It is described as an "aching" pain. He is a steel polisher, full time.

A: 1. Cubital tunnel, right elbow—354.2.

P: 1. Start pt. on Ibuprofen one × 3 days.
   2. Obtain EMG of the right extremity.
   3. Return in 1 week to discuss results.
   4. Off of work until further notice.
   5. Refer to Mannie Mends, MD, for possible surgical repair of the ulnar nerve.
   6. Please bill his workers' compensation. His info is as follows:
      Capital Workers' Compensation Insurance Co.
      40 Hurt Rd.
      Capital City, NY 12345
      Claim#WCZR5742
   7. Phil Wells, MD state license#-MD-123456-L

_____

Phil Wells, MD
Family Practice
NPI: 1234567890

CASE 18-1

Patient Name Zoe Rocco

Capital City Medical
123 Unknown Boulevard, Capital City, NY 12345-2222

Date of Service
09-20-20XX

New Patient			Other Invasive/Noninvasive			Laboratory	
Problem Focused	99201		Arthrocentesis/Aspiration/Injection			Amylase	82150
Expanded Problem, Focused	99202		Small Joint	20600		B12	82607
Detailed	99203	X	Interm Joint	20605		CBC & Diff	85025
Comprehensive	99204		Major Joint	20610		Comp Metabolic Panel	80053
Comprehensive/High Complex	99205		Other Invasive/Noninvasive			Chlamydia Screen	87110
Well Exam Infant (up to 12 mos.)	99381		Audiometry	92552		Cholesterol	82465
Well Exam 1–4 yrs.	99382		Cast Application			Digoxin	80162
Well Exam 5–11 yrs.	99383		Location Long Short			Electrolytes	80051
Well Exam 12–17 yrs.	99384		Catheterization	51701		Ferritin	82728
Well Exam 18–39 yrs.	99385		Circumcision	54150		Folate	82746
Well Exam 40–64 yrs.	99386		Colposcopy	57452		GC Screen	87070
			Colposcopy w/Biopsy	57454		Glucose	82947
			Cryosurgery Premalignant Lesion			Glucose 1 HR	82950
			Location (s):			Glycosylated HGB A1C	83036
Established Patient			Cryosurgery Warts			HCT	85014
Post-Op Follow Up Visit	99024		Location (s):			HDL	83718
Minimum	99211		Curettement Lesion			Hep BSAG	87340
Problem Focused	99212		Single	11055		Hepatitis panel, acute	80074
Expanded Problem Focused	99213		2–4	11056		HGB	85018
Detailed	99214		>4	11057		HIV	86703
Comprehensive/High Complex	99215		Diaphragm Fitting	57170		Iron & TIBC	83550
Well Exam Infant (up to 12 mos.)	99391		Ear Irrigation	69210		Kidney Profile	80069
Well exam 1–4 yrs.	99392		ECG	93000		Lead	83655
Well Exam 5–11 yrs.	99393		Endometrial Biopsy	58100		Liver Profile	80076
Well Exam 12–17 yrs.	99394		Exc. Lesion Malignant			Mono Test	86308
Well Exam 18–39 yrs.	99395		Benign			Pap Smear	88155
Well Exam 40–64 yrs.	99396		Location			Pregnancy Test	84703
Obstetrics			Exc. Skin Tags (1–15)	11200		Obstetric Panel	80055
Total OB Care	59400		Each Additional 10	11201		Pro Time	85610
Injections			Fracture Treatment			PSA	84153
Administration Sub. / IM	90772		Loc			RPR	86592
Drug			w/Reduc	w/o Reduc		Sed. Rate	85651
Dosage			I & D Abscess Single/Simple	10060		Stool Culture	87045
Allergy	95115		Multiple or Comp	10061		Stool O & P	87177
Cocci Skin Test	86490		I & D Pilonidal Cyst Simple	10080		Strep Screen	87880
DPT	90701		Pilonidal Cyst Complex	10081		Theophylline	80198
Hemophilus	90646		IV Therapy—To One Hour	90760		Thyroid Uptake	84479
Influenza	90658		Each Additional Hour	90761		TSH	84443
MMR	90707		Laceration Repair			Urinalysis	81000
OPV	90712		Location Size Simp/Comp			Urine Culture	87088
Pneumovax	90732		Laryngoscopy	31505		Drawing Fee	36415
TB Skin Test	86580		Oximetry	94760		Specimen Collection	99000
TD	90718		Punch Biopsy			**Other:**	
Unlisted Immun	90749		Rhythm Strip	93040			
Tetanus Toxoid	90703		Treadmill	93015			
Vaccine/Toxoid Admin <8 Yr Old w/ Counseling	90465		Trigger Point or Tendon Sheath Inj.	20550			
Vaccine/Toxoid Administration for Adult	90471		Tympanometry	92567			

Diagnosis/ICD-9: **354.2**

I acknowledge receipt of medical services and authorize the release of any medical information necessary to process this claim for healthcare payment only. I do authorize payment to the provider.

Total Estimated Charges: _____

Payment Amount: _____

Patient Signature _Zoe Rocco_____

Next Appointment: _____

Figure 18-1

Capital City Medical
Fee Schedule

New Patient OV		Punch Biopsy various codes	$80
Problem Focused 99201	$45	Nebulizer various codes	$45
Expanded Problem Focused 99202	$65	Cast Application various codes	$85
Detailed 99203	$85	Laryngoscopy 31505	$255
Comprehensive 99204	$105	Audiometry 92552	$85
Comprehensive/High Complex 99205	$115	Tympanometry 92567	$85
Well Exam infant (less than 1 year) 99381	$45	Ear Irrigation 69210	$25
Well Exam 1–4 yrs. 99382	$50	Diaphragm Fitting 57170	$30
Well Exam 5–11 yrs. 99383	$55	IV Therapy (up to one hour) 90760	$65
Well Exam 12–17 yrs. 99384	$65	Each additional hour 90761	$50
Well Exam 18–39 yrs. 99385	$85	Oximetry 94760	$10
Well Exam 40–64 yrs. 99386	$105	ECG 93000	$75
Established Patient OV		Holter Monitor various codes	$170
Post Op Follow Up Visit 99024	$0	Rhythm Strip 93040	$60
Minimum 99211	$35	Treadmill 93015	$375
Problem Focused 99212	$45	Cocci Skin Test 86490	$20
Expanded Problem Focused 99213	$55	X-ray, spine, chest, bone—any area various codes	$275
Detailed 99214	$65	Avulsion Nail 11730	$200
Comprehensive/High Complex 99215	$75	**Laboratory**	
Well exam infant (less than 1 year) 99391	$35	Amylase 82150	$40
Well Exam 1–4 yrs. 99392	$40	B12 82607	$30
Well Exam 5–11 yrs. 99393	$45	CBC & Diff 85025	$95
Well Exam 12–17 yrs. 99394	$55	Comp Metabolic Panel 80053	$75
Well Exam 18–39 yrs. 99395	$65	Chlamydia Screen 87110	$70
Well Exam 40–64 yrs. 99396	$75	Cholestrerol 82465	$75
Obstetrics		Digoxin 80162	$40
Total OB Care 59400	$1700	Electrolytes 80051	$70
Injections		Estrogen, Total 82672	$50
Administration 90772	$10	Ferritin 82728	$40
Allergy 95115	$35	Folate 82746	$30
DPT 90701	$50	GC Screen 87070	$60
Drug various codes	$35	Glucose 82947	$35
Influenza 90658	$25	Glycosylated HGB A1C 83036	$45
MMR 90707	$50	HCT 85014	$30
OPV 90712	$40	HDL 83718	$35
Pneumovax 90732	$35	HGB 85018	$30
TB Skin Test 86580	$15	Hep BSAG 83740	$40
TD 90718	$40	Hepatitis panel, acute 80074	$95
Tetanus Toxoid 90703	$40	HIV 86703	$100
Vaccine/Toxoid Administration for Younger Than 8 Years Old w/ counseling 90465	$10	Iron & TIBC 83550	$45
		Kidney Profile 80069	$95
Vaccine/Toxoid Administration for Adult 90471	$10	Lead 83665	$55
Arthrocentesis/Aspiration/Injection		Lipase 83690	$40
Small Joint 20600	$50	Lipid Panel 80061	$95
Interm Joint 20605	$60	Liver Profile 80076	$95
Major Joint 20610	$70	Mono Test 86308	$30
Trigger Point/Tendon Sheath Inj. 20550	$90	Pap Smear 88155	$90
Other Invasive/Noninvasive Procedures		Pap Collection/Supervision 88142	$95
Catheterization 51701	$55	Pregnancy Test 84703	$90
Circumcision 54150	$150	Obstetric Panel 80055	$85
Colposcopy 57452	$225	Pro Time 85610	$50
Colposcopy w/Biopsy 57454	$250	PSA 84153	$50
Cryosurgery Premalignant Lesion various codes	$160	RPR 86592	$55
Endometrial Biopsy 58100	$190	Sed. Rate 85651	$50
Excision Lesion Malignant various codes	$145	Stool Culture 87045	$80
Excision Lesion Benign various codes	$125	Stool O & P 87177	$105
Curettement Lesion		Strep Screen 87880	$35
Single 11055	$70	Theophylline 80198	$40
2–4 11056	$80	Thyroid Uptake 84479	$75
>4 11057	$90	TSH 84443	$50
Excision Skin Tags (1–15) 11200	$55	Urinalysis 81000	$35
Each Additional 10 11201	$30	Urine Culture 87088	$80
I & D Abscess Single/Simple 10060	$75	Drawing Fee 36415	$15
Multiple/Complex 10061	$95	Specimen Collection 99000	$10
I & D Pilonidal Cyst Simple 10080	$105		
I & D Pilonidal Cyst Complex 10081	$130		
Laceration Repair various codes	$60		

(1500)

HEALTH INSURANCE CLAIM FORM
APPROVED BY NATIONAL UNIFORM CLAIM COMMITTEE 08/05

PICA ▢▢ | PICA ▢▢

1. MEDICARE ▢ (Medicare #) **MEDICAID** ▢ (Medicaid #) **TRICARE CHAMPUS** ▢ (Sponsor's SSN) **CHAMPVA** ▢ (Member ID#) **GROUP HEALTH PLAN** ▢ (SSN or ID) **FECA BLK LUNG** ▢ (SSN) **OTHER** ▢ (ID)

1a. INSURED'S I.D. NUMBER (For Program in Item 1)

2. PATIENT'S NAME (Last Name, First Name, Middle Initial)

3. PATIENT'S BIRTH DATE MM | DD | YY **SEX** M▢ F▢

4. INSURED'S NAME (Last Name, First Name, Middle Initial)

5. PATIENT'S ADDRESS (No., Street)

6. PATIENT RELATIONSHIP TO INSURED Self▢ Spouse▢ Child▢ Other▢

7. INSURED'S ADDRESS (No, Street)

CITY   **STATE**

8. PATIENT STATUS Single▢ Married▢ Other▢ Employed▢ Full-Time Student▢ Part-Time Student▢

CITY   **STATE**

ZIP CODE **TELEPHONE (Include Area Code)** ( )

ZIP CODE **TELEPHONE (Include Area Code)** ( )

9. OTHER INSURED'S NAME (Last Name, First Name, Middle Initial)

10. IS PATIENT'S CONDITION RELATED TO:

11. INSURED'S POLICY GROUP OR FECA NUMBER

a. OTHER INSURED'S POLICY OR GROUP NUMBER

a. EMPLOYMENT? (Current or Previous) ▢YES ▢NO

a. INSURED'S DATE OF BIRTH MM | DD | YY **SEX** M▢ F▢

b. OTHER INSURED'S DATE OF BIRTH MM | DD | YY **SEX** M▢ F▢

b. AUTO ACCIDENT? **PLACE (State)** ▢YES ▢NO

b. EMPLOYER'S NAME OR SCHOOL NAME

c. EMPLOYER'S NAME OR SCHOOL NAME

c. OTHER ACCIDENT? ▢YES ▢NO

c. INSURANCE PLAN NAME OR PROGRAM NAME

d. INSURANCE PLAN NAME OR PROGRAM NAME

10d. RESERVED FOR LOCAL USE

d. IS THERE ANOTHER HEALTH BENEFIT PLAN? ▢YES ▢NO If yes, return to and complete item 9 a-d.

READ BACK OF FORM BEFORE COMPLETING & SIGNING THIS FORM.
12. PATIENT'S OR AUTHORIZED PERSON'S SIGNATURE I authorize the release of any medical or other information necessary to process this claim. I also request payment of government benefits either to myself or to the party who accepts assignment below.

SIGNED _____ DATE _____

13. INSURED'S OR AUTHORIZED PERSON'S SIGNATURE I authorize payment of medical benefits to the undersigned physician or supplier for services described below.

SIGNED _____

14. DATE OF CURRENT: MM | DD | YY ILLNESS (First symptom) OR INJURY (Accident) OR PREGNANCY (LMP)

15. IF PATIENT HAS HAD SAME OR SIMILAR ILLNESS, GIVE FIRST DATE MM | DD | YY

16. DATES PATIENT UNABLE TO WORK IN CURRENT OCCUPATION FROM MM | DD | YY TO MM | DD | YY

17. NAME OF REFERRING PHYSICIAN OR OTHER SOURCE 17a. 17b. NPI

18. HOSPITALIZATION DATES RELATED TO CURRENT SERVICES FROM MM | DD | YY TO MM | DD | YY

19. RESERVED FOR LOCAL USE

20. OUTSIDE LAB? ▢YES ▢NO **$ CHARGES**

21. DIAGNOSIS OR NATURE OF ILLNESS OR INJURY (Relate Items 1,2,3 or 4 to Item 24E by Line)
1. |___.___| 3. |___.___|
2. |___.___| 4. |___.___|

22. MEDICAID RESUBMISSION CODE | ORIGINAL REF. NO.

23. PRIOR AUTHORIZATION NUMBER

24. A. DATE(S) OF SERVICE		B.	C.	D. PROCEDURES, SERVICES, OR SUPPLIES	E.	F.	G.	H.	I.	J.
From MM DD YY	To MM DD YY	PLACE OF SERVICE	EMG	(Explain Unusual Circumstances) CPT/HCPCS | MODIFIER	DIAGNOSIS POINTER	$ CHARGES	DAYS OR UNITS	EPSDT Family Plan	ID. QUAL.	RENDERING PROVIDER ID. #
1									NPI	
2									NPI	
3									NPI	
4									NPI	
5									NPI	
6									NPI	

25. FEDERAL TAX I.D. NUMBER SSN EIN ▢▢

26. PATIENT'S ACCOUNT NO.

27. ACCEPT ASSIGNMENT? (For govt. claims, see back) ▢YES ▢NO

28. TOTAL CHARGE $

29. AMOUNT PAID $

30. BALANCE DUE $

31. SIGNATURE OF PHYSICIAN OR SUPPLIER INCLUDING DEGREES OR CREDENTIALS (I certify that the statements on the reverse apply to this bill and are made a part thereof.)

SIGNED _____ DATE _____

32. SERVICE FACILITY LOCATION INFORMATION
a. NPI   b.

33. BILLING PROVIDER INFO & PH. # ( )
a. NPI   b.

APPROVED OMB 0938-0999 FORM CMS-1500 (08/05)

Figure 18-2

b. Using the source documents, the Capital City Medical Fee Schedule (Figure 18-3), and the blank CMS-1500 form provided (Figure 18-4), complete the following case study for patient Fritz Patrick (Case 18-2):

CASE 18-2

Capital City Medical—123 Unknown Boulevard, Capital City, NY 12345-2222 (555) 555-1234	Patient Information Form
Phil Wells, MD, Mannie Mends, MD, Bette R. Soone, MD	Tax ID: 75-0246810
	Group NPI: 1513171216

Patient Information:

Name: (Last, First) Patrick, Fritz ☒ Male ☐ Female Birth Date: 02/22/1959

Address: 795 Moon Rd, Township, NY 12345 Phone: (555) 555-9909

Social Security Number: 271-88-4567 Full-Time Student: ☐ Yes ☒ No

Marital Status: ☒ Single ☐ Married ☐ Divorced ☐ Other

Employment:

Employer: Retired Phone: ( )

Address:

Condition Related to: ☐ Auto Accident ☒ Employment ☐ Other Accident

Date of Accident: State:

Emergency Contact: Phone: ( )

Primary Insurance: Black Lung Workers' Compensation Phone: ( )

Address: 88 Injury Center, Capital City, NY 12345

Insurance Policyholder's Name: ☐ M ☐ F DOB:

Address:

Phone: Relationship to Insured: ☒ Self ☐ Spouse ☐ Child ☐ Other

Employer: Phone: ( )

Employer's Address:

Policy/ID No: 271884567 Group No: Percent Covered: % Copay Amt: $

Secondary Insurance: Phone: ( )

Address:

Insurance Policyholder's Name: ☐ M ☐ F DOB:

Address:

Phone: Relationship to Insured: ☐ Self ☐ Spouse ☐ Child ☐ Other

Employer: Phone: ( )

Employer's Address:

Policy/ID No: Group No: Percent Covered: % Copay Amt: $

Reason for Visit: I am here for a follow-up on coal dust in my lungs.

Known Allergies:

Referred by:

CASE 18-2
SOAP

11/16/20XX
Assignment of Benefits: Y
Signature on File: Y
Referring Physician: N

S: Fritz Patrick presents in the office today for a checkup on his black lung disease.
Q: He has no new complaints. He does use oxygen and his nebulizer as directed. He presents as stable.
A: 1. Pneumoconiosis (coal miners)—500.
P: 1. Continue meds and oxygen.
    2. Return in 3 months.
    3. Phil Wells, MD state license#-MD-123456-L

_____

Phil Wells, MD
Family Practice
NPI: 1234567890

CASE 18-2

Patient Name Fritz Patrick

Capital City Medical
123 Unknown Boulevard, Capital City, NY 12345-2222

Date of Service
11-18-20XX

New Patient			Arthrocentesis/Aspiration/Injection			Laboratory	
Problem Focused	99201		Small Joint		20600	Amylase	82150
Expanded Problem, Focused	99202		Interm Joint		20605	B12	82607
Detailed	99203		Major Joint		20610	CBC & Diff	85025
Comprehensive	99204		**Other Invasive/Noninvasive**			Comp Metabolic Panel	80053
Comprehensive/High Complex	99205		Audiometry		92552	Chlamydia Screen	87110
Well Exam Infant (up to 12 mos.)	99381		Cast Application			Cholesterol	82465
Well Exam 1–4 yrs.	99382		Location Long Short			Digoxin	80162
Well Exam 5–11 yrs.	99383		Catheterization		51701	Electrolytes	80051
Well Exam 12–17 yrs.	99384		Circumcision		54150	Ferritin	82728
Well Exam 18–39 yrs.	99385		Colposcopy		57452	Folate	82746
Well Exam 40–64 yrs.	99386		Colposcopy w/Biopsy		57454	GC Screen	87070
			Cryosurgery Premalignant Lesion			Glucose	82947
			Location (s):			Glucose 1 HR	82950
			Cryosurgery Warts			Glycosylated HGB A1C	83036
Established Patient			Location (s):			HCT	85014
Post-Op Follow Up Visit	99024		Curettement Lesion			HDL	83718
Minimum	99211		Single		11055	Hep BSAG	87340
Problem Focused	99212	X	2–4		11056	Hepatitis panel, acute	80074
Expanded Problem Focused	99213		>4		11057	HGB	85018
Detailed	99214		Diaphragm Fitting		57170	HIV	86703
Comprehensive/High Complex	99215		Ear Irrigation		69210	Iron & TIBC	83550
Well Exam Infant (up to 12 mos.)	99391		ECG		93000	Kidney Profile	80069
Well exam 1–4 yrs.	99392		Endometrial Biopsy		58100	Lead	83655
Well Exam 5–11 yrs.	99393		Exc. Lesion Malignant			Liver Profile	80076
Well Exam 12–17 yrs.	99394		Benign			Mono Test	86308
Well Exam 18–39 yrs.	99395		Location			Pap Smear	88155
Well Exam 40–64 yrs.	99396		Exc. Skin Tags (1–15)		11200	Pregnancy Test	84703
Obstetrics			Each Additional 10		11201	Obstetric Panel	80055
Total OB Care	59400		Fracture Treatment			Pro Time	85610
Injections			Loc			PSA	84153
Administration Sub. / IM	90772		w/Reduc w/o Reduc			RPR	86592
Drug			I & D Abscess Single/Simple		10060	Sed. Rate	85651
Dosage			Multiple or Comp		10061	Stool Culture	87045
Allergy	95115		I & D Pilonidal Cyst Simple		10080	Stool O & P	87177
Cocci Skin Test	86490		Pilonidal Cyst Complex		10081	Strep Screen	87880
DPT	90701		IV Therapy—To One Hour		90760	Theophylline	80198
Hemophilus	90646		Each Additional Hour		90761	Thyroid Uptake	84479
Influenza	90658		Laceration Repair			TSH	84443
MMR	90707		Location Size Simp/Comp			Urinalysis	81000
OPV	90712		Laryngoscopy		31505	Urine Culture	87088
Pneumovax	90732		Oximetry		94760	Drawing Fee	36415
TB Skin Test	86580		Punch Biopsy			Specimen Collection	99000
TD	90718		Rhythm Strip		93040	**Other:**	
Unlisted Immun	90749		Treadmill		93015		
Tetanus Toxoid	90703		Trigger Point or Tendon Sheath Inj.		20550		
Vaccine/Toxoid Admin <8 Yr Old w/ Counseling	90465		Tympanometry		92567		
Vaccine/Toxoid Administration for Adult	90471						

Diagnosis/ICD-9: **500**

I acknowledge receipt of medical services and authorize the release of any medical information necessary to process this claim for healthcare payment only. I do authorize payment to the provider.

Patient Signature Fritz Patrick

Total Estimated Charges: _____

Payment Amount: _____

Next Appointment: _____

Figure 18-3

Capital City Medical
Fee Schedule

New Patient OV			Punch Biopsy various codes	$80
Problem Focused 99201	$45		Nebulizer various codes	$45
Expanded Problem Focused 99202	$65		Cast Application various codes	$85
Detailed 99203	$85		Laryngoscopy 31505	$255
Comprehensive 99204	$105		Audiometry 92552	$85
Comprehensive/High Complex 99205	$115		Tympanometry 92567	$85
Well Exam infant (less than 1 year) 99381	$45		Ear Irrigation 69210	$25
Well Exam 1–4 yrs. 99382	$50		Diaphragm Fitting 57170	$30
Well Exam 5–11 yrs. 99383	$55		IV Therapy (up to one hour) 90760	$65
Well Exam 12–17 yrs. 99384	$65		Each additional hour 90761	$50
Well Exam 18–39 yrs. 99385	$85		Oximetry 94760	$10
Well Exam 40–64 yrs. 99386	$105		ECG 93000	$75
Established Patient OV			Holter Monitor various codes	$170
Post Op Follow Up Visit 99024	$0		Rhythm Strip 93040	$60
Minimum 99211	$35		Treadmill 93015	$375
Problem Focused 99212	$45		Cocci Skin Test 86490	$20
Expanded Problem Focused 99213	$55		X-ray, spine, chest, bone—any area various codes	$275
Detailed 99214	$65		Avulsion Nail 11730	$200
Comprehensive/High Complex 99215	$75		**Laboratory**	
Well exam infant (less than 1 year) 99391	$35		Amylase 82150	$40
Well Exam 1–4 yrs. 99392	$40		B12 82607	$30
Well Exam 5–11 yrs. 99393	$45		CBC & Diff 85025	$95
Well Exam 12–17 yrs. 99394	$55		Comp Metabolic Panel 80053	$75
Well Exam 18–39 yrs. 99395	$65		Chlamydia Screen 87110	$70
Well Exam 40–64 yrs. 99396	$75		Cholestrerol 82465	$75
Obstetrics			Digoxin 80162	$40
Total OB Care 59400	$1700		Electrolytes 80051	$70
Injections			Estrogen, Total 82672	$50
Administration 90772	$10		Ferritin 82728	$40
Allergy 95115	$35		Folate 82746	$30
DPT 90701	$50		GC Screen 87070	$60
Drug various codes	$35		Glucose 82947	$35
Influenza 90658	$25		Glycosylated HGB A1C 83036	$45
MMR 90707	$50		HCT 85014	$30
OPV 90712	$40		HDL 83718	$35
Pneumovax 90732	$35		HGB 85018	$30
TB Skin Test 86580	$15		Hep BSAG 83740	$40
TD 90718	$40		Hepatitis panel, acute 80074	$95
Tetanus Toxoid 90703	$40		HIV 86703	$100
Vaccine/Toxoid Administration for Younger			Iron & TIBC 83550	$45
Than 8 Years Old w/ counseling 90465	$10		Kidney Profile 80069	$95
Vaccine/Toxoid Administration for Adult 90471	$10		Lead 83665	$55
Arthrocentesis/Aspiration/Injection			Lipase 83690	$40
Small Joint 20600	$50		Lipid Panel 80061	$95
Interm Joint 20605	$60		Liver Profile 80076	$95
Major Joint 20610	$70		Mono Test 86308	$30
Trigger Point/Tendon Sheath Inj. 20550	$90		Pap Smear 88155	$90
Other Invasive/Noninvasive Procedures			Pap Collection/Supervision 88142	$95
Catheterization 51701	$55		Pregnancy Test 84703	$90
Circumcision 54150	$150		Obstetric Panel 80055	$85
Colposcopy 57452	$225		Pro Time 85610	$50
Colposcopy w/Biopsy 57454	$250		PSA 84153	$50
Cryosurgery Premalignant Lesion various codes	$160		RPR 86592	$55
Endometrial Biopsy 58100	$190		Sed. Rate 85651	$50
Excision Lesion Malignant various codes	$145		Stool Culture 87045	$80
Excision Lesion Benign various codes	$125		Stool O & P 87177	$105
Curettement Lesion			Strep Screen 87880	$35
Single 11055	$70		Theophylline 80198	$40
2–4 11056	$80		Thyroid Uptake 84479	$75
>4 11057	$90		TSH 84443	$50
Excision Skin Tags (1–15) 11200	$55		Urinalysis 81000	$35
Each Additional 10 11201	$30		Urine Culture 87088	$80
I & D Abscess Single/Simple 10060	$75		Drawing Fee 36415	$15
Multiple/Complex 10061	$95		Specimen Collection 99000	$10
I & D Pilonidal Cyst Simple 10080	$105			
I & D Pilonidal Cyst Complex 10081	$130			
Laceration Repair various codes	$60			

1500

HEALTH INSURANCE CLAIM FORM
APPROVED BY NATIONAL UNIFORM CLAIM COMMITTEE 08/05

☐☐☐PICA

1. MEDICARE	MEDICAID	TRICARE CHAMPUS	CHAMPVA	GROUP HEALTH PLAN	FECA BLK LUNG	OTHER	1a. INSURED'S I.D. NUMBER (For Program in Item 1)
☐(Medicare #)	☐(Medicaid #)	☐(Sponsor's SSN)	☐(Member ID#)	☐(SSN or ID)	☐(SSN)	☐(ID)	

2. PATIENT'S NAME (Last Name, First Name, Middle Initial)

3. PATIENT'S BIRTH DATE MM | DD | YY   SEX   M☐   F☐

4. INSURED'S NAME (Last Name, First Name, Middle Initial)

5. PATIENT'S ADDRESS (No., Street)

6. PATIENT RELATIONSHIP TO INSURED
Self☐   Spouse☐   Child☐   Other☐

7. INSURED'S ADDRESS (No, Street)

CITY   STATE

8. PATIENT STATUS
Single☐   Married☐   Other☐
Full-Time   Part-Time
Employed☐   Student☐   Student☐

CITY   STATE

ZIP CODE   TELEPHONE (Include Area Code)
(   )

ZIP CODE   TELEPHONE (Include Area Code)
(   )

9. OTHER INSURED'S NAME (Last Name, First Name, Middle Initial)

10. IS PATIENT'S CONDITION RELATED TO:

11. INSURED'S POLICY GROUP OR FECA NUMBER

a. OTHER INSURED'S POLICY OR GROUP NUMBER

a. EMPLOYMENT? (Current or Previous)
☐YES   ☐NO

a. INSURED'S DATE OF BIRTH MM | DD | YY   SEX   M☐   F☐

b. OTHER INSURED'S DATE OF BIRTH MM | DD | YY   SEX   M☐   F☐

b. AUTO ACCIDENT?   PLACE (State)
☐YES   ☐NO   └___┘

b. EMPLOYER'S NAME OR SCHOOL NAME

c. EMPLOYER'S NAME OR SCHOOL NAME

c. OTHER ACCIDENT?
☐YES   ☐NO

c. INSURANCE PLAN NAME OR PROGRAM NAME

d. INSURANCE PLAN NAME OR PROGRAM NAME

10d. RESERVED FOR LOCAL USE

d. IS THERE ANOTHER HEALTH BENEFIT PLAN?
☐YES   ☐NO   If yes, return to and complete item 9 a-d.

READ BACK OF FORM BEFORE COMPLETING & SIGNING THIS FORM.
12. PATIENT'S OR AUTHORIZED PERSON'S SIGNATURE I authorize the release of any medical or other information necessary to process this claim. I also request payment of government benefits either to myself or to the party who accepts assignment below.

SIGNED _____   DATE _____

13. INSURED'S OR AUTHORIZED PERSON'S SIGNATURE I authorize payment of medical benefits to the undersigned physician or supplier for services described below.

SIGNED _____

14. DATE OF CURRENT: ILLNESS (First symptom) OR
MM | DD | YY   INJURY (Accident) OR
PREGNANCY (LMP)

15. IF PATIENT HAS HAD SAME OR SIMILAR ILLNESS, GIVE FIRST DATE   MM | DD | YY

16. DATES PATIENT UNABLE TO WORK IN CURRENT OCCUPATION
FROM   MM | DD | YY   TO   MM | DD | YY

17. NAME OF REFERRING PHYSICIAN OR OTHER SOURCE

17a.
17b. | NPI

18. HOSPITALIZATION DATES RELATED TO CURRENT SERVICES
FROM   MM | DD | YY   TO   MM | DD | YY

19. RESERVED FOR LOCAL USE

20. OUTSIDE LAB? $ CHARGES
☐YES   ☐NO

21. DIAGNOSIS OR NATURE OF ILLNESS OR INJURY (Relate Items 1,2,3 or 4 to Item 24E by Line)
1. |___.___   3. |___.___
2. |___.___   4. |___.___

22. MEDICAID RESUBMISSION
CODE   ORIGINAL REF. NO.

23. PRIOR AUTHORIZATION NUMBER

24. A. DATE(S) OF SERVICE		B. PLACE OF SERVICE	C. EMG	D. PROCEDURES, SERVICES, OR SUPPLIES (Explain Unusual Circumstances)		E. DIAGNOSIS POINTER	F. $ CHARGES	G. DAYS OR UNITS	H. EPSDT Family Plan	I. ID. QUAL.	J. RENDERING PROVIDER ID. #
From MM DD YY	To MM DD YY			CPT/HCPCS	MODIFIER						
1										NPI	
2										NPI	
3										NPI	
4										NPI	
5										NPI	
6										NPI	

25. FEDERAL TAX I.D. NUMBER   SSN EIN
☐☐

26. PATIENT'S ACCOUNT NO.

27. ACCEPT ASSIGNMENT? (For govt. claims, see back)
☐YES   ☐NO

28. TOTAL CHARGE $

29. AMOUNT PAID $

30. BALANCE DUE $

31. SIGNATURE OF PHYSICIAN OR SUPPLIER INCLUDING DEGREES OR CREDENTIALS
(I certify that the statements on the reverse apply to this bill and are made a part thereof.)

SIGNED _____   DATE _____

32. SERVICE FACILITY LOCATION INFORMATION

a. NPI   b.

33. BILLING PROVIDER INFO & PH. # (   )

a. NPI   b.

NUCC Instruction Manual available at: www.nucc.org
WCMS-1500CS

APPROVED OMB 0938-0999 FORM CMS-1500 (08/05)

Right margin, top to bottom: CARRIER — PATIENT AND INSURED INFORMATION — PHYSICIAN OR SUPPLIER INFORMATION

Left margin: SECOND FOLD — WHCF-10-ENV-SS — FIRST FOLD WHCF-10-ENV / WHCF-10-ENV-SS

Figure 18-4

c. Using the source documents, the Capital City Medical Fee Schedule (Figure 18-5), and the blank CMS-1500 form provided (Figure 18-6), complete the following case study for patient Nick Orelli (Case 18-3):

CASE 18-3

Capital City Medical—123 Unknown Boulevard, Capital City, NY 12345-2222 (555) 555-1234	Patient Information Form
Phil Wells, MD, Mannie Mends, MD, Bette R. Soone, MD	Tax ID: 75-0246810 Group NPI: 1513171216

Patient Information:

Name: (Last, First) Orelli, Nick   ☒ Male   ☐ Female   Birth Date: 07/15/1964

Address: 41 Sixth Ave, Capital City, NY 12345   Phone: (555) 555-1867

Social Security Number: 387-81-5185   Full-Time Student: ☐ Yes   ☒ No

Marital Status: ☐ Single   ☒ Married   ☐ Divorced   ☐ Other

Employment:

Employer: Metal Recycle Co.   Phone: (555) 555-8438

Address: 2934 Balph Rd, Township, NY 12345

Condition Related to: ☐ Auto Accident   ☒ Employment   ☐ Other Accident

Date of Accident: 05/04/20XX   State: NY

Emergency Contact: _____ **Phone: ( )** _____

Primary Insurance: Employees Workers' Compensation Insurance Co.   Phone: ( ) _____

Address: 1408 Baker Rd, Capital City, NY 12345

Insurance Policyholder's Name: _____ ☐ M ☐ F DOB: _____

Address: _____

Phone: _____ Relationship to Insured: ☒ Self ☐ Spouse ☐ Child ☐ Other

Employer: _____ Phone: ( ) _____

Employer's Address: _____

Policy/ID No: WCN06496   Group No: _____ Percent Covered: ____% Copay Amt: $_____

Secondary Insurance: _____ Phone: ( ) _____

Address: _____

Insurance Policyholder's Name: same _____ ☐ M ☐ F DOB: _____

Address: _____

Phone: _____ Relationship to Insured: ☐ Self ☐ Spouse ☐ Child ☐ Other

Employer: _____ Phone: ( ) _____

Employer's Address: _____

Policy/ID No: _____ Group No: _____ Percent Covered: ____% Copay Amt: $_____

Reason for Visit: I burned my hand at work while welding.

Known Allergies: _____

Referred by: _____

CASE 18-3
SOAP

05/04/20XX
Assignment of Benefits: Y
Signature on File: Y
Referring Physician: N

S: Nick Orelli is being seen for a burn on his left hand today. He was welding at work when his arm slipped, causing his welding torch to burn his left hand.

O: The exam reveals rubor on the back of his left hand. The area is blistered. It does not look infected at this time. He denies any other burns.

A: 1. Burn, back of left hand, 2nd degree—944.26.
2. Welding torch burn—E898.1.

P: 1. Start oral antibiotics.
2. Antibiotic ointment twice daily.
3. Keep area clean and dry.
4. Change dressing twice a day, or if dirty or wet.
5. Return to office if infection occurs.
6. Return to work 05/08/20XX if there are no complications.
7. Please bill his workers' compensation. His info is as follows:
Employees' Workers' Compensation Insurance Co.
1408 Baker Road
Capital City, NY 12345
Claim#WCNO6496
8. Phil Wells, MD state license#-MD-123456-L

_____

Phil Wells, MD
Family Practice
NPI: 1234567890

CASE 18-3

Patient Name <u>Nick Orelli</u>

Capital City Medical
123 Unknown Boulevard, Capital City, NY 12345-2222

Date of Service
<u>05-04-20XX</u>

New Patient			Other Invasive/Noninvasive			Laboratory	
Problem Focused	99201		Arthrocentesis/Aspiration/Injection			Amylase	82150
Expanded Problem, Focused	99202		Small Joint	20600		B12	82607
Detailed	99203		Interm Joint	20605		CBC & Diff	85025
Comprehensive	99204		Major Joint	20610		Comp Metabolic Panel	80053
Comprehensive/High Complex	99205		**Other Invasive/Noninvasive**			Chlamydia Screen	87110
Well Exam Infant (up to 12 mos.)	99381		Audiometry	92552		Cholesterol	82465
Well Exam 1–4 yrs.	99382		Cast Application			Digoxin	80162
Well Exam 5–11 yrs.	99383		Location Long Short			Electrolytes	80051
Well Exam 12–17 yrs.	99384		Catheterization	51701		Ferritin	82728
Well Exam 18–39 yrs.	99385		Circumcision	54150		Folate	82746
Well Exam 40–64 yrs.	99386		Colposcopy	57452		GC Screen	87070
			Colposcopy w/Biopsy	57454		Glucose	82947
			Cryosurgery Premalignant Lesion			Glucose 1 HR	82950
			Location (s):			Glycosylated HGB A1C	83036
Established Patient			Cryosurgery Warts			HCT	85014
Post-Op Follow Up Visit	99024		Location (s):			HDL	83718
Minimum	99211		Curettement Lesion			Hep BSAG	87340
Problem Focused	99212		Single	11055		Hepatitis panel, acute	80074
Expanded Problem Focused	99213	X	2–4	11056		HGB	85018
Detailed	99214		>4	11057		HIV	86703
Comprehensive/High Complex	99215		Diaphragm Fitting	57170		Iron & TIBC	83550
Well Exam Infant (up to 12 mos.)	99391		Ear Irrigation	69210		Kidney Profile	80069
Well exam 1–4 yrs.	99392		ECG	93000		Lead	83655
Well Exam 5–11 yrs.	99393		Endometrial Biopsy	58100		Liver Profile	80076
Well Exam 12–17 yrs.	99394		Exc. Lesion Malignant			Mono Test	86308
Well Exam 18–39 yrs.	99395		Benign			Pap Smear	88155
Well Exam 40–64 yrs.	99396		Location			Pregnancy Test	84703
Obstetrics			Exc. Skin Tags (1–15)	11200		Obstetric Panel	80055
Total OB Care	59400		Each Additional 10	11201		Pro Time	85610
Injections			Fracture Treatment			PSA	84153
Administration Sub. / IM	90772		Loc			RPR	86592
Drug			w/Reduc	w/o Reduc		Sed. Rate	85651
Dosage			I & D Abscess Single/Simple	10060		Stool Culture	87045
Allergy	95115		Multiple or Comp	10061		Stool O & P	87177
Cocci Skin Test	86490		I & D Pilonidal Cyst Simple	10080		Strep Screen	87880
DPT	90701		Pilonidal Cyst Complex	10081		Theophylline	80198
Hemophilus	90646		IV Therapy—To One Hour	90760		Thyroid Uptake	84479
Influenza	90658		Each Additional Hour	90761		TSH	84443
MMR	90707		Laceration Repair			Urinalysis	81000
OPV	90712		Location Size Simp/Comp			Urine Culture	87088
Pneumovax	90732		Laryngoscopy	31505		Drawing Fee	36415
TB Skin Test	86580		Oximetry	94760		Specimen Collection	99000
TD	90718		Punch Biopsy			**Other:**	
Unlisted Immun	90749		Rhythm Strip	93040			
Tetanus Toxoid	90703		Treadmill	93015			
Vaccine/Toxoid Admin <8 Yr Old w/ Counseling	90465		Trigger Point or Tendon Sheath Inj.	20550			
Vaccine/Toxoid Administration for Adult	90471		Tympanometry	92567			

Diagnosis/ICD-9: **500**

I acknowledge receipt of medical services and authorize the release of any medical information necessary to process this claim for healthcare payment only. I do authorize payment to the provider.

Patient Signature <u>Nick Orelli</u>

Total Estimated Charges: _____

Payment Amount: _____

Next Appointment: _____

Figure 18-5

Capital City Medical
Fee Schedule

New Patient OV		Punch Biopsy various codes	$80	
Problem Focused 99201	$45	Nebulizer various codes	$45	
Expanded Problem Focused 99202	$65	Cast Application various codes	$85	
Detailed 99203	$85	Laryngoscopy 31505	$255	
Comprehensive 99204	$105	Audiometry 92552	$85	
Comprehensive/High Complex 99205	$115	Tympanometry 92567	$85	
Well Exam infant (less than 1 year) 99381	$45	Ear Irrigation 69210	$25	
Well Exam 1–4 yrs. 99382	$50	Diaphragm Fitting 57170	$30	
Well Exam 5–11 yrs. 99383	$55	IV Therapy (up to one hour) 90760	$65	
Well Exam 12–17 yrs. 99384	$65	Each additional hour 90761	$50	
Well Exam 18–39 yrs. 99385	$85	Oximetry 94760	$10	
Well Exam 40–64 yrs. 99386	$105	ECG 93000	$75	
Established Patient OV		Holter Monitor various codes	$170	
Post Op Follow Up Visit 99024	$0	Rhythm Strip 93040	$60	
Minimum 99211	$35	Treadmill 93015	$375	
Problem Focused 99212	$45	Cocci Skin Test 86490	$20	
Expanded Problem Focused 99213	$55	X-ray, spine, chest, bone—any area various codes	$275	
Detailed 99214	$65	Avulsion Nail 11730	$200	
Comprehensive/High Complex 99215	$75	**Laboratory**		
Well exam infant (less than 1 year) 99391	$35	Amylase 82150	$40	
Well Exam 1–4 yrs. 99392	$40	B12 82607	$30	
Well Exam 5–11 yrs. 99393	$45	CBC & Diff 85025	$95	
Well Exam 12–17 yrs. 99394	$55	Comp Metabolic Panel 80053	$75	
Well Exam 18–39 yrs. 99395	$65	Chlamydia Screen 87110	$70	
Well Exam 40–64 yrs. 99396	$75	Cholestrerol 82465	$75	
Obstetrics		Digoxin 80162	$40	
Total OB Care 59400	$1700	Electrolytes 80051	$70	
Injections		Estrogen, Total 82672	$50	
Administration 90772	$10	Ferritin 82728	$40	
Allergy 95115	$35	Folate 82746	$30	
DPT 90701	$50	GC Screen 87070	$60	
Drug various codes	$35	Glucose 82947	$35	
Influenza 90658	$25	Glycosylated HGB A1C 83036	$45	
MMR 90707	$50	HCT 85014	$30	
OPV 90712	$40	HDL 83718	$35	
Pneumovax 90732	$35	HGB 85018	$30	
TB Skin Test 86580	$15	Hep BSAG 83740	$40	
TD 90718	$40	Hepatitis panel, acute 80074	$95	
Tetanus Toxoid 90703	$40	HIV 86703	$100	
Vaccine/Toxoid Administration for Younger		Iron & TIBC 83550	$45	
Than 8 Years Old w/ counseling 90465	$10	Kidney Profile 80069	$95	
Vaccine/Toxoid Administration for Adult 90471	$10	Lead 83665	$55	
Arthrocentesis/Aspiration/Injection		Lipase 83690	$40	
Small Joint 20600	$50	Lipid Panel 80061	$95	
Interm Joint 20605	$60	Liver Profile 80076	$95	
Major Joint 20610	$70	Mono Test 86308	$30	
Trigger Point/Tendon Sheath Inj. 20550	$90	Pap Smear 88155	$90	
Other Invasive/Noninvasive Procedures		Pap Collection/Supervision 88142	$95	
Catheterization 51701	$55	Pregnancy Test 84703	$90	
Circumcision 54150	$150	Obstetric Panel 80055	$85	
Colposcopy 57452	$225	Pro Time 85610	$50	
Colposcopy w/Biopsy 57454	$250	PSA 84153	$50	
Cryosurgery Premalignant Lesion various codes	$160	RPR 86592	$55	
Endometrial Biopsy 58100	$190	Sed. Rate 85651	$50	
Excision Lesion Malignant various codes	$145	Stool Culture 87045	$80	
Excision Lesion Benign various codes	$125	Stool O & P 87177	$105	
Curettement Lesion		Strep Screen 87880	$35	
Single 11055	$70	Theophylline 80198	$40	
2–4 11056	$80	Thyroid Uptake 84479	$75	
>4 11057	$90	TSH 84443	$50	
Excision Skin Tags (1–15) 11200	$55	Urinalysis 81000	$35	
Each Additional 10 11201	$30	Urine Culture 87088	$80	
I & D Abscess Single/Simple 10060	$75	Drawing Fee 36415	$15	
Multiple/Complex 10061	$95	Specimen Collection 99000	$10	
I & D Pilonidal Cyst Simple 10080	$105			
I & D Pilonidal Cyst Complex 10081	$130			
Laceration Repair various codes	$60			

HEALTH INSURANCE CLAIM FORM
APPROVED BY NATIONAL UNIFORM CLAIM COMMITTEE 08/05

☐☐ PICA

1. MEDICARE	MEDICAID	TRICARE CHAMPUS	CHAMPVA	GROUP HEALTH PLAN	FECA BLK LUNG	OTHER
☐ (Medicare #)	☐ (Medicaid #)	☐ (Sponsor's SSN)	☐ (Member ID#)	☐ (SSN or ID)	☐ (SSN)	☐ (ID)

1a. INSURED'S I.D. NUMBER (For Program in Item 1)

2. PATIENT'S NAME (Last Name, First Name, Middle Initial)

3. PATIENT'S BIRTH DATE SEX
MM ╎ DD ╎ YY
M ☐ F ☐

4. INSURED'S NAME (Last Name, First Name, Middle Initial)

5. PATIENT'S ADDRESS (No, Street)

6. PATIENT RELATIONSHIP TO INSURED
Self ☐ Spouse ☐ Child ☐ Other ☐

7. INSURED'S ADDRESS (No, Street)

CITY   STATE

8. PATIENT STATUS
Single ☐ Married ☐ Other ☐
Full-Time   Part-Time
Employed ☐ Student ☐ Student ☐

CITY   STATE

ZIP CODE   TELEPHONE (Include Area Code)
( )

ZIP CODE   TELEPHONE (Include Area Code)
( )

9. OTHER INSURED'S NAME (Last Name, First Name, Middle Initial)

10. IS PATIENT'S CONDITION RELATED TO:

11. INSURED'S POLICY GROUP OR FECA NUMBER

a. OTHER INSURED'S POLICY OR GROUP NUMBER

a. EMPLOYMENT? (Current or Previous)
☐ YES ☐ NO

a. INSURED'S DATE OF BIRTH   SEX
MM ╎ DD ╎ YY
M ☐ F ☐

b. OTHER INSURED'S DATE OF BIRTH SEX
MM ╎ DD ╎ YY
M ☐ F ☐

b. AUTO ACCIDENT?   PLACE (State)
☐ YES ☐ NO

b. EMPLOYER'S NAME OR SCHOOL NAME

c. EMPLOYER'S NAME OR SCHOOL NAME

c. OTHER ACCIDENT?
☐ YES ☐ NO

c. INSURANCE PLAN NAME OR PROGRAM NAME

d. INSURANCE PLAN NAME OR PROGRAM NAME

10d. RESERVED FOR LOCAL USE

d. IS THERE ANOTHER HEALTH BENEFIT PLAN?
☐ YES ☐ NO If yes, return to and complete item 9 a-d.

READ BACK OF FORM BEFORE COMPLETING & SIGNING THIS FORM.
12. PATIENT'S OR AUTHORIZED PERSON'S SIGNATURE I authorize the release of any medical or other information necessary to process this claim. I also request payment of government benefits either to myself or to the party who accepts assignment below.

SIGNED _____ DATE _____

13. INSURED'S OR AUTHORIZED PERSON'S SIGNATURE I authorize payment of medical benefits to the undersigned physician or supplier for services described below.

SIGNED _____

14. DATE OF CURRENT: ILLNESS (First symptom) OR INJURY (Accident) OR PREGNANCY (LMP)
MM ╎ DD ╎ YY

15. IF PATIENT HAS HAD SAME OR SIMILAR ILLNESS, GIVE FIRST DATE MM ╎ DD ╎ YY

16. DATES PATIENT UNABLE TO WORK IN CURRENT OCCUPATION
FROM MM ╎ DD ╎ YY TO MM ╎ DD ╎ YY

17. NAME OF REFERRING PHYSICIAN OR OTHER SOURCE

17a.
17b. NPI

18. HOSPITALIZATION DATES RELATED TO CURRENT SERVICES
FROM MM ╎ DD ╎ YY TO MM ╎ DD ╎ YY

19. RESERVED FOR LOCAL USE

20. OUTSIDE LAB? $ CHARGES
☐ YES ☐ NO

21. DIAGNOSIS OR NATURE OF ILLNESS OR INJURY (Relate Items 1,2,3 or 4 to Item 24E by Line)
1. ╎_____   3. ╎_____
2. ╎_____   4. ╎_____

22. MEDICAID RESUBMISSION
CODE   ORIGINAL REF. NO.

23. PRIOR AUTHORIZATION NUMBER

24. A. DATE(S) OF SERVICE		B. PLACE OF SERVICE	C. EMG	D. PROCEDURES, SERVICES, OR SUPPLIES (Explain Unusual Circumstances)		E. DIAGNOSIS POINTER	F. $ CHARGES	G. DAYS OR UNITS	H. EPSDT Family Plan	I. ID. QUAL.	J. RENDERING PROVIDER ID. #
From MM DD YY	To MM DD YY			CPT/HCPCS	MODIFIER						
1										NPI	
2										NPI	
3										NPI	
4										NPI	
5										NPI	
6										NPI	

25. FEDERAL TAX I.D. NUMBER SSN EIN
☐ ☐

26. PATIENT'S ACCOUNT NO.

27. ACCEPT ASSIGNMENT? (For govt. claims, see back)
☐ YES ☐ NO

28. TOTAL CHARGE $

29. AMOUNT PAID $

30. BALANCE DUE $

31. SIGNATURE OF PHYSICIAN OR SUPPLIER INCLUDING DEGREES OR CREDENTIALS
(I certify that the statements on the reverse apply to this bill and are made a part thereof.)

SIGNED _____ DATE _____

32. SERVICE FACILITY LOCATION INFORMATION

a. NPI   b.

33. BILLING PROVIDER INFO & PH. # ( )

a. NPI   b.

NUCC Instruction Manual available at: www.nucc.org
WCMS-1500CS

APPROVED OMB 0938-0999 FORM CMS-1500 (08/05)

CARRIER

PATIENT AND INSURED INFORMATION

PHYSICIAN OR SUPPLIER INFORMATION

SECOND FOLD

FIRST FOLD WHCF-10-ENV / WHCF-10-ENV-SS

Figure 18-6

d. Using the source documents, the Capital City Medical Fee Schedule (Figure 18-7), and the blank CMS-1500 form provided (Figure 18-8), complete the following case study for patient Gloria McMannis (Case 18-4):

CASE 18-4

Capital City Medical—123 Unknown Boulevard, Capital City, NY 12345-2222 (555) 555-1234	Patient Information Form
Phil Wells, MD, Mannie Mends, MD, Bette R. Soone, MD	Tax ID: 75-0246810
	Group NPI: 1513171216

Patient Information:

Name: (Last, First) McMannis, Gloria ☐ Male ☒ Female Birth Date: 11/09/1961

Address: 53 Homer St, Township, NY 12345 Phone: (555) 555-8613

Social Security Number: 695-08-2865 Full-Time Student: ☐ Yes ☒ No

Marital Status: ☒ Single ☐ Married ☐ Divorced ☐ Other

Employment:

Employer: Furniture Plus Phone: (555) 555-5316

Address: 4592 Capital Square, Capital City, NY 12345

Condition Related to: ☐ Auto Accident ☒ Employment ☐ Other Accident

Date of Accident: 08/12/20XX State: Capital City

Emergency Contact: _____ **Phone: ( )** _____

Primary Insurance: State Workers' Compensation Insurance Co. Phone: ( ) _____

Address: 88 Injury Center, Capital City, NY 12345

Insurance Policyholder's Name: _____ ☐ M ☐ F DOB: _____

Address: _____

Phone: _____ Relationship to Insured: ☒ Self ☐ Spouse ☐ Child ☐ Other

Employer: _____ Phone: ( ) _____

Employer's Address: _____

Policy/ID No: WCGMO802 Group No: _____ Percent Covered: ____% Copay Amt: $____

Secondary Insurance: _____ Phone: ( ) _____

Address: _____

Insurance Policyholder's Name: _____ ☐ M ☐ F DOB: _____

Address: _____

Phone: _____ Relationship to Insured: ☐ Self ☐ Spouse ☐ Child ☐ Other

Employer: _____ Phone: ( ) _____

Employer's Address: _____

Policy/ID No: _____ Group No: _____ Percent Covered: ____% Copay Amt: $____

Reason for Visit: I hurt my back at work today while moving a couch.

Known Allergies: _____

Referred by: _____

CASE 18-4
SOAP

08/12/20XX
Assignment of Benefits: Y
Signature on File: Y
Referring Physician: N

S: New patient Gloria McMannis hurt her lower back at work today, while helping another employee move a couch.

O: Pt. complains of pain in the lumber region. It is tender to the touch. She states that the pain is an "8." The skin shows no bruising or lesions. She was wearing a lifting belt. Lumbar spine X-ray today shows swelling. There is no evidence of herniation or fracture.

A: 1. Back strain, lumber—847.2.
　　2. Injury during lifting/moving—E927.

P: 1. Naproxen 2 times/day.
　　2. Heating pad as needed.
　　3. Appointment in 1 week.
　　4. Return to work 08/15/20XX, only under light duty.
　　5. Please bill her workers' compensation. Her info is as follows:
　　　State Workers' Compensation Insurance Co.
　　　88 Injury Center
　　　Capital City, NY 12345
　　　Claim#WCGM0802
　　6. Phil Wells, MD state license#-MD-123456-L

_____

Phil Wells, MD
Family Practice
NPI: 1234567890

CASE 18-4

Patient Name Gloria McMannis

Capital City Medical
123 Unknown Boulevard, Capital City, NY 12345-2222

Date of Service
08-12-20XX

New Patient			Other Invasive/Noninvasive			Laboratory	
Problem Focused	99201		Arthrocentesis/Aspiration/Injection			Amylase	82150
Expanded Problem, Focused	99202		Small Joint	20600		B12	82607
Detailed	99203	X	Interm Joint	20605		CBC & Diff	85025
Comprehensive	99204		Major Joint	20610		Comp Metabolic Panel	80053
Comprehensive/High Complex	99205		**Other Invasive/Noninvasive**			Chlamydia Screen	87110
Well Exam Infant (up to 12 mos.)	99381		Audiometry	92552		Cholesterol	82465
Well Exam 1–4 yrs.	99382		Cast Application			Digoxin	80162
Well Exam 5–11 yrs.	99383		Location Long Short			Electrolytes	80051
Well Exam 12–17 yrs.	99384		Catheterization	51701		Ferritin	82728
Well Exam 18–39 yrs.	99385		Circumcision	54150		Folate	82746
Well Exam 40–64 yrs.	99386		Colposcopy	57452		GC Screen	87070
			Colposcopy w/Biopsy	57454		Glucose	82947
			Cryosurgery Premalignant Lesion			Glucose 1 HR	82950
			Location (s):			Glycosylated HGB A1C	83036
Established Patient			Cryosurgery Warts			HCT	85014
Post-Op Follow Up Visit	99024		Location (s):			HDL	83718
Minimum	99211		Curettement Lesion			Hep BSAG	87340
Problem Focused	99212		Single	11055		Hepatitis panel, acute	80074
Expanded Problem Focused	99213		2–4	11056		HGB	85018
Detailed	99214		>4	11057		HIV	86703
Comprehensive/High Complex	99215		Diaphragm Fitting	57170		Iron & TIBC	83550
Well Exam Infant (up to 12 mos.)	99391		Ear Irrigation	69210		Kidney Profile	80069
Well exam 1–4 yrs.	99392		ECG	93000		Lead	83655
Well Exam 5–11 yrs.	99393		Endometrial Biopsy	58100		Liver Profile	80076
Well Exam 12–17 yrs.	99394		Exc. Lesion Malignant			Mono Test	86308
Well Exam 18–39 yrs.	99395		Benign			Pap Smear	88155
Well Exam 40–64 yrs.	99396		Location			Pregnancy Test	84703
Obstetrics			Exc. Skin Tags (1–15)	11200		Obstetric Panel	80055
Total OB Care	59400		Each Additional 10	11201		Pro Time	85610
Injections			Fracture Treatment			PSA	84153
Administration Sub. / IM	90772		Loc			RPR	86592
Drug			w/Reduc w/o Reduc			Sed. Rate	85651
Dosage			I & D Abscess Single/Simple	10060		Stool Culture	87045
Allergy	95115		Multiple or Comp	10061		Stool O & P	87177
Cocci Skin Test	86490		I & D Pilonidal Cyst Simple	10080		Strep Screen	87880
DPT	90701		Pilonidal Cyst Complex	10081		Theophylline	80198
Hemophilus	90646		IV Therapy—To One Hour	90760		Thyroid Uptake	84479
Influenza	90658		Each Additional Hour	90761		TSH	84443
MMR	90707		Laceration Repair			Urinalysis	81000
OPV	90712		Location Size Simp/Comp			Urine Culture	87088
Pneumovax	90732		Laryngoscopy	31505		Drawing Fee	36415
TB Skin Test	86580		Oximetry	94760		Specimen Collection	99000
TD	90718		Punch Biopsy			**Other:**	
Unlisted Immun	90749		Rhythm Strip	93040		X-Ray L-Spine	72100	X
Tetanus Toxoid	90703		Treadmill	93015			
Vaccine/Toxoid Admin <8 Yr Old w/ Counseling	90465		Trigger Point or Tendon Sheath Inj.	20550			
Vaccine/Toxoid Administration for Adult	90471		Tympanometry	92567			

Diagnosis/ICD-9: **847.2, E927**

I acknowledge receipt of medical services and authorize the release of any medical information necessary to process this claim for healthcare payment only. I do authorize payment to the provider.

Total Estimated Charges: _____

Payment Amount: _____

Patient Signature *Gloria McMannis*

Next Appointment: _____

Figure 18-7

Capital City Medical
Fee Schedule

New Patient OV			Punch Biopsy various codes	$80
Problem Focused 99201	$45		Nebulizer various codes	$45
Expanded Problem Focused 99202	$65		Cast Application various codes	$85
Detailed 99203	$85		Laryngoscopy 31505	$255
Comprehensive 99204	$105		Audiometry 92552	$85
Comprehensive/High Complex 99205	$115		Tympanometry 92567	$85
Well Exam infant (less than 1 year) 99381	$45		Ear Irrigation 69210	$25
Well Exam 1–4 yrs. 99382	$50		Diaphragm Fitting 57170	$30
Well Exam 5–11 yrs. 99383	$55		IV Therapy (up to one hour) 90760	$65
Well Exam 12–17 yrs. 99384	$65		Each additional hour 90761	$50
Well Exam 18–39 yrs. 99385	$85		Oximetry 94760	$10
Well Exam 40–64 yrs. 99386	$105		ECG 93000	$75
Established Patient OV			Holter Monitor various codes	$170
Post Op Follow Up Visit 99024	$0		Rhythm Strip 93040	$60
Minimum 99211	$35		Treadmill 93015	$375
Problem Focused 99212	$45		Cocci Skin Test 86490	$20
Expanded Problem Focused 99213	$55		X-ray, spine, chest, bone—any area various codes	$275
Detailed 99214	$65		Avulsion Nail 11730	$200
Comprehensive/High Complex 99215	$75		**Laboratory**	
Well exam infant (less than 1 year) 99391	$35		Amylase 82150	$40
Well Exam 1–4 yrs. 99392	$40		B12 82607	$30
Well Exam 5–11 yrs. 99393	$45		CBC & Diff 85025	$95
Well Exam 12–17 yrs. 99394	$55		Comp Metabolic Panel 80053	$75
Well Exam 18–39 yrs. 99395	$65		Chlamydia Screen 87110	$70
Well Exam 40–64 yrs. 99396	$75		Cholestrerol 82465	$75
Obstetrics			Digoxin 80162	$40
Total OB Care 59400	$1700		Electrolytes 80051	$70
Injections			Estrogen, Total 82672	$50
Administration 90772	$10		Ferritin 82728	$40
Allergy 95115	$35		Folate 82746	$30
DPT 90701	$50		GC Screen 87070	$60
Drug various codes	$35		Glucose 82947	$35
Influenza 90658	$25		Glycosylated HGB A1C 83036	$45
MMR 90707	$50		HCT 85014	$30
OPV 90712	$40		HDL 83718	$35
Pneumovax 90732	$35		HGB 85018	$30
TB Skin Test 86580	$15		Hep BSAG 83740	$40
TD 90718	$40		Hepatitis panel, acute 80074	$95
Tetanus Toxoid 90703	$40		HIV 86703	$100
Vaccine/Toxoid Administration for Younger			Iron & TIBC 83550	$45
Than 8 Years Old w/ counseling 90465	$10		Kidney Profile 80069	$95
Vaccine/Toxoid Administration for Adult 90471	$10		Lead 83665	$55
Arthrocentesis/Aspiration/Injection			Lipase 83690	$40
Small Joint 20600	$50		Lipid Panel 80061	$95
Interm Joint 20605	$60		Liver Profile 80076	$95
Major Joint 20610	$70		Mono Test 86308	$30
Trigger Point/Tendon Sheath Inj. 20550	$90		Pap Smear 88155	$90
Other Invasive/Noninvasive Procedures			Pap Collection/Supervision 88142	$95
Catheterization 51701	$55		Pregnancy Test 84703	$90
Circumcision 54150	$150		Obstetric Panel 80055	$85
Colposcopy 57452	$225		Pro Time 85610	$50
Colposcopy w/Biopsy 57454	$250		PSA 84153	$50
Cryosurgery Premalignant Lesion various codes	$160		RPR 86592	$55
Endometrial Biopsy 58100	$190		Sed. Rate 85651	$50
Excision Lesion Malignant various codes	$145		Stool Culture 87045	$80
Excision Lesion Benign various codes	$125		Stool O & P 87177	$105
Curettement Lesion			Strep Screen 87880	$35
Single 11055	$70		Theophylline 80198	$40
2–4 11056	$80		Thyroid Uptake 84479	$75
>4 11057	$90		TSH 84443	$50
Excision Skin Tags (1–15) 11200	$55		Urinalysis 81000	$35
Each Additional 10 11201	$30		Urine Culture 87088	$80
I & D Abscess Single/Simple 10060	$75		Drawing Fee 36415	$15
Multiple/Complex 10061	$95		Specimen Collection 99000	$10
I & D Pilonidal Cyst Simple 10080	$105			
I & D Pilonidal Cyst Complex 10081	$130			
Laceration Repair various codes	$60			

HEALTH INSURANCE CLAIM FORM

APPROVED BY NATIONAL UNIFORM CLAIM COMMITTEE 08/05

☐☐☐PICA   PICA☐☐☐

1. MEDICARE	MEDICAID	TRICARE CHAMPUS	CHAMPVA	GROUP HEALTH PLAN	FECA BLK LUNG	OTHER	1a. INSURED'S I.D. NUMBER	(For Program in Item 1)
☐(Medicare #)	☐(Medicaid #)	☐(Sponsor's SSN)	☐(Member ID#)	☐(SSN or ID)	☐(SSN)	☐(ID)		

2. PATIENT'S NAME (Last Name, First Name, Middle Initial)	3. PATIENT'S BIRTH DATE SEX	4. INSURED'S NAME (Last Name, First Name, Middle Initial)
	MM ⋮ DD ⋮ YY M☐ F☐	

5. PATIENT'S ADDRESS (No., Street)	6. PATIENT RELATIONSHIP TO INSURED	7. INSURED'S ADDRESS (No., Street)
	Self☐ Spouse☐ Child☐ Other☐	
CITY STATE	8. PATIENT STATUS	CITY STATE
	Single☐ Married☐ Other☐	
ZIP CODE TELEPHONE (Include Area Code) ( )	Full-Time Part-Time Employed☐ Student☐ Student☐	ZIP CODE TELEPHONE (Include Area Code) ( )

9. OTHER INSURED'S NAME (Last Name, First Name, Middle Initial)	10. IS PATIENT'S CONDITION RELATED TO:	11. INSURED'S POLICY GROUP OR FECA NUMBER
a. OTHER INSURED'S POLICY OR GROUP NUMBER	a. EMPLOYMENT? (Current or Previous) ☐YES ☐NO	a. INSURED'S DATE OF BIRTH SEX MM ⋮ DD ⋮ YY M☐ F☐
b. OTHER INSURED'S DATE OF BIRTH SEX MM ⋮ DD ⋮ YY M☐ F☐	b. AUTO ACCIDENT? PLACE (State) ☐YES ☐NO L⎯⎯⎯	b. EMPLOYER'S NAME OR SCHOOL NAME
c. EMPLOYER'S NAME OR SCHOOL NAME	c. OTHER ACCIDENT? ☐YES ☐NO	c. INSURANCE PLAN NAME OR PROGRAM NAME
d. INSURANCE PLAN NAME OR PROGRAM NAME	10d. RESERVED FOR LOCAL USE	d. IS THERE ANOTHER HEALTH BENEFIT PLAN? ☐YES ☐NO If yes, return to and complete item 9 a-d.

READ BACK OF FORM BEFORE COMPLETING & SIGNING THIS FORM.	13. INSURED'S OR AUTHORIZED PERSON'S SIGNATURE I authorize payment of medical benefits to the undersigned physician or supplier for services described below.
12. PATIENT'S OR AUTHORIZED PERSON'S SIGNATURE I authorize the release of any medical or other information necessary to process this claim. I also request payment of government benefits either to myself or to the party who accepts assignment below.	
SIGNED ⎯⎯⎯⎯ DATE⎯⎯⎯⎯	SIGNED ⎯⎯⎯⎯

14. DATE OF CURRENT: ILLNESS (First symptom) OR INJURY (Accident) OR PREGNANCY (LMP) MM ⋮ DD ⋮ YY	15. IF PATIENT HAS HAD SAME OR SIMILAR ILLNESS, GIVE FIRST DATE MM ⋮ DD ⋮ YY	16. DATES PATIENT UNABLE TO WORK IN CURRENT OCCUPATION MM ⋮ DD ⋮ YY MM ⋮ DD ⋮ YY FROM TO
17. NAME OF REFERRING PHYSICIAN OR OTHER SOURCE	17a. ⎯⎯⎯ 17b. NPI	18. HOSPITALIZATION DATES RELATED TO CURRENT SERVICES MM ⋮ DD ⋮ YY MM ⋮ DD ⋮ YY FROM TO
19. RESERVED FOR LOCAL USE		20. OUTSIDE LAB? $ CHARGES ☐YES ☐NO
21. DIAGNOSIS OR NATURE OF ILLNESS OR INJURY (Relate Items 1,2,3 or 4 to Item 24E by Line) 1. L⎯⎯.⎯⎯ 3. L⎯⎯.⎯⎯ 2. L⎯⎯.⎯⎯ 4. L⎯⎯.⎯⎯		22. MEDICAID RESUBMISSION CODE ⎯⎯ ORIGINAL REF. NO. ⎯⎯ 23. PRIOR AUTHORIZATION NUMBER

24. A. DATE(S) OF SERVICE		B. PLACE OF SERVICE	C. EMG	D. PROCEDURES, SERVICES, OR SUPPLIES (Explain Unusual Circumstances)		E. DIAGNOSIS POINTER	F. $ CHARGES	G. DAYS OR UNITS	H. EPSDT Family Plan	I. ID. QUAL.	J. RENDERING PROVIDER ID. #
From MM DD YY	To MM DD YY			CPT/HCPCS	MODIFIER						
1										NPI	
2										NPI	
3										NPI	
4										NPI	
5										NPI	
6										NPI	

25. FEDERAL TAX I.D. NUMBER SSN EIN ☐☐	26. PATIENT'S ACCOUNT NO.	27. ACCEPT ASSIGNMENT? (For govt. claims, see back) ☐YES ☐NO	28. TOTAL CHARGE $	29. AMOUNT PAID $	30. BALANCE DUE $
31. SIGNATURE OF PHYSICIAN OR SUPPLIER INCLUDING DEGREES OR CREDENTIALS (I certify that the statements on the reverse apply to this bill and are made a part thereof.) SIGNED ⎯⎯ DATE ⎯⎯	32. SERVICE FACILITY LOCATION INFORMATION a. NPI b.	33. BILLING PROVIDER INFO & PH. # ( ) a. NPI b.			

APPROVED OMB 0938-0999 FORM CMS-1500 (08/05)

Figure 18-8

e. Using the source documents, the Capital City Medical Fee Schedule (Figure 18-9), and the blank CMS-1500 form provided (Figure 18-10), complete the following case study for patient Sasha Janiels (Case 18-5):

CASE 18-5

Capital City Medical—123 Unknown Boulevard, Capital City,	Patient Information Form
NY 12345-2222 (555) 555-1234	Tax ID: 75-0246810
Phil Wells, MD, Mannie Mends, MD, Bette R. Soone, MD	Group NPI: 1513171216

Patient Information:

Name: (Last, First) Janiels, Sasha ___ ❑ Male ☒ Female Birth Date: 12/21/1958

Address: 981 Cross Rd, Capital City, NY 12345 Phone: (555) 555-1615

Social Security Number: 355-46-1161 Full-Time Student: ❑ Yes ☒ No

Marital Status: ❑ Single ☒ Married ❑ Divorced ❑ Other

Employment:

Employer: Capital City General Hospital Phone: (555) 555-1000

Address: 1000 Cherry St, Capital City, NY 12345

Condition Related to: ❑ Auto Accident ☒ Employment ❑ Other Accident

Date of Accident: 06/26/20XX State: NY

Emergency Contact: ___ **Phone: ( )** ___

Primary Insurance: State Workers' Compensation Insurance Co. Phone: ( ) ___

Address: 88 Injury Center, Capital City, NY 12345

Insurance Policyholder's Name: ___ ❑ M ❑ F DOB: ___

Address: ___

Phone: ___ Relationship to Insured: ☒ Self ❑ Spouse ❑ Child ❑ Other

Employer: ___ Phone: ( ) ___

Employer's Address: ___

Policy/ID No: WCSJ1111 Group No: ___ Percent Covered: ___% Copay Amt: $___

Secondary Insurance: ___ Phone: ( ) ___

Address: ___

Insurance Policyholder's Name: ___ ❑ M ❑ F DOB: ___

Address: ___

Phone: ___ Relationship to Insured: ❑ Self ❑ Spouse ❑ Child ❑ Other

Employer: ___ Phone: ( ) ___

Employer's Address: ___

Policy/ID No: ___ Group No: ___ Percent Covered: ___% Copay Amt: $___

Reason for Visit: I accidentally had a fingerstick today after administering an injection.

Known Allergies: ___

Referred by: ___

CASE 18-5
SOAP

06/26/20XX
Assignment of Benefits: Y
Signature on File: Y
Referring Physician: N

S: Sasha Janiels is being seen today due to a needlestick accident after administering an injection of codeine to a patient. It is not known whether the patient has any bloodborne disease.

O: Pt. has a hypodermic needle puncture on her right middle finger. There is no infection at the site. Pt. has no history of any bloodborne diseases. All other systems are unremarkable. Mood and affect are anxious, but pleasant. This is normal, due to this recent event.

A: 1. Wound, hypodermic needle puncture of right middle finger—883.0.
2. Accidental needlestick—E920.5.

P: 1. HIV test today and in 6 months; Hepatitis panel today.
2. Follow up in 10 days for results.
3. May return to work tomorrow.
4. Please bill her workers' compensation. Her info is as follows:
   State Workers' Compensation Insurance Co.
   88 Injury Center
   Capital City, NY 12345
   Claim#WCSJ1111
5. Phil Wells, MD state license#-MD-123456-L

_____

Phil Wells, MD
Family Practice
NPI: 1234567890

CASE 18-5

Patient Name <u>Sasha Janiels</u>

Capital City Medical
123 Unknown Boulevard, Capital City, NY 12345-2222

Date of Service
<u>06-26-20XX</u>

New Patient			Arthrocentesis/Aspiration/Injection		Laboratory		
Problem Focused	99201		Arthrocentesis/Aspiration/Injection		Amylase	82150	
Expanded Problem, Focused	99202		Small Joint	20600	B12	82607	
Detailed	99203		Interm Joint	20605	CBC & Diff	85025	
Comprehensive	99204		Major Joint	20610	Comp Metabolic Panel	80053	
Comprehensive/High Complex	99205		**Other Invasive/Noninvasive**		Chlamydia Screen	87110	
Well Exam Infant (up to 12 mos.)	99381		Audiometry	92552	Cholesterol	82465	
Well Exam 1–4 yrs.	99382		Cast Application		Digoxin	80162	
Well Exam 5–11 yrs.	99383		Location Long Short		Electrolytes	80051	
Well Exam 12–17 yrs.	99384		Catheterization	51701	Ferritin	82728	
Well Exam 18–39 yrs.	99385		Circumcision	54150	Folate	82746	
Well Exam 40–64 yrs.	99386		Colposcopy	57452	GC Screen	87070	
			Colposcopy w/Biopsy	57454	Glucose	82947	
			Cryosurgery Premalignant Lesion		Glucose 1 HR	82950	
			Location (s):		Glycosylated HGB A1C	83036	
Established Patient			Cryosurgery Warts		HCT	85014	
Post-Op Follow Up Visit	99024		Location (s):		HDL	83718	
Minimum	99211		Curettement Lesion		Hep BSAG	87340	
Problem Focused	99212		Single	11055	Hepatitis panel, acute	80074	X
Expanded Problem Focused	99213	X	2–4	11056	HGB	85018	
Detailed	99214		>4	11057	HIV	86703	X
Comprehensive/High Complex	99215		Diaphragm Fitting	57170	Iron & TIBC	83550	
Well Exam Infant (up to 12 mos.)	99391		Ear Irrigation	69210	Kidney Profile	80069	
Well exam 1–4 yrs.	99392		ECG	93000	Lead	83655	
Well Exam 5–11 yrs.	99393		Endometrial Biopsy	58100	Liver Profile	80076	
Well Exam 12–17 yrs.	99394		Exc. Lesion Malignant		Mono Test	86308	
Well Exam 18–39 yrs.	99395		Benign		Pap Smear	88155	
Well Exam 40–64 yrs.	99396		Location		Pregnancy Test	84703	
Obstetrics			Exc. Skin Tags (1–15)	11200	Obstetric Panel	80055	
Total OB Care	59400		Each Additional 10	11201	Pro Time	85610	
Injections			Fracture Treatment		PSA	84153	
Administration Sub. / IM	90772		Loc		RPR	86592	
Drug			w/Reduc w/o Reduc		Sed. Rate	85651	
Dosage			I & D Abscess Single/Simple	10060	Stool Culture	87045	
Allergy	95115		Multiple or Comp	10061	Stool O & P	87177	
Cocci Skin Test	86490		I & D Pilonidal Cyst Simple	10080	Strep Screen	87880	
DPT	90701		Pilonidal Cyst Complex	10081	Theophylline	80198	
Hemophilus	90646		IV Therapy—To One Hour	90760	Thyroid Uptake	84479	
Influenza	90658		Each Additional Hour	90761	TSH	84443	
MMR	90707		Laceration Repair		Urinalysis	81000	
OPV	90712		Location Size Simp/Comp		Urine Culture	87088	
Pneumovax	90732		Laryngoscopy	31505	Drawing Fee	36415	X
TB Skin Test	86580		Oximetry	94760	Specimen Collection	99000	
TD	90718		Punch Biopsy		**Other:**		
Unlisted Immun	90749		Rhythm Strip	93040			
Tetanus Toxoid	90703		Treadmill	93015			
Vaccine/Toxoid Admin <8 Yr Old w/ Counseling	90465		Trigger Point or Tendon Sheath Inj.	20550			
Vaccine/Toxoid Administration for Adult	90471		Tympanometry	92567			

Diagnosis/ICD-9: **883.0, E920.5**

I acknowledge receipt of medical services and authorize the release of any medical information necessary to process this claim for healthcare payment only. I do authorize payment to the provider.

Patient Signature <u>Sasha Janiels</u>

Total Estimated Charges: _____

Payment Amount: _____

Next Appointment: _____

Figure 18-9

Capital City Medical
Fee Schedule

New Patient OV			Punch Biopsy various codes	$80
Problem Focused 99201	$45		Nebulizer various codes	$45
Expanded Problem Focused 99202	$65		Cast Application various codes	$85
Detailed 99203	$85		Laryngoscopy 31505	$255
Comprehensive 99204	$105		Audiometry 92552	$85
Comprehensive/High Complex 99205	$115		Tympanometry 92567	$85
Well Exam infant (less than 1 year) 99381	$45		Ear Irrigation 69210	$25
Well Exam 1–4 yrs. 99382	$50		Diaphragm Fitting 57170	$30
Well Exam 5–11 yrs. 99383	$55		IV Therapy (up to one hour) 90760	$65
Well Exam 12–17 yrs. 99384	$65		Each additional hour 90761	$50
Well Exam 18–39 yrs. 99385	$85		Oximetry 94760	$10
Well Exam 40–64 yrs. 99386	$105		ECG 93000	$75
Established Patient OV			Holter Monitor various codes	$170
Post Op Follow Up Visit 99024	$0		Rhythm Strip 93040	$60
Minimum 99211	$35		Treadmill 93015	$375
Problem Focused 99212	$45		Cocci Skin Test 86490	$20
Expanded Problem Focused 99213	$55		X-ray, spine, chest, bone—any area various codes	$275
Detailed 99214	$65		Avulsion Nail 11730	$200
Comprehensive/High Complex 99215	$75		**Laboratory**	
Well exam infant (less than 1 year) 99391	$35		Amylase 82150	$40
Well Exam 1–4 yrs. 99392	$40		B12 82607	$30
Well Exam 5–11 yrs. 99393	$45		CBC & Diff 85025	$95
Well Exam 12–17 yrs. 99394	$55		Comp Metabolic Panel 80053	$75
Well Exam 18–39 yrs. 99395	$65		Chlamydia Screen 87110	$70
Well Exam 40–64 yrs. 99396	$75		Cholestrerol 82465	$75
Obstetrics			Digoxin 80162	$40
Total OB Care 59400	$1700		Electrolytes 80051	$70
Injections			Estrogen, Total 82672	$50
Administration 90772	$10		Ferritin 82728	$40
Allergy 95115	$35		Folate 82746	$30
DPT 90701	$50		GC Screen 87070	$60
Drug various codes	$35		Glucose 82947	$35
Influenza 90658	$25		Glycosylated HGB A1C 83036	$45
MMR 90707	$50		HCT 85014	$30
OPV 90712	$40		HDL 83718	$35
Pneumovax 90732	$35		HGB 85018	$30
TB Skin Test 86580	$15		Hep BSAG 83740	$40
TD 90718	$40		Hepatitis panel, acute 80074	$95
Tetanus Toxoid 90703	$40		HIV 86703	$100
Vaccine/Toxoid Administration for Younger			Iron & TIBC 83550	$45
Than 8 Years Old w/ counseling 90465	$10		Kidney Profile 80069	$95
Vaccine/Toxoid Administration for Adult 90471	$10		Lead 83665	$55
Arthrocentesis/Aspiration/Injection			Lipase 83690	$40
Small Joint 20600	$50		Lipid Panel 80061	$95
Interm Joint 20605	$60		Liver Profile 80076	$95
Major Joint 20610	$70		Mono Test 86308	$30
Trigger Point/Tendon Sheath Inj. 20550	$90		Pap Smear 88155	$90
Other Invasive/Noninvasive Procedures			Pap Collection/Supervision 88142	$95
Catheterization 51701	$55		Pregnancy Test 84703	$90
Circumcision 54150	$150		Obstetric Panel 80055	$85
Colposcopy 57452	$225		Pro Time 85610	$50
Colposcopy w/Biopsy 57454	$250		PSA 84153	$50
Cryosurgery Premalignant Lesion various codes	$160		RPR 86592	$55
Endometrial Biopsy 58100	$190		Sed. Rate 85651	$50
Excision Lesion Malignant various codes	$145		Stool Culture 87045	$80
Excision Lesion Benign various codes	$125		Stool O & P 87177	$105
Curettement Lesion			Strep Screen 87880	$35
Single 11055	$70		Theophylline 80198	$40
2–4 11056	$80		Thyroid Uptake 84479	$75
>4 11057	$90		TSH 84443	$50
Excision Skin Tags (1–15) 11200	$55		Urinalysis 81000	$35
Each Additional 10 11201	$30		Urine Culture 87088	$80
I & D Abscess Single/Simple 10060	$75		Drawing Fee 36415	$15
Multiple/Complex 10061	$95		Specimen Collection 99000	$10
I & D Pilonidal Cyst Simple 10080	$105			
I & D Pilonidal Cyst Complex 10081	$130			
Laceration Repair various codes	$60			

HEALTH INSURANCE CLAIM FORM

APPROVED BY NATIONAL UNIFORM CLAIM COMMITTEE 08/05

PICA   PICA

1. MEDICARE MEDICAID TRICARE CHAMPVA GROUP HEALTH PLAN FECA BLK LUNG OTHER	1a. INSURED'S I.D. NUMBER (For Program in Item 1)

CHAMPUS

☐(Medicare #)   ☐(Medicaid #)   ☐(Sponsor's SSN)   ☐(Member ID#)   ☐(SSN or ID)   ☐(SSN)   ☐(ID)

2. PATIENT'S NAME (Last Name, First Name, Middle Initial)

3. PATIENT'S BIRTH DATE   SEX
MM   DD   YY   M☐   F☐

4. INSURED'S NAME (Last Name, First Name, Middle Initial)

5. PATIENT'S ADDRESS (No., Street)

6. PATIENT RELATIONSHIP TO INSURED
Self☐   Spouse☐   Child☐   Other☐

7. INSURED'S ADDRESS (No, Street)

CITY   STATE

8. PATIENT STATUS
Single☐   Married☐   Other☐

CITY   STATE

ZIP CODE   TELEPHONE (Include Area Code)
( )

Full-Time   Part-Time
Employed☐   Student☐   Student☐

ZIP CODE   TELEPHONE (Include Area Code)
( )

9. OTHER INSURED'S NAME (Last Name, First Name, Middle Initial)

10. IS PATIENT'S CONDITION RELATED TO:

11. INSURED'S POLICY GROUP OR FECA NUMBER

a. OTHER INSURED'S POLICY OR GROUP NUMBER

a. EMPLOYMENT? (Current or Previous)
☐YES   ☐NO

a. INSURED'S DATE OF BIRTH   SEX
MM   DD   YY   M☐   F☐

b. OTHER INSURED'S DATE OF BIRTH   SEX
MM   DD   YY   M☐   F☐

b. AUTO ACCIDENT?   PLACE (State)
☐YES   ☐NO

b. EMPLOYER'S NAME OR SCHOOL NAME

c. EMPLOYER'S NAME OR SCHOOL NAME

c. OTHER ACCIDENT?
☐YES   ☐NO

c. INSURANCE PLAN NAME OR PROGRAM NAME

d. INSURANCE PLAN NAME OR PROGRAM NAME

10d. RESERVED FOR LOCAL USE

d. IS THERE ANOTHER HEALTH BENEFIT PLAN?
☐YES   ☐NO   If yes, return to and complete item 9 a-d.

READ BACK OF FORM BEFORE COMPLETING & SIGNING THIS FORM.

12. PATIENT'S OR AUTHORIZED PERSON'S SIGNATURE I authorize the release of any medical or other information necessary to process this claim. I also request payment of government benefits either to myself or to the party who accepts assignment below.

SIGNED _____ DATE _____

13. INSURED'S OR AUTHORIZED PERSON'S SIGNATURE I authorize payment of medical benefits to the undersigned physician or supplier for services described below.

SIGNED _____

14. DATE OF CURRENT: ILLNESS (First symptom) OR
MM   DD   YY   INJURY (Accident) OR PREGNANCY (LMP)

15. IF PATIENT HAS HAD SAME OR SIMILAR ILLNESS, GIVE FIRST DATE   MM   DD   YY

16. DATES PATIENT UNABLE TO WORK IN CURRENT OCCUPATION
MM   DD   YY   MM   DD   YY
FROM   TO

17. NAME OF REFERRING PHYSICIAN OR OTHER SOURCE

17a.
17b. NPI

18. HOSPITALIZATION DATES RELATED TO CURRENT SERVICES
MM   DD   YY   MM   DD   YY
FROM   TO

19. RESERVED FOR LOCAL USE

20. OUTSIDE LAB? $ CHARGES
☐YES   ☐NO

21. DIAGNOSIS OR NATURE OF ILLNESS OR INJURY (Relate Items 1,2,3 or 4 to Item 24E by Line)

1. |___.___   3. |___.___

2. |___.___   4. |___.___

22. MEDICAID RESUBMISSION
CODE   ORIGINAL REF. NO.

23. PRIOR AUTHORIZATION NUMBER

24. A. DATE(S) OF SERVICE		B. PLACE OF SERVICE	C. EMG	D. PROCEDURES, SERVICES, OR SUPPLIES (Explain Unusual Circumstances)		E. DIAGNOSIS POINTER	F. $ CHARGES	G. DAYS OR UNITS	H. EPSDT Family Plan	I. ID. QUAL.	J. RENDERING PROVIDER ID. #
From MM DD YY	To MM DD YY			CPT/HCPCS	MODIFIER						
1										NPI	
2										NPI	
3										NPI	
4										NPI	
5										NPI	
6										NPI	

25. FEDERAL TAX I.D. NUMBER   SSN EIN
☐ ☐

26. PATIENT'S ACCOUNT NO.

27. ACCEPT ASSIGNMENT? (For govt. claims, see back)
☐YES   ☐NO

28. TOTAL CHARGE
$

29. AMOUNT PAID
$

30. BALANCE DUE
$

31. SIGNATURE OF PHYSICIAN OR SUPPLIER INCLUDING DEGREES OR CREDENTIALS
(I certify that the statements on the reverse apply to this bill and are made a part thereof.)

SIGNED _____ DATE _____

32. SERVICE FACILITY LOCATION INFORMATION

a. NPI   b.

33. BILLING PROVIDER INFO & PH. # ( )

a. NPI   b.

NUCC Instruction Manual available at: www.nucc.org
WCMS-1500CS0

APPROVED OMB 0938-0999 FORM CMS-1500 (08/05)

Side labels: CARRIER — PATIENT AND INSURED INFORMATION — PHYSICIAN OR SUPPLIER INFORMATION
SECOND FOLD — FIRST FOLD WHCF-10-ENV / WHCF-10-ENV-SS

Figure 18-10

REVIEW QUESTIONS

MATCHING

Choose the correct answer, and place its corresponding letter in the space provided.

a. occupational diseases and illnesses
b. impairment
c. FECA
d. OSHA
e. independent review

1. _____ Act that provides millions of workers with workers' compensation benefits
2. _____ Process of checking over healthcare services for the purpose of medical necessity
3. _____ Health problems due to exposure to a health hazard in the workplace (also known as nontraumatic injuries/illnesses)
4. _____ Enforces a safe working environment for employees
5. _____ Permanent physical damage to a worker's body resulting from a work-related injury/illness

MULTIPLE CHOICE

Circle the letter of the choice that best completes the statement or answers the question.

1. Which of the following is considered workers' compensation fraud?
   a. A worker who gets paid "under the table" while receiving workers' compensation benefits
   b. Boilerplate medical reports
   c. Product switching
   d. All of the above

2. Once an injured worker has been examined by a designated physician, which of the following is (are) the only person(s) involved in the case who is (are) allowed to have direct communication with this physician?
   a. The injured worker
   b. Representatives of the workers' compensation carrier
   c. The worker's attorney
   d. All of the above

3. Which of the following is considered a work-related injury?
   a. Repetitive motions such as typing
   b. Lung problems due to dust
   c. Loss of hearing due to loud noises
   d. All of the above

4. Which of the following is (are) *not* considered a work-related injury?
   a. A work injury that requires vocational rehabilitation
   b. A work injury that does not result in a disability
   c. An injury to a worker by another worker due to a personal conflict
   d. Both a and b

5. Which of the following can refer to a treating physician/physician of record?

    a. An injured worker's PCP who has been approved by the workers' compensation carrier

    b. A designated physician

    c. One who helps to resolve a worker's compensation claim dispute

    d. All of the above

SHORT ANSWER

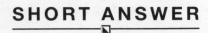

Provide the correct response to each of the following questions:

1. List the four types of worker's compensation income benefits.

    1. _____

    2. _____

    3. _____

    4. _____

2. What is the time limit for an injured worker or insurance carrier to dispute the maximum medical improvement date or the impairment rating?

    _____

3. What are the four types of workers' compensation benefits?

    1. _____

    _____

    2. _____

    _____

    3. _____

    _____

    4. _____

4. a. What important steps should be taken to ensure that a workers' compensation medical chart and related information are easily identified and retrieved?

    _____

    _____

    _____

    b. What important documentation should be included in an injured worker's medical chart?

    _____

    _____

    _____

5. Name the six reasons for termination of temporary partial and temporary permanent disability benefits.

    1. _____

    2. _____

    3. _____

4. _____

5. _____

6. _____

TRUE/FALSE

Identify each statement as true (T) or false (F).

1. _____ The medical office specialist does not need a workers' compensation case number to file a claim with the workers' compensation plan.

2. _____ An occupational injury/illness may develop over time.

3. _____ Temporary disability benefits will not be terminated if benefits are exhausted.

4. _____ An injured worker does not have to file a report of injury/illness with his/her employer for workers' compensation benefits to become effective.

5. _____ Each state governs and administers its own workers' compensation program.

CHAPTER 19
Electronic Medical Claims Processing

CHAPTER OBJECTIVES

Upon completion of this chapter in your student text, you should be able to do the following:

1. Enter all patient demographic information and post charges, payments, and adjustments, using medical practice management software.
2. Print a walkout receipt for each patient who has charges posted to his or her account.
3. Balance the batch at the end of each day.
4. Print insurance claim forms for the patients who are covered by insurance.

CHAPTER OUTLINE

Simulation Instructions

KEY TERMS

Using the highlighted terms and glossary in the textbook, define the following terms:

1. batching out _____
2. charges _____
3. commands _____
4. payments _____
5. transactions _____
6. walkout receipt _____

CRITICAL THINKING QUESTIONS

Using the knowledge you have gained from reading the textbook, apply critical thinking skills to answer the following questions.

1. You are the medical office specialist responsible for payment posting. Your job consists of accounts receivable duties. What are the seven functions of your job?

   1. _____

   2. _____

   3. _____

   4. _____

   5. _____

   6. _____

   7. _____

2. In your own words, describe how to "batch out" at the end of the day.

   _____

   _____

   _____

   _____

   _____

   _____

   _____

   _____

   _____

3. Answer the following questions related to entering information into the MPM software:

   a. The information needed for you to post transaction information is found on what two important medical forms?

   _____

   _____

   b. While entering a patient's employment information into the computer, you notice that this employer is not listed in your software. What should you do?

   _____

   _____

   _____

c. While entering a patient's insurance information into the computer, you notice that the insurance carrier is listed in the practice software, but the address that is on the back of the patient's insurance card is not the same as the address listed in the computer practice software. Is it acceptable to choose the carrier with the inaccurate address? Why or why not?

_____

_____

_____

_____

d. Joseph Fairmont is a new patient with your office. Where in the computer would you enter his demographics?

_____

_____

4. Joseph Fairmont is being seen for a sore throat and sneezing. Where in the computer would you enter the reason for his visit?

_____

_____

5. Discuss how to enter a new patient into the system.

_____

_____

PRACTICE EXERCISES

1. Utilizing the information provided in Chapter 19 and Appendix I of your student textbook, enter the case information for each of the given case studies into medical practice management software and prepare a CMS-1500 claim form. Complete the cases on the basis of the following assumptions:

   - All patients have release of information and assignment of benefit signatures on file.
   - All providers are participating and accept assignment.
   - The group practice is the billing entity.
   - The national transition to NPI numbers is complete, and legacy PINs of individual payers are no longer used. If legacy PINs are still being used by selected payers in your region, your instructor may provide legacy PINS in addition to the NPI.
   - 2012 ICD-9-CM and CPT codes are used.
   - Use eight-digit dates for birthdates. Use six-digit dates for all other dates.
   - All street names should be entered with standard postal abbreviations, even if they are spelled out on the source documents.
   - Enter ICD-9 codes in the order in which they appear on the encounter form.
   - When entering CPT codes, enter the E/M code first. Enter remaining codes in descending price order.

   a. Using the source documents provided, complete the given case study for patient Spencer Gerard (Case 19-1) by entering the case information into medical practice management software. Prepare a CMS-1500 claim form.

CASE 19-1

Capital City Medical—123 Unknown Boulevard, Capital City, NY 12345-2222 (555) 555-1234 Phil Wells, MD, Mannie Mends, MD, Bette R. Soone, MD	Patient Information Form Tax ID: 75-0246810 Group NPI: 1513171216

Patient Information:

Name: (Last, First) <u>Gerard, Spencer</u>   ☒ Male   ☐ Female   Birth Date: <u>10/05/1942</u>

Address: <u>91 W. Willow Rd., Township, NY 12345</u>   Phone: (555) <u>555-6001</u>

Social Security Number: <u>296-17-4004</u>   Full-Time Student: ☐ Yes   ☒ No

Marital Status: ☐ Single   ☒ Married   ☐ Divorced   ☐ Other

- -

Employment:

Employer: <u>Retired</u>   Phone: ( ) _____

Address: _____

Condition Related to: ☐ Auto Accident   ☐ Employment   ☐ Other Accident

Date of Accident: _____   State: _____

Emergency Contact: _____   **Phone: ( )** _____

- -

Primary Insurance: <u>Medicare</u>   Phone: ( ) _____

Address: <u>P. O Box 9834, Capital City, NY 12345</u>

Insurance Policyholder's Name: <u>Same</u>   ☐ M   ☐ F   DOB: _____

Address: _____

Phone: _____   Relationship to Insured: ☒ Self   ☐ Spouse   ☐ Child   ☐ Other

Employer: _____   Phone: ( ) _____

Employer's Address: _____

Policy/ID No: <u>754369782A</u>   Group No: _____   Percent Covered: <u>80</u> % Copay Amt: $ _____

- -

Secondary Insurance: _____   Phone: ( ) _____

Address: _____

Insurance Policyholder's Name: _____   ☐ M   ☐ F   DOB: _____

Address: _____

Phone: _____   Relationship to Insured: ☐ Self   ☐ Spouse   ☐ Child   ☐ Other

Employer: _____   Phone: ( ) _____

Employer's Address: _____

Policy/ID No: _____   Group No: _____   Percent Covered: ___% Copay Amt: $ _____

- -

Reason for Visit: <u>I am here for a follow-up to being in the hospital for shingles.</u>

Known Allergies: _____

Referred by: _____

CASE 19-1
SOAP

07/16/20XX
Assignment of Benefits: Y
Signature on File: Y
Referring Physician: N

S: Spencer Gerard is here for a follow-up on his COPD, which he was hospitalized for from 7/5/XX to 7/7/XX. DOO 7/5/XX.
O: Patient is doing very well. His breathing has improved since discharge. Good breath sounds bilaterally.
A: 1. COPD-496
P: 1. Continue breathing treatments and use inhaler daily.
　　2. Return in 1 month for recheck.

_____

Phil Wells, MD
Family Practice
NPI: 1234567890

CASE 19-1

Patient Name Spencer Gerard

Capital City Medical
123 Unknown Boulevard, Capital City, NY 12345-2222

Date of Service
07-16-20XX

New Patient			Arthrocentesis/Aspiration/Injection			Laboratory	
Problem Focused	99201		Arthrocentesis/Aspiration/Injection			Amylase	82150
Expanded Problem, Focused	99202		Small Joint	20600		B12	82607
Detailed	99203		Interm Joint	20605		CBC & Diff	85025
Comprehensive	99204		Major Joint	20610		Comp Metabolic Panel	80053
Comprehensive/High Complex	99205		**Other Invasive/Noninvasive**			Chlamydia Screen	87110
Well Exam Infant (up to 12 mos.)	99381		Audiometry	92552		Cholesterol	82465
Well Exam 1–4 yrs.	99382		Cast Application			Digoxin	80162
Well Exam 5–11 yrs.	99383		Location Long Short			Electrolytes	80051
Well Exam 12–17 yrs.	99384		Catheterization	51701		Ferritin	82728
Well Exam 18–39 yrs.	99385		Circumcision	54150		Folate	82746
Well Exam 40–64 yrs.	99386		Colposcopy	57452		GC Screen	87070
			Colposcopy w/Biopsy	57454		Glucose	82947
			Cryosurgery Premalignant Lesion			Glucose 1 HR	82950
			Location (s):			Glycosylated HGB A1C	83036
Established Patient			Cryosurgery Warts			HCT	85014
Post-Op Follow Up Visit	99024		Location (s):			HDL	83718
Minimum	99211		Curettement Lesion			Hep BSAG	87340
Problem Focused	99212	X	Single	11055		Hepatitis panel, acute	80074
Expanded Problem Focused	99213		2–4	11056		HGB	85018
Detailed	99214		>4	11057		HIV	86703
Comprehensive/High Complex	99215		Diaphragm Fitting	57170		Iron & TIBC	83550
Well Exam Infant (up to 12 mos.)	99391		Ear Irrigation	69210		Kidney Profile	80069
Well exam 1–4 yrs.	99392		ECG	93000		Lead	83655
Well Exam 5–11 yrs.	99393		Endometrial Biopsy	58100		Liver Profile	80076
Well Exam 12–17 yrs.	99394		Exc. Lesion Malignant			Mono Test	86308
Well Exam 18–39 yrs.	99395		Benign			Pap Smear	88155
Well Exam 40–64 yrs.	99396		Location			Pregnancy Test	84703
Obstetrics			Exc. Skin Tags (1–15)	11200		Obstetric Panel	80055
Total OB Care	59400		Each Additional 10	11201		Pro Time	85610
Injections			Fracture Treatment			PSA	84153
Administration Sub. / IM	90772		Loc			RPR	86592
Drug			w/Reduc w/o Reduc			Sed. Rate	85651
Dosage			I & D Abscess Single/Simple	10060		Stool Culture	87045
Allergy	95115		Multiple or Comp	10061		Stool O & P	87177
Cocci Skin Test	86490		I & D Pilonidal Cyst Simple	10080		Strep Screen	87880
DPT	90701		Pilonidal Cyst Complex	10081		Theophylline	80198
Hemophilus	90646		IV Therapy—To One Hour	90760		Thyroid Uptake	84479
Influenza	90658		Each Additional Hour	90761		TSH	84443
MMR	90707		Laceration Repair			Urinalysis	81000
OPV	90712		Location Size Simp/Comp			Urine Culture	87088
Pneumovax	90732		Laryngoscopy	31505		Drawing Fee	36415
TB Skin Test	86580		Oximetry	94760		Specimen Collection	99000
TD	90718		Punch Biopsy			**Other:**	
Unlisted Immun	90749		Rhythm Strip	93040			
Tetanus Toxoid	90703		Treadmill	93015			
Vaccine/Toxoid Admin <8 Yr Old w/ Counseling	90465		Trigger Point or Tendon Sheath Inj.	20550			
Vaccine/Toxoid Administration for Adult	90471		Tympanometry	92567			

Diagnosis/ICD-9: **053.9**

I acknowledge receipt of medical services and authorize the release of any medical information necessary to process this claim for healthcare payment only. I do authorize payment to the provider.

Total Estimated Charges: _____

Payment Amount: _____

Patient Signature *Gerard Spencer* _____

Next Appointment: _____

b. Using the source documents provided, complete the given casestudy for patient Cindy Ettinger (Case 19-2) by entering the case information into medical practice management software. Prepare a CMS-1500 claim form.

CASE 19-2

Capital City Medical—123 Unknown Boulevard, Capital City, NY 12345-2222 (555) 555-1234	Patient Information Form
	Tax ID: 75-0246810
Phil Wells, MD, Mannie Mends, MD, Bette R. Soone, MD	Group NPI: 1513171216

Patient Information:

Name: (Last, First) Ettinger, Cindy ___ ☐ Male ☒ Female Birth Date: 08/04/1982

Address: 6312 Glass Ave, Capital City, NY 12345 ___ Phone: (555) 555-6693

Social Security Number: 654-27-9356 ___ Full-Time Student: ☐ Yes ☒ No

Marital Status: ☐ Single ☒ Married ☐ Divorced ☐ Other

Employment:

Employer: ___ Phone: ( ) ___

Address: ___

Condition Related to: ☐ Auto Accident ☐ Employment ☐ Other Accident

Date of Accident: ___ State: ___

Emergency Contact: ___ Phone: ( ) ___

Primary Insurance: Blue Cross Blue Shield ___ Phone: ( ) ___

Address: 379 Blue Plaza, Capital City, NY 12345

Insurance Policyholder's Name: Glenn Ettinger ___ ☒ M ☐ F DOB: 09/11/1982

Address: Same

Phone: ___ Relationship to Insured: ☐ Self ☒ Spouse ☐ Child ☐ Other

Employer: Spike Fabrication ___ Phone: (555) 555-1881

Employer's Address: 21 Blue Highway Ext, Capital City, NY 12345

Policy/ID No: YYJ29633879 ___ Group No: 238647 Percent Covered: ___% Copay Amt: $25.00

Secondary Insurance: ___ Phone: ( ) ___

Address: ___

Insurance Policyholder's Name: ___ ☐ M ☐ F DOB: ___

Address: ___

Phone: ___ Relationship to Insured: ☐ Self ☐ Spouse ☐ Child ☐ Other

Employer: ___ Phone: ( ) ___

Employer's Address: ___

Policy/ID No: ___ Group No: ___ Percent Covered: ___% Copay Amt: $ ___

Reason for Visit: Itchy rash on arms that looks infected.

Known Allergies: ___

Referred by: ___

CASE 19-2
SOAP

12/24/20XX
Assignment of Benefits: Y
Signature on File: Y
Referring Physician: N

S: Cindy Ettinger is a new patient presenting with an itchy rash on both forearms. It started yesterday.

O: On exam, the rash presents as pustules. Pt. says that she was cleaning out her attic on Sunday, but denies being around anyone with this rash. The rest of the ROS is unremarkable.

A: 1. Scabies—133.0.

P: 1. Start medication.
2. Keep area clean and dry.
3. Avoid contact with furniture and other people for the next week.
4. Wash clothes and bedding daily.
5. Return in 1 week.

_____

Phil Wells, MD
Family Practice
NPI: 1234567890

CASE 19-2

Patient Name Cindy Ettinger

Capital City Medical
123 Unknown Boulevard, Capital City, NY 12345-2222

Date of Service
12-24-20XX

New Patient			Arthrocentesis/Aspiration/Injection			Laboratory	
Problem Focused	99201		Arthrocentesis/Aspiration/Injection			Amylase	82150
Expanded Problem, Focused	99202		Small Joint	20600		B12	82607
Detailed	99203	X	Interm Joint	20605		CBC & Diff	85025
Comprehensive	99204		Major Joint	20610		Comp Metabolic Panel	80053
Comprehensive/High Complex	99205		**Other Invasive/Noninvasive**			Chlamydia Screen	87110
Well Exam Infant (up to 12 mos.)	99381		Audiometry	92552		Cholesterol	82465
Well Exam 1–4 yrs.	99382		Cast Application			Digoxin	80162
Well Exam 5–11 yrs.	99383		Location Long Short			Electrolytes	80051
Well Exam 12–17 yrs.	99384		Catheterization	51701		Ferritin	82728
Well Exam 18–39 yrs.	99385		Circumcision	54150		Folate	82746
Well Exam 40–64 yrs.	99386		Colposcopy	57452		GC Screen	87070
			Colposcopy w/Biopsy	57454		Glucose	82947
			Cryosurgery Premalignant Lesion			Glucose 1 HR	82950
			Location (s):			Glycosylated HGB A1C	83036
			Cryosurgery Warts			HCT	85014
Established Patient			Location (s):			HDL	83718
Post-Op Follow Up Visit	99024		Curettement Lesion			Hep BSAG	87340
Minimum	99211		Single	11055		Hepatitis panel, acute	80074
Problem Focused	99212		2–4	11056		HGB	85018
Expanded Problem Focused	99213		>4	11057		HIV	86703
Detailed	99214		Diaphragm Fitting	57170		Iron & TIBC	83550
Comprehensive/High Complex	99215		Ear Irrigation	69210		Kidney Profile	80069
Well Exam Infant (up to 12 mos.)	99391		ECG	93000		Lead	83655
Well exam 1–4 yrs.	99392		Endometrial Biopsy	58100		Liver Profile	80076
Well Exam 5–11 yrs.	99393		Exc. Lesion Malignant			Mono Test	86308
Well Exam 12–17 yrs.	99394		Benign			Pap Smear	88155
Well Exam 18–39 yrs.	99395		Location			Pregnancy Test	84703
Well Exam 40–64 yrs.	99396		Exc. Skin Tags (1–15)	11200		Obstetric Panel	80055
Obstetrics			Each Additional 10	11201		Pro Time	85610
Total OB Care	59400		Fracture Treatment			PSA	84153
Injections			Loc			RPR	86592
Administration Sub. / IM	90772		w/Reduc w/o Reduc			Sed. Rate	85651
Drug			I & D Abscess Single/Simple	10060		Stool Culture	87045
Dosage			Multiple or Comp	10061		Stool O & P	87177
Allergy	95115		I & D Pilonidal Cyst Simple	10080		Strep Screen	87880
Cocci Skin Test	86490		Pilonidal Cyst Complex	10081		Theophylline	80198
DPT	90701		IV Therapy—To One Hour	90760		Thyroid Uptake	84479
Hemophilus	90646		Each Additional Hour	90761		TSH	84443
Influenza	90658		Laceration Repair			Urinalysis	81000
MMR	90707		Location Size Simp/Comp			Urine Culture	87088
OPV	90712		Laryngoscopy	31505		Drawing Fee	36415
Pneumovax	90732		Oximetry	94760		Specimen Collection	99000
TB Skin Test	86580		Punch Biopsy			**Other:**	
TD	90718		Rhythm Strip	93040			
Unlisted Immun	90749		Treadmill	93015			
Tetanus Toxoid	90703		Trigger Point or Tendon Sheath Inj.	20550			
Vaccine/Toxoid Admin <8 Yr Old w/ Counseling	90465		Tympanometry	92567			
Vaccine/Toxoid Administration for Adult	90471						

Diagnosis/ICD-9: **133.0**

I acknowledge receipt of medical services and authorize the release of any medical information necessary to process this claim for healthcare payment only. I do authorize payment to the provider.

Total Estimated Charges: _____

Payment Amount: _____

Patient Signature _Cindy Ettinger_

Next Appointment: _____

c. Using the source documents provided, complete the given case study for patient Reggie Dexter (Case 19-3) by entering the case information into medical practice management software. Prepare a CMS-1500 claim form.

CASE 19-3

Capital City Medical—123 Unknown Boulevard, Capital City, NY 12345-2222 (555) 555-1234	Patient Information Form
	Tax ID: 75-0246810
Phil Wells, MD, Mannie Mends, MD, Bette R. Soone, MD	Group NPI: 1513171216

Patient Information:

Name: (Last, First) Dexter, Reggie ☒ Male ☐ Female Birth Date: 05/17/1987

Address: 627 Sutton Way, Capital City, NY 12345 Phone: (555) 555-8840

Social Security Number: 833-88-4332 Full-Time Student: ☐ Yes ☒ No

Marital Status: ☒ Single ☐ Married ☐ Divorced ☐ Other

Employment:

Employer: _____ Phone: ( ) _____

Address: _____

Condition Related to: ☐ Auto Accident ☐ Employment ☐ Other Accident

Date of Accident: _____ State: _____

Emergency Contact: _____ **Phone: ( )** _____

Primary Insurance: Medicaid Phone: ( ) _____

Address: 4875 Capital Blvd, Capital City, NY 12345

Insurance Policyholder's Name: Same ☐ M ☐ F DOB: _____

Address: _____

Phone: _____ Relationship to Insured: ☒ Self ☐ Spouse ☐ Child ☐ Other

Employer: _____ Phone: ( ) _____

Employer's Address: _____

Policy/ID No: 0054631658763 Group No: ____ Percent Covered: ____% Copay Amt: $5.00

Secondary Insurance: _____ Phone: ( ) _____

Address: _____

Insurance Policyholder's Name: _____ ☐ M ☐ F DOB: _____

Address: _____

Phone: _____ Relationship to Insured: ☐ Self ☐ Spouse ☐ Child ☐ Other

Employer: _____ Phone: ( ) _____

Employer's Address: _____

Policy/ID No: _____ Group No: ____ Percent Covered: ____% Copay Amt: $____

Reason for Visit: Pt. is here for a URI.

Known Allergies: _____

Referred by: _____

CASE 19-3
SOAP

03/02/20XX
Assignment of Benefits: Y
Signature on File: Y
Referring Physician: N

S: New patient Reggie Dexter is brought here today by his sister Marie. He has been complaining of a sore throat and sneezing.

O: Pt. says that he has been sick for 3 days. T: 98.4°F. He does have nasal congestion. He has recently entered a camp for young adults with Down syndrome. He loves it. He has made new friends there. Chest is clear. Throat shows a little redness.

A: 1. Upper respiratory tract infection—465.9.

P: 1. Nasonex q.d.
    2. Stay home from camp for at least 2 days.
    3. Liquid diet for the next 24 hours.
    4. Use humidifier.
    5. Return p.r.n.

_____

Phil Wells, MD
Family Practice
NPI: 1234567890

CASE 19-3

Patient Name Reggie Dexter

Capital City Medical
123 Unknown Boulevard, Capital City, NY 12345-2222

Date of Service
03-02-20XX

New Patient			Arthrocentesis/Aspiration/Injection			Laboratory	
Problem Focused	99201		Small Joint	20600		Amylase	82150
Expanded Problem, Focused	99202		Small Joint	20600		B12	82607
Detailed	99203	X	Interm Joint	20605		CBC & Diff	85025
Comprehensive	99204		Major Joint	20610		Comp Metabolic Panel	80053
Comprehensive/High Complex	99205		**Other Invasive/Noninvasive**			Chlamydia Screen	87110
Well Exam Infant (up to 12 mos.)	99381		Audiometry	92552		Cholesterol	82465
Well Exam 1–4 yrs.	99382		Cast Application			Digoxin	80162
Well Exam 5–11 yrs.	99383		Location Long Short			Electrolytes	80051
Well Exam 12–17 yrs.	99384		Catheterization	51701		Ferritin	82728
Well Exam 18–39 yrs.	99385		Circumcision	54150		Folate	82746
Well Exam 40–64 yrs.	99386		Colposcopy	57452		GC Screen	87070
			Colposcopy w/Biopsy	57454		Glucose	82947
			Cryosurgery Premalignant Lesion			Glucose 1 HR	82950
			Location (s):			Glycosylated HGB A1C	83036
Established Patient			Cryosurgery Warts			HCT	85014
Post-Op Follow Up Visit	99024		Location (s):			HDL	83718
Minimum	99211		Curettement Lesion			Hep BSAG	87340
Problem Focused	99212		Single	11055		Hepatitis panel, acute	80074
Expanded Problem Focused	99213		2–4	11056		HGB	85018
Detailed	99214		>4	11057		HIV	86703
Comprehensive/High Complex	99215		Diaphragm Fitting	57170		Iron & TIBC	83550
Well Exam Infant (up to 12 mos.)	99391		Ear Irrigation	69210		Kidney Profile	80069
Well exam 1–4 yrs.	99392		ECG	93000		Lead	83655
Well Exam 5–11 yrs.	99393		Endometrial Biopsy	58100		Liver Profile	80076
Well Exam 12–17 yrs.	99394		Exc. Lesion Malignant			Mono Test	86308
Well Exam 18–39 yrs.	99395		Benign			Pap Smear	88155
Well Exam 40–64 yrs.	99396		Location			Pregnancy Test	84703
Obstetrics			Exc. Skin Tags (1–15)	11200		Obstetric Panel	80055
Total OB Care	59400		Each Additional 10	11201		Pro Time	85610
Injections			Fracture Treatment			PSA	84153
Administration Sub. / IM	90772		Loc			RPR	86592
Drug			w/Reduc w/o Reduc			Sed. Rate	85651
Dosage			I & D Abscess Single/Simple	10060		Stool Culture	87045
Allergy	95115		Multiple or Comp	10061		Stool O & P	87177
Cocci Skin Test	86490		I & D Pilonidal Cyst Simple	10080		Strep Screen	87880
DPT	90701		Pilonidal Cyst Complex	10081		Theophylline	80198
Hemophilus	90646		IV Therapy—To One Hour	90760		Thyroid Uptake	84479
Influenza	90658		Each Additional Hour	90761		TSH	84443
MMR	90707		Laceration Repair			Urinalysis	81000
OPV	90712		Location Size Simp/Comp			Urine Culture	87088
Pneumovax	90732		Laryngoscopy	31505		Drawing Fee	36415
TB Skin Test	86580		Oximetry	94760		Specimen Collection	99000
TD	90718		Punch Biopsy			**Other:**	
Unlisted Immun	90749		Rhythm Strip	93040			
Tetanus Toxoid	90703		Treadmill	93015			
Vaccine/Toxoid Admin <8 Yr Old w/ Counseling	90465		Trigger Point or Tendon Sheath Inj.	20550			
Vaccine/Toxoid Administration for Adult	90471		Tympanometry	92567			

Diagnosis/ICD-9: **465.0**

I acknowledge receipt of medical services and authorize the release of any medical information necessary to process this claim for healthcare payment only. I do authorize payment to the provider.

Patient Signature _Reggie Dexter_

Total Estimated Charges: _____

Payment Amount: _____

Next Appointment: _____

d. Using the source documents provided, complete the given case study for patient Christian Monaco (Case 19-4) by entering the case information into medical practice management software. Prepare a CMS-1500 claim form.

CASE 19-4

Capital City Medical—123 Unknown Boulevard, Capital City, NY 12345-2222 (555) 555-1234	Patient Information Form
Phil Wells, MD, Mannie Mends, MD, Bette R. Soone, MD	Tax ID: 75-0246810
	Group NPI: 1513171216

Patient Information:

Name: (Last, First) Monaco, Christian   ☒ Male   ❑ Female   Birth Date: 12/31/1965

Address: 9 Fording Rd, Capital City, NY 12345   Phone: (555) 555-5654

Social Security Number: 719-60-7197   Full-Time Student: ❑ Yes   ☒ No

Marital Status: ❑ Single   ☒ Married   ❑ Divorced   ❑ Other

Employment:

Employer: Monaco Paving   Phone: (555) 555-5654

Address: 9 Fording Rd, Capital City, NY 12345

Condition Related to: ❑ Auto Accident   ❑ Employment   ❑ Other Accident

Date of Accident: _____ State: _____

Emergency Contact: _____ **Phone: ( )** _____

Primary Insurance: Aetna   Phone: ( ) _____

Address: 1625 Healthcare Bldg, Capital City, NY 12345

Insurance Policyholder's Name: Same   ❑ M ❑ F DOB: _____

Address: _____

Phone: _____ Relationship to Insured: ☒ Self ❑ Spouse ❑ Child ❑ Other

Employer: _____ Phone: ( ) _____

Employer's Address: _____

Policy/ID No: 43216932   Group No: 0687 Percent Covered: ____% Copay Amt: $ 20.00

Secondary Insurance: _____ Phone: ( ) _____

Address: _____

Insurance Policyholder's Name: _____   ❑ M ❑ F DOB: _____

Address: _____

Phone: _____ Relationship to Insured: ❑ Self ❑ Spouse ❑ Child ❑ Other

Employer: _____ Phone: ( ) _____

Employer's Address: _____

Policy/ID No: _____ Group No: ____ Percent Covered: ____% Copay Amt: $____

Reason for Visit: I am here for a hiatal hernia.

Known Allergies: _____

Referred by: _____

CASE 19–4
SOAP

05/27/20XX
Assignment of Benefits: Y
Signature on File: Y
Referring Physician: N

S: Christian Monaco is being seen for his hiatal hernia. He has no new complaints.

O: Pt. states that he has had good response to Reglan. He has been avoiding trigger foods. Oropharynx is clear. Chest is clear to A&P. Bowel sounds are normal. Abdomen is soft, nontender.

A: 1. Hiatal hernia—553.3.

P: 1. Continue Reglan.
    2. Return in 4 months.

_____

Phil Wells, MD
Family Practice
NPI: 1234567890

CASE 19-4

Patient Name Christian Monaco

Capital City Medical
123 Unknown Boulevard, Capital City, NY 12345-2222

Date of Service
05-27-20XX

New Patient		Arthrocentesis/Aspiration/Injection		Laboratory	
Problem Focused	99201	Arthrocentesis/Aspiration/Injection		Amylase	82150
Expanded Problem, Focused	99202	Small Joint	20600	B12	82607
Detailed	99203	Interm Joint	20605	CBC & Diff	85025
Comprehensive	99204	Major Joint	20610	Comp Metabolic Panel	80053
Comprehensive/High Complex	99205	**Other Invasive/Noninvasive**		Chlamydia Screen	87110
Well Exam Infant (up to 12 mos.)	99381	Audiometry	92552	Cholesterol	82465
Well Exam 1–4 yrs.	99382	Cast Application		Digoxin	80162
Well Exam 5–11 yrs.	99383	Location Long Short		Electrolytes	80051
Well Exam 12–17 yrs.	99384	Catheterization	51701	Ferritin	82728
Well Exam 18–39 yrs.	99385	Circumcision	54150	Folate	82746
Well Exam 40–64 yrs.	99386	Colposcopy	57452	GC Screen	87070
		Colposcopy w/Biopsy	57454	Glucose	82947
		Cryosurgery Premalignant Lesion		Glucose 1 HR	82950
		Location (s):		Glycosylated HGB A1C	83036
Established Patient		Cryosurgery Warts		HCT	85014
Post-Op Follow Up Visit	99024	Location (s):		HDL	83718
Minimum	99211	Curettement Lesion		Hep BSAG	87340
Problem Focused	99212 X	Single	11055	Hepatitis panel, acute	80074
Expanded Problem Focused	99213	2–4	11056	HGB	85018
Detailed	99214	>4	11057	HIV	86703
Comprehensive/High Complex	99215	Diaphragm Fitting	57170	Iron & TIBC	83550
Well Exam Infant (up to 12 mos.)	99391	Ear Irrigation	69210	Kidney Profile	80069
Well exam 1–4 yrs.	99392	ECG	93000	Lead	83655
Well Exam 5–11 yrs.	99393	Endometrial Biopsy	58100	Liver Profile	80076
Well Exam 12–17 yrs.	99394	Exc. Lesion Malignant		Mono Test	86308
Well Exam 18–39 yrs.	99395	Benign		Pap Smear	88155
Well Exam 40–64 yrs.	99396	Location		Pregnancy Test	84703
Obstetrics		Exc. Skin Tags (1–15)	11200	Obstetric Panel	80055
Total OB Care	59400	Each Additional 10	11201	Pro Time	85610
Injections		Fracture Treatment		PSA	84153
Administration Sub. / IM	90772	Loc		RPR	86592
Drug		w/Reduc w/o Reduc		Sed. Rate	85651
Dosage		I & D Abscess Single/Simple	10060	Stool Culture	87045
Allergy	95115	Multiple or Comp	10061	Stool O & P	87177
Cocci Skin Test	86490	I & D Pilonidal Cyst Simple	10080	Strep Screen	87880
DPT	90701	Pilonidal Cyst Complex	10081	Theophylline	80198
Hemophilus	90646	IV Therapy—To One Hour	90760	Thyroid Uptake	84479
Influenza	90658	Each Additional Hour	90761	TSH	84443
MMR	90707	Laceration Repair		Urinalysis	81000
OPV	90712	Location Size Simp/Comp		Urine Culture	87088
Pneumovax	90732	Laryngoscopy	31505	Drawing Fee	36415
TB Skin Test	86580	Oximetry	94760	Specimen Collection	99000
TD	90718	Punch Biopsy		**Other:**	
Unlisted Immun	90749	Rhythm Strip	93040		
Tetanus Toxoid	90703	Treadmill	93015		
Vaccine/Toxoid Admin <8 Yr Old w/ Counseling	90465	Trigger Point or Tendon Sheath Inj.	20550		
Vaccine/Toxoid Administration for Adult	90471	Tympanometry	92567		

Diagnosis/ICD-9: **553.3**

I acknowledge receipt of medical services and authorize the release of any medical information necessary to process this claim for healthcare payment only. I do authorize payment to the provider.

Total Estimated Charges: _____

Payment Amount: _____

Patient Signature *Christian Monaco*

Next Appointment: _____

e. Using the source documents provided, complete the given case study for patient Edie Everly (Case 19-5) by entering the case information into medical practice management software. Prepare a CMS-1500 claim form.

CASE 19-5

Capital City Medical—123 Unknown Boulevard, Capital City, NY 12345-2222 (555) 555-1234	Patient Information Form
Phil Wells, MD, Mannie Mends, MD, Bette R. Soone, MD	Tax ID: 75-0246810
	Group NPI: 1513171216

Patient Information:

Name: (Last, First) Everly, Edie ☐ Male ☒ Female Birth Date: 10/01/1994

Address: 13 Church St, Township, NY 12345 Phone: (555) 555-1858

Social Security Number: 369-96-3000 Full-Time Student: ☒ Yes ☐ No

Marital Status: ☒ Single ☐ Married ☐ Divorced ☐ Other

Employment:

Employer: _____ Phone: ( ) _____

Address: _____

Condition Related to: ☐ Auto Accident ☐ Employment ☐ Other Accident

Date of Accident: _____ State: _____

Emergency Contact: _____ **Phone: ( )** _____

Primary Insurance: Aetna Phone: ( ) _____

Address: 1625 Healthcare Bldg, Capital City, NY 12345

Insurance Policyholder's Name: Lori Everly ☐ M ☒ F DOB: 06/20/1972

Address: Same

Phone: _____ Relationship to Insured: ☐ Self ☐ Spouse ☒ Child ☐ Other

Employer: Westview Management Corp. Phone: (555) 555-9444

Employer's Address: 910 Harding Rd, Township, NY 12345

Policy/ID No: 852013315 Group No: 2157 Percent Covered: ___% Copay Amt: $ 30.00

Secondary Insurance: Blue Cross Blue Shield Phone: ( ) _____

Address: 379 Blue Plaza, Capital City, NY 12345

Insurance Policyholder's Name: Kurt Everly ☒ M ☐ F DOB: 10/29/1972

Address: Same

Phone: _____ Relationship to Insured: ☐ Self ☐ Spouse ☒ Child ☐ Other

Employer: Capital City Morgue Phone: (555) 555-3323

Employer's Address: 2300 City Bldg, Capital City, NY 12345

Policy/ID No: YYJ199699828 Group No: 752771 Percent Covered: ___% Copay Amt: $25.00

Reason for Visit: My daughter seems to have an infected toenail.

Known Allergies: _____

Referred by: _____

CASE 19-5
SOAP

07/05/20XX
Assignment of Benefits: Y
Signature on File: Y
Referring Physician: N

S: New patient Edie Everly is in the office today because of an infected nail of the great toe on her left foot. She says that it hurts really bad.

O: The toenail is infected. It is tender to the touch. All other toenails are normal. She admits to walking outside barefoot all the time. Liver enzymes are normal; cleared for medication therapy.

A: 1. Onychomycosis—110.1.

P: 1. Lamasil one daily for 12 weeks.
2. Return in 1 month.
3. Lab work before next appointment to evaluate liver enzymes.
4. Wear shoes outdoors.

_____

Phil Wells, MD
Family Practice
NPI: 1234567890

CASE 19-5

Patient Name Edie Everly

Capital City Medical
123 Unknown Boulevard, Capital City, NY 12345-2222

Date of Service
07-05-20XX

New Patient			Other Invasive/Noninvasive			Laboratory		
Problem Focused	99201		Arthrocentesis/Aspiration/Injection			Amylase	82150	
Expanded Problem, Focused	99202		Small Joint	20600		B12	82607	
Detailed	99203	X	Interm Joint	20605		CBC & Diff	85025	
Comprehensive	99204		Major Joint	20610		Comp Metabolic Panel	80053	
Comprehensive/High Complex	99205		**Other Invasive/Noninvasive**			Chlamydia Screen	87110	
Well Exam Infant (up to 12 mos.)	99381		Audiometry	92552		Cholesterol	82465	
Well Exam 1–4 yrs.	99382		Cast Application			Digoxin	80162	
Well Exam 5–11 yrs.	99383		Location Long Short			Electrolytes	80051	
Well Exam 12–17 yrs.	99384		Catheterization	51701		Ferritin	82728	
Well Exam 18–39 yrs.	99385		Circumcision	54150		Folate	82746	
Well Exam 40–64 yrs.	99386		Colposcopy	57452		GC Screen	87070	
			Colposcopy w/Biopsy	57454		Glucose	82947	
			Cryosurgery Premalignant Lesion			Glucose 1 HR	82950	
			Location (s):			Glycosylated HGB A1C	83036	
Established Patient			Cryosurgery Warts			HCT	85014	
Post-Op Follow Up Visit	99024		Location (s):			HDL	83718	
Minimum	99211		Curettement Lesion			Hep BSAG	87340	
Problem Focused	99212		Single	11055		Hepatitis panel, acute	80074	
Expanded Problem Focused	99213		2–4	11056		HGB	85018	
Detailed	99214		>4	11057		HIV	86703	
Comprehensive/High Complex	99215		Diaphragm Fitting	57170		Iron & TIBC	83550	
Well Exam Infant (up to 12 mos.)	99391		Ear Irrigation	69210		Kidney Profile	80069	
Well exam 1–4 yrs.	99392		ECG	93000		Lead	83655	
Well Exam 5–11 yrs.	99393		Endometrial Biopsy	58100		Liver Profile	80076	X
Well Exam 12–17 yrs.	99394		Exc. Lesion Malignant			Mono Test	86308	
Well Exam 18–39 yrs.	99395		Benign			Pap Smear	88155	
Well Exam 40–64 yrs.	99396		Location			Pregnancy Test	84703	
Obstetrics			Exc. Skin Tags (1–15)	11200		Obstetric Panel	80055	
Total OB Care	59400		Each Additional 10	11201		Pro Time	85610	
Injections			Fracture Treatment			PSA	84153	
Administration Sub. / IM	90772		Loc			RPR	86592	
Drug			w/Reduc	w/o Reduc		Sed. Rate	85651	
Dosage			I & D Abscess Single/Simple	10060		Stool Culture	87045	
Allergy	95115		Multiple or Comp	10061		Stool O & P	87177	
Cocci Skin Test	86490		I & D Pilonidal Cyst Simple	10080		Strep Screen	87880	
DPT	90701		Pilonidal Cyst Complex	10081		Theophylline	80198	
Hemophilus	90646		IV Therapy—To One Hour	90760		Thyroid Uptake	84479	
Influenza	90658		Each Additional Hour	90761		TSH	84443	
MMR	90707		Laceration Repair			Urinalysis	81000	
OPV	90712		Location Size Simp/Comp			Urine Culture	87088	
Pneumovax	90732		Laryngoscopy	31505		Drawing Fee	36415	X
TB Skin Test	86580		Oximetry	94760		Specimen Collection	99000	
TD	90718		Punch Biopsy			**Other:**		
Unlisted Immun	90749		Rhythm Strip	93040				
Tetanus Toxoid	90703		Treadmill	93015				
Vaccine/Toxoid Admin <8 Yr Old w/ Counseling	90465		Trigger Point or Tendon Sheath Inj.	20550				
Vaccine/Toxoid Administration for Adult	90471		Tympanometry	92567				

Diagnosis/ICD-9: **110.1**

I acknowledge receipt of medical services and authorize the release of any medical information necessary to process this claim for healthcare payment only. I do authorize payment to the provider.

Total Estimated Charges: _____

Payment Amount: _____

Patient Signature Edie Everly _____

Next Appointment: _____

REVIEW QUESTIONS

MATCHING

Choose the correct answer and place its corresponding letter in the space provided.

a. walkout receipt
b. day sheet
c. aging report
d. superbill
e. transactions

1. _____ Form that lists both procedure and diagnosis codes, charges, rendering physician, and a return appointment for a patient
2. _____ Lists outstanding accounts
3. _____ Records of charges, payments, and adjustments
4. _____ Lists all patient transactions for a specific day
5. _____ Form printed out for each patient, listing each patient's posted charges

MULTIPLE CHOICE

Circle the letter of the choice that best completes the statement or answers the question.

1. What information is used to enter the diagnosis code and code any procedures?
   a. Patient SOAP note
   b. Patient information form
   c. Superbill
   d. Both a and b

2. Which form is used to post insurance payments and any adjustments?
   a. Superbill
   b. Ledger
   c. Explanation of benefits
   d. Day sheet

3. If the patient and guarantor are two different people, you should _____.
   a. add the patient to the patient/guarantor list
   b. add the patient and guarantor to the patient/guarantor list
   c. add the guarantor to the patient/guarantor list
   d. None of the above

4. Which report reflecting all posting activity is run at the end of the day?
   a. Day sheet
   b. Ledger
   c. Walkout receipt
   d. Encounter form

5. A patient's signature for authorization of insurance payments to be made directly to the provider would be found on which form?
   a. Encounter form
   b. Registration form
   c. Explanation of benefits
   d. All of the above

SHORT ANSWER

Provide the correct response to each of the following questions.

1. To obtain the total charges for the day you must add up the _____,
_____, and _____.

2. After you have completed the day's batch, you then need to create what important forms to bill the insurance carriers?
   _____

3. What are four different provider ID numbers that can be used in the MPM system?

   1. _____
   2. _____
   3. _____
   4. _____

4. What menu option in the MPM system allows you to access and run reports?
   _____

5. What is the superbill used for?
   _____

TRUE/FALSE

Identify each statement as true (T) or false (F).

1. _____ An insurance claim can still be submitted even before a batch is complete.
2. _____ Correcting an error in a patient's account will automatically update the claim form.
3. _____ The MPM system does not have any shortcut buttons.
4. _____ You do not have to note the relationship of the patient to the insured in the MPM software.
5. _____ All procedure and diagnosis codes will already be listed in the MPM system.

Tests

TEST 1: IDENTIFY THE CORRECT DIAGNOSTIC CODE

Directions: Accurately code each given diagnosis with the correct ICD-9-CM and/or ICD-10-CM/PCS code(s). Determine the correct number of codes for each scenario. Code E codes where applicable.

1. Admission for radiation (block delivery)

   ICD-9-CM Code(s) _____ ICD-10-CM Code(s) _____

2. Alcoholism complicating pregnancy (not yet delivered)

   ICD-9-CM Code(s) _____ ICD-10-CM Code(s) _____

3. Aplastic anemia due to red cell aplasia (adult, acquired)

   ICD-9-CM Code(s) _____ ICD-10-CM Code(s) _____

4. Abdominal aortic aneurysm

   ICD-9-CM Code(s) _____ ICD-10-CM Code(s) _____

5. Childhood asthma

   ICD-9-CM Code(s) _____ ICD-10-CM Code(s) _____

6. Birthing injury to eye

   ICD-9-CM Code(s) _____ ICD-10-CM Code(s) _____

7. Sinus bradycardia

   ICD-9-CM Code(s) _____ ICD-10-CM Code(s) _____

8. Chlamydial balanitis

   ICD-9-CM Code(s) _____ ICD-10-CM Code(s) _____

9. Second-degree and third-degree burn to back due to fall into campfire in fire ring

   ICD-9-CM Code(s) _____ ICD-10-CM Code(s) _____

10. Routine follow-up for postpartum care

    ICD-9-CM Code(s) _____ ICD-10-CM Code(s) _____

11. Breech Cesarean delivery

    ICD-9-CM Code(s) _____ ICD-10-CM Code(s) _____

12. Sacral decubitus

    ICD-9-CM Code(s) _____ ICD-10-CM Code(s) _____

13. Hereditary macular degeneration

    ICD-9-CM Code(s) _____ ICD-10-CM Code(s) _____

14. Diabetes Mellitus II with cataracts

    ICD-9-CM Code(s) _____ ICD-10-CM Code(s) _____

15. Rash from allergic reaction to initial dose of penicillin

    ICD-9-CM Code(s) _____ ICD-10-CM Code(s) _____

16. Post-op pulmonary embolism

    ICD-9-CM Code(s) _____ ICD-10-CM Code(s) _____

17. Congestive heart failure

   ICD-9-CM Code(s) _____ ICD-10-CM Code(s) _____

18. Abnormal protein findings in urine

   ICD-9-CM Code(s) _____ ICD-10-CM Code(s) _____

19. Denture fitting

   ICD-9-CM Code(s) _____ ICD-10-CM Code(s) _____

20. Fracture, neck of humerus due to roller skating accident

   ICD-9-CM Code(s) _____ ICD-10-CM Code(s) _____

21. Tension headache

   ICD-9-CM Code(s) _____ ICD-10-CM Code(s) _____

22. History of penicillin allergy

   ICD-9-CM Code(s) _____ ICD-10-CM Code(s) _____

23. Family history of polycystic kidney disease

   ICD-9-CM Code(s) _____ ICD-10-CM Code(s) _____

24. History of noncompliance to medical treatment

   ICD-9-CM Code(s) _____ ICD-10-CM Code(s) _____

25. Benign orthostatic hypertension

   ICD-9-CM Code(s) _____ ICD-10-CM Code(s) _____

26. Late effect, traumatic arthritis due to old ankle sprain

   ICD-9-CM Code(s) _____ ICD-10-CM Code(s) _____

27. Primary neoplasm of stomach with secondary neoplasm of the spine

   ICD-9-CM Code(s) _____ ICD-10-CM Code(s) _____

28. Outcome, delivery of twins, both born alive

   ICD-9-CM Code(s) _____ ICD-10-CM Code(s) _____

29. Melanoma on the back

   ICD-9-CM Code(s) _____ ICD-10-CM Code(s) _____

30. Respiratory arrest after accidental overdose of dilaudid by nurse

   ICD-9-CM Code(s) _____ ICD-10-CM Code(s) _____

31. Food poisoning due to salmonella with gastroenteritis

   ICD-9-CM Code(s) _____ ICD-10-CM Code(s) _____

32. Late effect of facial droop due to cerebrovascular accident suffered 3 months ago

   ICD-9-CM Code(s) _____ ICD-10-CM Code(s) _____

33. End-stage kidney disease

   ICD-9-CM Code(s) _____ ICD-10-CM Code(s) _____

TEST 2: CODING HOSPITAL PROCEDURES

Directions: Using the ICD-9-CM manual, Volume 3, and the ICD-10-PCS manual accurately code the following hospital procedures, determining the correct number of codes for each scenario:

1. Laparoscopic ablation of liver lesion

   ICD-9 Code _____ ICD-10 Code _____

2. Small intestine to anus anastomosis

   ICD-9 Code _____ ICD-10 Code _____

3. Appendicocecostomy

   ICD-9 Code _____ ICD-10 Code _____

4. Arthroplasty of wrist, total

   ICD-9 Code _____ ICD-10 Code _____

5. Brush lung biopsy

   ICD-9 Code _____ ICD-10 Code _____

6. Blood transfusion (platelets)

   ICD-9 Code _____ ICD-10 Code _____

7. Cardiopulmonary bypass, open

   ICD-9 Code _____ ICD-10 Code _____

8. Atrial cardioversion

   ICD-9 Code _____ ICD-10 Code _____

9. Swan-Ganz catheterization

   ICD-9 Code _____ ICD-10 Code _____

10. Chemotherapy for cancer

    ICD-9 Code _____ ICD-10 Code _____

11. Vacuum extraction delivery with episiotomy

    ICD-9 Code _____ ICD-10 Code _____

12. Destruction of prostatic lesion by transurethral needle ablation

    ICD-9 Code _____ ICD-10 Code _____

13. EKG

    ICD-9 Code _____ ICD-10 Code _____

14. Steroid injection

    ICD-9 Code _____ ICD-10 Code _____

15. Laryngotracheoscopy

    ICD-9 Code _____ ICD-10 Code _____

16. Laparoscopic lysis of abdominal adhesions

    ICD-9 Code _____ ICD-10 Code _____

17. Mammoplasty with augmentation for left breast implant

    ICD-9 Code _____ ICD-10 Code _____

18. Femoral phlebography

    ICD-9 Code _____ ICD-10 Code _____

19. X-ray of left knee

ICD-9 Code _____ ICD-10 Code _____

20. Cranial cavity catheterization

ICD-9 Code _____ ICD-10 Code _____

21. Partial ascending colon resection

ICD-9 Code _____ ICD-10 Code _____

22. Bone CT scan

ICD-9 Code _____ ICD-10 Code _____

23. Nasolacrimal duct syringing with tube insertion

ICD-9 Code _____ ICD-10 Code _____

24. Cardiac stress test, treadmill

ICD-9 Code _____ ICD-10 Code _____

25. Retrograde pyelogram

ICD-9 Code _____ ICD-10 Code _____

TEST 3: CODING OUTPATIENT PROCEDURES AND DIAGNOSES

Directions: Using the ICD-9-CM, the ICD-10-CM/PCS, and the CPT® manuals, accurately code each given outpatient procedure and diagnosis. Include CPT modifiers as necessary. (These codes do not require an E/M code.)

1. A 17-year-old male has had chronic tonsillitis with adenitis since he was a toddler. He undergoes a tonsillectomy with adenectomy without any complications.

   Diagnosis code(s) ICD-9: _____

   Diagnosis code(s) ICD-10: _____

   Procedure code(s) _____

2. An attending technician performs a sleep study on a patient who has not been sleeping well. The test reveals obstructive sleep apnea.

   Diagnosis code(s) ICD-9: _____

   Diagnosis code(s) ICD-10: _____

   Procedure code(s) _____

3. During a physical examination, a patient's EKG reveals premature atrial contractions (PACs).

   Diagnosis code(s) ICD-9: _____

   Diagnosis code(s) ICD-10: _____

   Procedure code(s) _____

4. A transurethral resection of the prostate is performed by an assistant surgeon on a patient with prostate cancer, primary. The surgery is performed by the electrosurgical technique.

   Diagnosis code(s) ICD-9: _____

   Diagnosis code(s) ICD-10: _____

   Procedure code(s) _____

5. A female patient is admitted to the hospital for a right and left bundle branch block (R&L BBB). A dual chamber pacemaker with epicardial electrodes is inserted by endoscopy. The patient tolerates the procedure well. The cardiovascular surgeon informs the patient that he only performed the surgery, and that she is to follow up with her regular consulting cardiologist for postoperative care.

   Diagnosis code(s) ICD-9: _____

   Diagnosis code(s) ICD-10: _____

   Procedure code(s) _____

6. Mrs. Packard is in the office today for her monthly vitamin B12 injection. She has a vitamin B12 deficiency.

   Diagnosis code(s) ICD-9: _____

   Diagnosis code(s) ICD-10: _____

   Procedure code(s) _____

7. A patient presents with shortness of breath (SOB) and chest pain (CP). The EKG that is done in the office shows no abnormalities. The patient is sent home with a 24-hour Holter monitor that was also normal. The next day, a stress exercise conducted in the physician's office is stopped due to the occurrence of chest pain. Code for all services.

   Diagnosis code(s) ICD-9: _____

   Diagnosis code(s) ICD-10: _____

   Procedure code(s) _____

8. Carolyn Ashbury has been having reflux esophagitis problems for 4 months. She has tried three different medicines that have provided no relief. Because Carolyn's mother had esophageal cancer, the physician performs a flexible esophagoscopy with biopsy.

Diagnosis code(s) ICD-9: _____

Diagnosis code(s) ICD-10: _____

Procedure code(s) _____

9. A patient has injured his ulnar nerve of the wrist and hand. Neuroplasty of the ulnar nerve is performed to free it of scar tissue.

Diagnosis code(s) ICD-9: _____

Diagnosis code(s) ICD-10: _____

Procedure code(s) _____

10. A patient with an acute recurrent myocardial infarction (MI) 1 week ago has a right heart catheterization. This procedure includes contrast injection for the heart catheter with supervision, interpretation, and report for the imaging.

Diagnosis code(s) ICD-9: _____

Diagnosis code(s) ICD-10: _____

Procedure code(s) _____

11. Douglas Fuller suffered a complicated forehead wound due to striking his head against the corner of his bedroom dresser. He has an adjacent skin tissue transfer of 3 sq. cm. to his forehead.

Diagnosis code(s) ICD-9: _____

Diagnosis code(s) ICD-10: _____

Procedure code(s) _____

12. A patient has simple destruction of vaginal venereal warts by laser surgery.

Diagnosis code(s) ICD-9: _____

Diagnosis code(s) ICD-10: _____

Procedure code(s) _____

13. Mr. Wallace has a repair to his diaphragm for a hiatal hernia. The procedure is done by thoracoabdominal approach.

Diagnosis code(s) ICD-9: _____

Diagnosis code(s) ICD-10: _____

Procedure code(s) _____

14. A patient is seen today for a psychological interview and evaluation. The patient has narcissistic personality disorder.

Diagnosis code(s) ICD-9: _____

Diagnosis code(s) ICD-10: _____

Procedure code(s) _____

15. A patient with acquired hydrocephalus undergoes Tokildsen operation to create a brain shunt.

Diagnosis code(s) ICD-9: _____

Diagnosis code(s) ICD-10: _____

Procedure code(s) _____

TEST 4: CODING OUTPATIENT RADIOLOGY AND/OR PATHOLOGY PROCEDURES AND DIAGNOSES

Directions: Using the ICD-9-CM, ICD-10-CM/PCS, and the CPT manuals, accurately code each given outpatient radiology and/or pathology procedure and diagnosis. Include CPT modifiers as necessary. (These codes do not require an E/M code.)

Radiology

1. A CT scan without contrast, followed by contrast, with 3-D rendering and postprocessing, is performed on a patient with clonic epilepsy.

   Diagnosis code(s) ICD-9: _____

   Diagnosis code(s) ICD-10: _____

   Procedure code(s) _____

2. A limited abdominal ultrasound (U/S) is performed on a patient with R upper quadrant abdominal pain.

   Diagnosis code(s) ICD-9: _____

   Diagnosis code(s) ICD-10: _____

   Procedure code(s) _____

3. Rebecca DeMarco undergoes a DXA scan to evaluate her total body composition. She is at postmenopausal status and is having an osteoporosis screen.

   Diagnosis code(s) ICD-9: _____

   Diagnosis code(s) ICD-10: _____

   Procedure code(s) _____

4. A B/L pulmonary angiography is performed to confirm an iatrogenic pulmonary embolism.

   Diagnosis code(s) ICD-9: _____

   Diagnosis code(s) ICD-10: _____

   Procedure code(s) _____

5. Lucas Andrews, who has been experiencing shoulder pain and limited ROM, is ordered an MRI of the left shoulder. Films show a left rotator cuff tear.

   Diagnosis code(s) ICD-9: _____

   Diagnosis code(s) ICD-10: _____

   Procedure code(s) _____

6. Eugene Vitale receives five radiation treatment management sessions for his papillary carcinoma thyroid cancer, in situ.

   Diagnosis code(s) ICD-9: _____

   Diagnosis code(s) ICD-10: _____

   Procedure code(s) _____

Laboratory/Pathology

7. During surgery, the pathologist receives a specimen of the descending colon. He freezes one block and separates two frozen sections to examine. He makes a diagnosis of primary carcinoma and calls up the result to the operating room.

   Diagnosis code(s) ICD-9: _____

   Diagnosis code(s) ICD-10: _____

   Procedure code(s) _____

8. Steven Palmer is seen today with complaints of frequent urination and excessive thirst. A urinalysis (U/A) dipstick and complete metabolic panel (CMP) are performed. Patient is ordered a glucose tolerance test, which will be performed by an outside lab.

   Diagnosis code(s) ICD-9: _____

   Diagnosis code(s) ICD-10: _____

   Procedure code(s) _____

9. A patient experiencing headaches and nausea is admitted for carbon monoxide poisoning due to a gas leak in her home gas pipes. A qualitative carbon monoxide level is drawn three times in one day.

   Diagnosis code(s) ICD-9: _____

   Diagnosis code(s) ICD-10: _____

   Procedure code(s) _____

10. A patient presents, complaining of the inability to stop bleeding. A platelet count assay, a partial thromboplastin time (PTT), and a clot factor VIII (vw factor, multimetric analysis) are drawn. Blood tests reveal hemophilia A.

    Diagnosis code(s) ICD-9: _____

    Diagnosis code(s) ICD-10: _____

    Procedure code(s) _____

11. A stool sample is tested for Helicobacter pylori (H. pylori). Positive test results confirm the infection.

    Diagnosis code(s) ICD-9: _____

    Diagnosis code(s) ICD-10: _____

    Procedure code(s) _____

12. Surgical pathology for sterilization by vasectomy is negative for disease process.

    Diagnosis code(s) ICD-9: _____

    Diagnosis code(s) ICD-10: _____

    Procedure code(s) _____

13. Surgical pathology of a bone marrow biopsy is ordered for a patient with leukocytosis and a family history of leukemia.

    Diagnosis code(s) ICD-9: _____

    Diagnosis code(s) ICD-10: _____

    Procedure code(s) _____

14. Blood typing for ABO, Rh, and MN is drawn for paternity testing.

    Diagnosis code(s) ICD-9: _____

    Diagnosis code(s) ICD-10: _____

    Procedure code(s) _____

TEST 5: CODING PROCEDURES AND DIAGNOSES, USING E/M CODES

Directions: Using the CPT, ICD-9-CM, and ICD-10-CM/PCS manuals, code each scenario with a diagnosis code and an E/M code. Code any applicable diagnoses and/or procedures. Include modifiers as appropriate.

1. Denise Cox sees her family physician for a routine checkup on hypothyroidism and migraines. She has no complaints. An EFP exam is performed, with the following results: Neck: Supple. Throat: No masses felt. BP: 108/74, P: 80. TSH is 2.4. Maxalt has reduced her migraine episodes. Increase Synthroid to 50 mcg. daily. MDM was of low complexity. Return in 3 months with another TSH. Total time spent: 15 minutes.

   Diagnosis code(s) ICD-9: _____

   Diagnosis code(s) ICD-10: _____

   E/M code_____

   Procedure code(s)_____

2. Leonard Black is seeing his new PCP today. He is a 35-year-old African American male who has recently moved to the area. He does have HTN, benign. He is currently taking Diovan 80 mg. daily. A full PE is conducted. On exam, BP: 124/80, P: 76. Wt: 186. Ht: 6'1". HEENT: Normocephalic, atraumatic. Ears clear bilaterally. Eyes: Ecteric. Sclera is white. Nose: Clear. Throat: No masses. Neck: No bruits. Chest: Clear to A&P. No wheezes, rales, or rhonchi. Cardiovascular: S1, S2 present. No murmur. Abdomen: Soft, nontender. No masses felt. GI: Pt. denies heartburn and nausea. Bowel sounds are normal. MS: Normal ROM. No pain or swelling present. Skin: No breaks or bruises. Neurologic: A&O 33. Deep tendon refluxes are symmetrical. Psychiatric: Mood and affect upbeat. Labs (in office): Urinalysis by dipstick is negative for any disease process. CBC, automated, and diff normal values. Fasting lab prescription given. Patient to return for fasting lab results in 1 month.

   Diagnosis code(s) ICD-9: _____

   Diagnosis code(s) ICD-10: _____

   E/M code_____

   Procedure code(s)_____

3. A patient who was admitted for osteomyelitis of the left thigh 2 days ago is seen by her attending physician. A problem-focused internal history and exam indicates that she is responding well to therapy.

   Diagnosis code(s) ICD-9: _____

   Diagnosis code(s) ICD-10: _____

   E/M code_____

   Procedure code(s)_____

4. Dr. Melvin Gregory spends 45 minutes preparing hospital discharge orders for his patient. The patient, who has suffered a CVA with cerebral infarct, will be transferred to skilled nursing.

   Diagnosis code(s) ICD-9: _____

   Diagnosis code(s) ICD-10: _____

   E/M code_____

   Procedure code(s)_____

5. Victoria Marshall is admitted to the hospital with acute cholecystitis and cholelithiasis. Her PCP orders Roger Marvin, M.D., General Surgeon, to evaluate Victoria's condition. He performs a comprehensive history and PE. MDM is MC. A recommendation for surgery is made to the PCP.

Diagnosis code(s) ICD-9: _____

Diagnosis code(s) ICD-10: _____

Procedure code(s)_____

E/M code_____

6. A patient with right heel pain is referred to an orthopedist. A detailed history reveals that the patient does have congenital flat feet. A detailed exam is performed. Right heel X-rays show the presence of a heel spur and plantar fasciitis. The patient is ordered orthotics. A prescription for Ibuprofen is given. MDM is LC. The patient is to return in 1 month for reevaluation. A report is dictated to the PCP.

Diagnosis code(s) ICD-9: _____

Diagnosis code(s) ICD-10: _____

E/M code_____

Procedure code(s)_____

7. A new patient, Ellen Armstrong, is being seen by Lois Garlock, M.D., Internal Medicine, for a rash on both forearms. In an EPF history, the patient states that the rash is itchy and has been spreading. She noticed the rash 2 days ago. An EPF examination is consistent with poison oak. The patient is administered Depo-Medrol injection. The patient also is given a prescription for hydrocortisone 2.5% to apply topically to the infected area 2 × daily. The patient is advised to keep the area clean and to change bedding often. MDM SF.

Diagnosis code(s) ICD-9: _____

Diagnosis code(s) ICD-10: _____

E/M code_____

Procedure code(s)_____

8. A physician delivers a total of 120 minutes of critical care for a patient in a hepatic coma.

Diagnosis code(s) ICD-9: _____

Diagnosis code(s) ICD-10: _____

E/M code_____

Procedure code(s)_____

TEST 6: EXPLANATION OF BENEFITS

◧

Directions: Using the information provided on the Explanation of Benefits form that follows, calculate the total insurance payment to the rendering physician, payment owed by the patient, and appropriate adjustments. In addition, calculate the totals for each column and complete the Patient Summary section.

Today's Date: 11/02/2011

Payer Name & Address, Telephone #

HealthCo
777 Corporate Way
Capital City, NY 12345

Provider's Name & Address

Phil Wells, M.D.
123 Unknown Boulevard
Capital City, NY 12345

This statement covers payments for the following patient(s):
Claim Detail Section (If there are numbers in the "SEE REMARKS" column, see the Remarks section for explanation.)

Patient Name: Depinto, Janice	**Patient Account #:** JD85235
Patient ID#: 710151933	**Insured's Name:** Depinto, Janice
Group #: 65257	
Provider Name: Phil Wells, M.D.	**Inventory #:** 11454 **Claim Control #:** 91075

Service Date(s)	Procedure	Charges	Adjustment	Allowed	Co-pay	Deduct/Not Covered	Coins	Paid Amt.	Provider Paid	Remarks
9/27/2011	99213	55.00		38.00	0.00	0.00		80%		CO 045
9/27/2011	85025	95.00		65.00	0.00	0.00		80%		CO 045
9/27/2011	81000	35.00		30.00	0.00	0.00		80%		CO 045
9/27/2011	36415	15.00		12.00	0.00	0.00		80%		CO 045
TOTALS										

BALANCE DUE FROM PATIENT: PT'S DED/NOT COV $_____

                                               PT'S COINS. $_____

045 Charges exceed contracted fee.
CO Contractual obligation—provider responsible

PAYMENT SUMMARY SECTION (TOTALS)

Charges	Adjustment	Allowed	Co-pay	Deduct/Not Covered	Coins	Total Paid

TEST 7: EXPLANATION OF BENEFITS

Directions: Using the information provided on the Explanation of Benefits form that follows, calculate the total insurance payment to the rendering physician, payment owed by the patient, and appropriate adjustments. In addition, calculate the totals for reach column and complete the Payment Summary section.

Today's Date: 03/20/2012

Payer Name & Address

| HealthCo |
| 777 Corporate Way |
| Capital City, NY 12345 |

Provider's Name & Address

| Phil Wells, M.D. |
| 123 Unknown Boulevard |
| Capital City, NY 12345 |

This statement covers payments for the following patient(s):

Claim Detail Section (If there are numbers in the "SEE REMARKS" column, see the Remarks section for explanation.)

Patient Name: Kendall, Marty	**Patient Account #:** MK65443	
Patient ID #: 685502020	**Insured's Name:** Kendall, Marty	
Group #: 86513		
Provider Name: Phil Wells, M.D.	**Inventory #:** 36374	**Claim Control #:** 75488

Service Date(s)	Procedure	Charges	Adjustment	Allowed	Co-pay	Deduct/Not Covered	Coins	Paid Amt.	Provider Paid	Remarks
02/16/2012	99202	65.00		50.00	0.00	50.00		80%		CO 045 PR 001
02/16/2012	93000	75.00		55.00	0.00			80%		CO 045
02/16/2012	85025	95.00		65.00	0.00			80%		CO 045
02/16/2012	36415	15.00		12.00	0.00			80%		CO 045
TOTALS										

BALANCE DUE FROM PATIENT:

PT'S DED/NOT COV $_____

PT'S COINS. $_____

045 Charges exceed contracted fee.
001 Deductible amount
PR Patient responsible
CO Contractual obligation—provider responsible

PAYMENT SUMMARY SECTION (TOTALS)

Charges	Adjustment	Allowed	Co-pay	Deduct/Not Covered	Coins	Total Paid

TEST 8: COMPLETE A MEDICARE CLAIM

Directions: Using the source documents provided for patient Elsie Spaulding and the Capital City Medical fee schedule (Figure 1), accurately complete a CMS-1500 claim form for Medicare. Use the blank CMS-1500 form provided (Figure 2).

Complete the case on the basis of the following criteria:

- All patients have release of information and assignment of benefit signatures on file.
- All providers are participating and accept assignment.
- The group practice is the billing entity.
- The national transition to NPI numbers is complete, and legacy PINs and UPINs are no longer used.
- 2012 ICD-9-CM, ICD-10-CM/PCS, and CPT codes are used.
- Use eight-digit dates for birthdates. Use six-digit dates for all other dates.
- All street names should be entered with standard postal abbreviations, even if they are spelled out on the source documents.
- Enter ICD-9 codes and ICD-10 codes in the order in which they are listed on the encounter form.
- When entering CPT codes, enter the E/M code first. Enter remaining codes in descending price order.

TEST 8

Capital City Medical—123 Unknown Boulevard, Capital City, NY 12345-2222 (555) 555-1234	Patient Information Form
Phil Wells, MD, Mannie Mends, MD, Bette R. Soone, MD	Tax ID: 75-0246810
	Group NPI: 1513171216

Patient Information:

Name: (Last, First) Spaulding, Elsie ☐ Male ☒ Female Birth Date: 04/26/1947

Address: 60 Pittsburgh Rd, Township, NY 12345 Phone: (555) 555-0082

Social Security Number: 949-29-7761 Full-Time Student: ☐ Yes ☒ No

Marital Status: ☐ Single ☒ Married ☐ Divorced ☐ Other

Employment:

Employer: Retired Phone: ( )

Address:

Condition Related to: ☐ Auto Accident ☐ Employment ☐ Other Accident

Date of Accident: State:

Emergency Contact: **Phone: ( )**

Primary Insurance: Medicare Phone: ( )

Address: P. O. Box 9834, Capital City, NY 12345

Insurance Policyholder's Name: Same ☐ M ☐ F DOB:

Address:

Phone: Relationship to Insured: ☐ Self ☐ Spouse ☐ Child ☐ Other

Employer: Phone: ( )

Employer's Address:

Policy/ID No: 698915517A Group No: Percent Covered: 80 % Copay Amt: $

Secondary Insurance: Phone: ( )

Address:

Insurance Policyholder's Name: ☐ M ☐ F DOB:

Address:

Phone: Relationship to Insured: ☐ Self ☐ Spouse ☐ Child ☐ Other

Employer: Phone: ( )

Employer's Address:

Policy/ID No: Group No: Percent Covered: % Copay Amt: $

Reason for Visit: Here for lower back pain

Known Allergies:

Referred by:

TEST 8
SOAP

11/04/20XX
Assignment of Benefits: Y
Signature on File: Y
Referring Physician: N

S: Elsie Spaulding is here to discuss the results of her spinal X-ray. She still has back pain constantly.

O: On exam, pt. still has lower back pain, especially with movement. X-ray shows degeneration in L4 1 L5 BP: 118/70, P: 68.

A: 1. Osteoarthritis lower back—715.18

P: 1. Start Celebrex 200mg one p.o. q.d.
2. Return in 1 month.

_____

Phil Wells, MD
Family Practice
NPI: 1234567890

TEST 8

Patient Name Elsie Spaulding

Capital City Medical
123 Unknown Boulevard, Capital City, NY 12345-2222

Date of Service 11-04-20XX

New Patient			Arthrocentesis/Aspiration/Injection			Laboratory	
Problem Focused	99201		Small Joint	20600		Amylase	82150
Expanded Problem, Focused	99202		Interm Joint	20605		B12	82607
Detailed	99203		Major Joint	20610		CBC & Diff	85025
Comprehensive	99204		**Other Invasive/Noninvasive**			Comp Metabolic Panel	80053
Comprehensive/High Complex	99205		Audiometry	92552		Chlamydia Screen	87110
Well Exam Infant (up to 12 mos.)	99381		Cast Application			Cholesterol	82465
Well Exam 1–4 yrs.	99382		Location Long Short			Digoxin	80162
Well Exam 5–11 yrs.	99383		Catheterization	51701		Electrolytes	80051
Well Exam 12–17 yrs.	99384		Circumcision	54150		Ferritin	82728
Well Exam 18–39 yrs.	99385		Colposcopy	57452		Folate	82746
Well Exam 40–64 yrs.	99386		Colposcopy w/Biopsy	57454		GC Screen	87070
			Cryosurgery Premalignant Lesion			Glucose	82947
			Location (s):			Glucose 1 HR	82950
						Glycosylated HGB A1C	83036
Established Patient			Cryosurgery Warts			HCT	85014
Post-Op Follow Up Visit	99024		Location (s):			HDL	83718
Minimum	99211		Curettement Lesion			Hep BSAG	87340
Problem Focused	99212		Single	11055		Hepatitis panel, acute	80074
Expanded Problem Focused	99213	X	2–4	11056		HGB	85018
Detailed	99214		>4	11057		HIV	86703
Comprehensive/High Complex	99215		Diaphragm Fitting	57170		Iron & TIBC	83550
Well Exam Infant (up to 12 mos.)	99391		Ear Irrigation	69210		Kidney Profile	80069
Well exam 1–4 yrs.	99392		ECG	93000		Lead	83655
Well Exam 5–11 yrs.	99393		Endometrial Biopsy	58100		Liver Profile	80076
Well Exam 12–17 yrs.	99394		Exc. Lesion Malignant			Mono Test	86308
Well Exam 18–39 yrs.	99395		Benign			Pap Smear	88155
Well Exam 40–64 yrs.	99396		Location			Pregnancy Test	84703
Obstetrics			Exc. Skin Tags (1–15)	11200		Obstetric Panel	80055
Total OB Care	59400		Each Additional 10	11201		Pro Time	85610
Injections			Fracture Treatment			PSA	84153
Administration Sub. / IM	90772		Loc			RPR	86592
Drug			w/Reduc w/o Reduc			Sed. Rate	85651
Dosage			I & D Abscess Single/Simple	10060		Stool Culture	87045
Allergy	95115		Multiple or Comp	10061		Stool O & P	87177
Cocci Skin Test	86490		I & D Pilonidal Cyst Simple	10080		Strep Screen	87880
DPT	90701		Pilonidal Cyst Complex	10081		Theophylline	80198
Hemophilus	90646		IV Therapy—To One Hour	90760		Thyroid Uptake	84479
Influenza	90658		Each Additional Hour	90761		TSH	84443
MMR	90707		Laceration Repair			Urinalysis	81000
OPV	90712		Location Size Simp/Comp			Urine Culture	87088
Pneumovax	90732		Laryngoscopy	31505		Drawing Fee	36415
TB Skin Test	86580		Oximetry	94760		Specimen Collection	99000
TD	90718		Punch Biopsy			**Other:**	
Unlisted Immun	90749		Rhythm Strip	93040			
Tetanus Toxoid	90703		Treadmill	93015			
Vaccine/Toxoid Admin <8 Yr Old w/ Counseling	90465		Trigger Point or Tendon Sheath Inj.	20550			
Vaccine/Toxoid Administration for Adult	90471		Tympanometry	92567			

Diagnosis/ICD-9: **715.18**

I acknowledge receipt of medical services and authorize the release of any
medical information necessary to process this claim for healthcare payment only. I do authorize payment to the provider.

Patient Signature *Elsie Spaulding*

Total Estimated Charges: _____

Payment Amount: _____

Next Appointment: _____

Figure 1

Capital City Medical
Fee Schedule

New Patient OV			Punch Biopsy various codes	$80
Problem Focused 99201	$45		Nebulizer various codes	$45
Expanded Problem Focused 99202	$65		Cast Application various codes	$85
Detailed 99203	$85		Laryngoscopy 31505	$255
Comprehensive 99204	$105		Audiometry 92552	$85
Comprehensive/High Complex 99205	$115		Tympanometry 92567	$85
Well Exam infant (less than 1 year) 99381	$45		Ear Irrigation 69210	$25
Well Exam 1–4 yrs. 99382	$50		Diaphragm Fitting 57170	$30
Well Exam 5–11 yrs. 99383	$55		IV Therapy (up to one hour) 90760	$65
Well Exam 12–17 yrs. 99384	$65		Each additional hour 90761	$50
Well Exam 18–39 yrs. 99385	$85		Oximetry 94760	$10
Well Exam 40–64 yrs. 99386	$105		ECG 93000	$75
Established Patient OV			Holter Monitor various codes	$170
Post Op Follow Up Visit 99024	$0		Rhythm Strip 93040	$60
Minimum 99211	$35		Treadmill 93015	$375
Problem Focused 99212	$45		Cocci Skin Test 86490	$20
Expanded Problem Focused 99213	$55		X-ray, spine, chest, bone—any area various codes	$275
Detailed 99214	$65		Avulsion Nail 11730	$200
Comprehensive/High Complex 99215	$75		**Laboratory**	
Well exam infant (less than 1 year) 99391	$35		Amylase 82150	$40
Well Exam 1–4 yrs. 99392	$40		B12 82607	$30
Well Exam 5–11 yrs. 99393	$45		CBC & Diff 85025	$95
Well Exam 12–17 yrs. 99394	$55		Comp Metabolic Panel 80053	$75
Well Exam 18–39 yrs. 99395	$65		Chlamydia Screen 87110	$70
Well Exam 40–64 yrs. 99396	$75		Cholestrerol 82465	$75
Obstetrics			Digoxin 80162	$40
Total OB Care 59400	$1700		Electrolytes 80051	$70
Injections			Estrogen, Total 82672	$50
Administration 90772	$10		Ferritin 82728	$40
Allergy 95115	$35		Folate 82746	$30
DPT 90701	$50		GC Screen 87070	$60
Drug various codes	$35		Glucose 82947	$35
Influenza 90658	$25		Glycosylated HGB A1C 83036	$45
MMR 90707	$50		HCT 85014	$30
OPV 90712	$40		HDL 83718	$35
Pneumovax 90732	$35		HGB 85018	$30
TB Skin Test 86580	$15		Hep BSAG 83740	$40
TD 90718	$40		Hepatitis panel, acute 80074	$95
Tetanus Toxoid 90703	$40		HIV 86703	$100
Vaccine/Toxoid Administration for Younger Than 8 Years Old w/ counseling 90465	$10		Iron & TIBC 83550	$45
			Kidney Profile 80069	$95
Vaccine/Toxoid Administration for Adult 90471	$10		Lead 83665	$55
Arthrocentesis/Aspiration/Injection			Lipase 83690	$40
Small Joint 20600	$50		Lipid Panel 80061	$95
Interm Joint 20605	$60		Liver Profile 80076	$95
Major Joint 20610	$70		Mono Test 86308	$30
Trigger Point/Tendon Sheath Inj. 20550	$90		Pap Smear 88155	$90
Other Invasive/Noninvasive Procedures			Pap Collection/Supervision 88142	$95
Catheterization 51701	$55		Pregnancy Test 84703	$90
Circumcision 54150	$150		Obstetric Panel 80055	$85
Colposcopy 57452	$225		Pro Time 85610	$50
Colposcopy w/Biopsy 57454	$250		PSA 84153	$50
Cryosurgery Premalignant Lesion various codes	$160		RPR 86592	$55
Endometrial Biopsy 58100	$190		Sed. Rate 85651	$50
Excision Lesion Malignant various codes	$145		Stool Culture 87045	$80
Excision Lesion Benign various codes	$125		Stool O & P 87177	$105
Curettement Lesion			Strep Screen 87880	$35
Single 11055	$70		Theophylline 80198	$40
2–4 11056	$80		Thyroid Uptake 84479	$75
>4 11057	$90		TSH 84443	$50
Excision Skin Tags (1–15) 11200	$55		Urinalysis 81000	$35
Each Additional 10 11201	$30		Urine Culture 87088	$80
I & D Abscess Single/Simple 10060	$75		Drawing Fee 36415	$15
Multiple/Complex 10061	$95		Specimen Collection 99000	$10
I & D Pilonidal Cyst Simple 10080	$105			
I & D Pilonidal Cyst Complex 10081	$130			
Laceration Repair various codes	$60			

Figure 2

The form contains the following text:

(1500)

HEALTH INSURANCE CLAIM FORM

APPROVED BY NATIONAL UNIFORM CLAIM COMMITTEE 08/05

PICA

1. MEDICARE   MEDICAID   TRICARE CHAMPUS   CHAMPVA   GROUP HEALTH PLAN   FECA BLK LUNG   OTHER   1a. INSURED'S I.D. NUMBER   (For Program in Item 1)

(Medicare #)   (Medicaid #)   (Sponsor's SSN)   (Member ID#)   (SSN or ID)   (SSN)   (ID)

2. PATIENT'S NAME (Last Name, First Name, Middle Initial)   3. PATIENT'S BIRTH DATE   SEX   4. INSURED'S NAME (Last Name, First Name, Middle Initial)

MM   DD   YY   M   F

5. PATIENT'S ADDRESS (No., Street)   6. PATIENT RELATIONSHIP TO INSURED   7. INSURED'S ADDRESS (No, Street)

Self   Spouse   Child   Other

CITY   STATE   8. PATIENT STATUS   CITY   STATE

Single   Married   Other

ZIP CODE   TELEPHONE (Include Area Code)   Full-Time   Part-Time   ZIP CODE   TELEPHONE (Include Area Code)

Employed   Student   Student   ( )

9. OTHER INSURED'S NAME (Last Name, First Name, Middle Initial)   10. IS PATIENT'S CONDITION RELATED TO: 11. INSURED'S POLICY GROUP OR FECA NUMBER

a. OTHER INSURED'S POLICY OR GROUP NUMBER   a. EMPLOYMENT? (Current or Previous)   a. INSURED'S DATE OF BIRTH   SEX

MM   DD   YY   M   F

YES   NO

b. OTHER INSURED'S DATE OF BIRTH   SEX   b. AUTO ACCIDENT?   PLACE (State)   b. EMPLOYER'S NAME OR SCHOOL NAME

MM   DD   YY   M   F   YES   NO

c. EMPLOYER'S NAME OR SCHOOL NAME   c. OTHER ACCIDENT?   c. INSURANCE PLAN NAME OR PROGRAM NAME

YES   NO

d. INSURANCE PLAN NAME OR PROGRAM NAME   10d. RESERVED FOR LOCAL USE   d. IS THERE ANOTHER HEALTH BENEFIT PLAN?

YES   NO   If yes, return to and complete item 9 a-d.

READ BACK OF FORM BEFORE COMPLETING & SIGNING THIS FORM.

12. PATIENT'S OR AUTHORIZED PERSON'S SIGNATURE I authorize the release of any medical or other information necessary to process this claim. I also request payment of government benefits either to myself or to the party who accepts assignment below.

SIGNED _____   DATE _____

13. INSURED'S OR AUTHORIZED PERSON'S SIGNATURE I authorize payment of medical benefits to the undersigned physician or supplier for services described below.

SIGNED _____

14. DATE OF CURRENT: ILLNESS (First symptom) OR INJURY (Accident) OR PREGNANCY (LMP)

MM   DD   YY

15. IF PATIENT HAS HAD SAME OR SIMILAR ILLNESS, GIVE FIRST DATE   MM   DD   YY

16. DATES PATIENT UNABLE TO WORK IN CURRENT OCCUPATION

FROM   MM   DD   YY   TO   MM   DD   YY

17. NAME OF REFERRING PHYSICIAN OR OTHER SOURCE   17a.   17b. NPI

18. HOSPITALIZATION DATES RELATED TO CURRENT SERVICES

FROM   MM   DD   YY   TO   MM   DD   YY

19. RESERVED FOR LOCAL USE   20. OUTSIDE LAB? $ CHARGES

YES   NO

21. DIAGNOSIS OR NATURE OF ILLNESS OR INJURY (Relate Items 1,2,3 or 4 to Item 24E by Line)

1. ___   3. ___

2. ___   4. ___

22. MEDICAID RESUBMISSION   CODE   ORIGINAL REF. NO.

23. PRIOR AUTHORIZATION NUMBER

24. A. DATE(S) OF SERVICE   B. PLACE OF SERVICE   C. EMG   D. PROCEDURES, SERVICES, OR SUPPLIES (Explain Unusual Circumstances) CPT/HCPCS   MODIFIER   E. DIAGNOSIS POINTER   F. $ CHARGES   G. DAYS OR UNITS   H. EPSDT Family Plan   I. ID. QUAL.   J. RENDERING PROVIDER ID. #

From   To
MM DD YY   MM DD YY

1   NPI
2   NPI
3   NPI
4   NPI
5   NPI
6   NPI

25. FEDERAL TAX I.D. NUMBER   SSN EIN   26. PATIENT'S ACCOUNT NO.   27. ACCEPT ASSIGNMENT? (For govt. claims, see back)   YES   NO   28. TOTAL CHARGE $ 29. AMOUNT PAID $ 30. BALANCE DUE $

31. SIGNATURE OF PHYSICIAN OR SUPPLIER INCLUDING DEGREES OR CREDENTIALS (I certify that the statements on the reverse apply to this bill and are made a part thereof.)

SIGNED _____   DATE _____

32. SERVICE FACILITY LOCATION INFORMATION

a. NPI   b.

33. BILLING PROVIDER INFO & PH. # ( )

a. NPI   b.

NUCC Instruction Manual available at: www.nucc.org   WCMS-1500CS

APPROVED OMB 0938-0999 FORM CMS-1500 (08/05)

Side labels: CARRIER, PATIENT AND INSURED INFORMATION, PHYSICIAN OR SUPPLIER INFORMATION, SECOND FOLD, FIRST FOLD WHCF-10-ENV / WHCF-10-ENV-SS

TEST 9: COMPLETE A MEDICAID CLAIM

Directions: Using the source documents provided for patient Ty Nelson and the Capital City Medical fee schedule (Figure 3), accurately complete a CMS-1500 claim form for Medicaid. Use the blank CMS-1500 claim form provided (Figure 4).

Complete the case on the basis of the following criteria:

- All patients have release of information and assignment of benefit signatures on file. Assignment of benefits is required by most states, for Medicaid. SOF is not required in Item 13.

- All providers accept assignment for Medicaid by law. Item 27 should not be marked.

- The group practice is the billing entity.

- The national transition to NPI numbers is complete, and legacy PINs of individual payers are no longer used. If legacy PINS are still being used by your state Medicaid program, your instructor may provide you with Medicaid PINs in addition to the NPI.

- 2012 ICD-9-CM, ICD-10-CM/PCS and CPT codes are used.

- Use eight-digit dates for birthdates. Use six-digit dates for all other dates.

- All street names should be entered with standard postal abbreviations, even if they are spelled out on the source documents.

- Enter the ICD-9 codes and ICD-10 codes in the order in which they appear on the encounter form.

- When entering CPT codes, enter the E/M code first. Enter remaining codes in descending price order.

TEST 9

Capital City Medical—123 Unknown Boulevard, Capital City, NY 12345-2222 (555) 555-1234

Phil Wells, MD, Mannie Mends, MD, Bette R. Soone, MD

Patient Information Form

Tax ID: 75-0246810

Group NPI: 1513171216

Patient Information:

Name: (Last, First) Nelson, Ty   ☒ Male   ☐ Female   Birth Date: 08/21/2006

Address: 518 Moon Ave, Capital City, NY 12345   Phone: (555) 555-8168

Social Security Number: 404-11-6786   Full-Time Student: ☒ Yes   ☐ No

Marital Status: ☒ Single   ☐ Married   ☐ Divorced   ☐ Other

Employment:

Employer: Retired   Phone: ( )

Address:

Condition Related to: ☐ Auto Accident   ☐ Employment   ☐ Other Accident

Date of Accident: _____ State: _____

Emergency Contact: _____ **Phone: ( )** _____

Primary Insurance: Medicaid   Phone: ( )

Address: 4875 Capital Blvd, Capital City, NY 12345

Insurance Policyholder's Name: Same   ☐ M ☐ F DOB: _____

Address: Same

Phone: _____ Relationship to Insured: ☒ Self ☐ Spouse ☐ Child ☐ Other

Employer: _____ Phone: ( ) _____

Employer's Address: _____

Policy/ID No: 8694631321   Group No: _____ Percent Covered: 80 % Copay Amt: $5.00

Secondary Insurance: _____ Phone: ( )

Address: _____

Insurance Policyholder's Name: _____ ☐ M ☐ F DOB: _____

Address: _____

Phone: _____ Relationship to Insured: ☐ Self ☐ Spouse ☐ Child ☐ Other

Employer: _____ Phone: ( ) _____

Employer's Address: _____

Policy/ID No: _____ Group No: _____ Percent Covered: ___% Copay Amt: $____

Reason for Visit: Annual checkup.

Known Allergies: _____

Referred by: _____

TEST 9
SOAP

08/30/20XX
Assignment of Benefits: Y
Signature on File: Y
Referring Physician: N

S: Ty Nelson is here for his annual well check. His mom says she has no new complaints for him.

O: Pt. has developed normally. Chest is clear to A&P. There is no lymphadenopathy present. He is alert and oriented ✕3.

A: 1. Well child—V20.2

P: 1. Return p.r.n.

_____

Phil Wells, MD
Family Practice
NPI: 1234567890

TEST 9

Patient Name Ty Nelson

Capital City Medical
123 Unknown Boulevard, Capital City, NY 12345-2222

Date of Service
08-30-20XX

New Patient			Other Invasive/Noninvasive		Laboratory	
Problem Focused	99201	Arthrocentesis/Aspiration/Injection		Amylase	82150
Expanded Problem, Focused	99202	Small Joint	20600	B12	82607
Detailed	99203	Interm Joint	20605	CBC & Diff	85025
Comprehensive	99204	Major Joint	20610	Comp Metabolic Panel	80053
Comprehensive/High Complex	99205	**Other Invasive/Noninvasive**		Chlamydia Screen	87110
Well Exam Infant (up to 12 mos.)	99381	Audiometry	92552	Cholesterol	82465
Well Exam 1–4 yrs.	99382	Cast Application		Digoxin	80162
Well Exam 5–11 yrs.	99383	Location Long Short		Electrolytes	80051
Well Exam 12–17 yrs.	99384	Catheterization	51701	Ferritin	82728
Well Exam 18–39 yrs.	99385	Circumcision	54150	Folate	82746
Well Exam 40–64 yrs.	99386	Colposcopy	57452	GC Screen	87070
		Colposcopy w/Biopsy	57454	Glucose	82947
		Cryosurgery Premalignant Lesion		Glucose 1 HR	82950
		Location (s):		Glycosylated HGB A1C	83036
Established Patient		Cryosurgery Warts		HCT	85014
Post-Op Follow Up Visit	99024	Location (s):		HDL	83718
Minimum	99211	Curettement Lesion		Hep BSAG	87340
Problem Focused	99212	Single	11055	Hepatitis panel, acute	80074
Expanded Problem Focused	99213	2–4	11056	HGB	85018
Detailed	99214	>4	11057	HIV	86703
Comprehensive/High Complex	99215	Diaphragm Fitting	57170	Iron & TIBC	83550
Well Exam Infant (up to 12 mos.)	99391	Ear Irrigation	69210	Kidney Profile	80069
Well exam 1–4 yrs.	99392	ECG	93000	Lead	83655
Well Exam 5–11 yrs.	99393 ☒	Endometrial Biopsy	58100	Liver Profile	80076
Well Exam 12–17 yrs.	99394	Exc. Lesion Malignant		Mono Test	86308
Well Exam 18–39 yrs.	99395	Benign		]Pap Smear	88155
Well Exam 40–64 yrs.	99396	Location		Pregnancy Test	84703
Obstetrics		Exc. Skin Tags (1–15)	11200	Obstetric Panel	80055
Total OB Care	59400	Each Additional 10	11201	Pro Time	85610
Injections		Fracture Treatment		PSA	84153
Administration Sub. / IM	90772	Loc		RPR	86592
Drug		w/Reduc w/o Reduc		Sed. Rate	85651
Dosage		I & D Abscess Single/Simple	10060	Stool Culture	87045
Allergy	95115	Multiple or Comp	10061	Stool O & P	87177
Cocci Skin Test	86490	I & D Pilonidal Cyst Simple	10080	Strep Screen	87880
DPT	90701	Pilonidal Cyst Complex	10081	Theophylline	80198
Hemophilus	90646	IV Therapy—To One Hour	90760	Thyroid Uptake	84479
Influenza	90658	Each Additional Hour	90761	TSH	84443
MMR	90707	Laceration Repair		Urinalysis	81000
OPV	90712	Location Size Simp/Comp		Urine Culture	87088
Pneumovax	90732	Laryngoscopy	31505	Drawing Fee	36415
TB Skin Test	86580	Oximetry	94760	Specimen Collection	99000
TD	90718	Punch Biopsy		**Other:**	
Unlisted Immun	90749	Rhythm Strip	93040		
Tetanus Toxoid	90703	Treadmill	93015		
Vaccine/Toxoid Admin <8 Yr Old w/ Counseling	90465	Trigger Point or Tendon Sheath Inj.	20550		
Vaccine/Toxoid Administration for Adult	90471	Tympanometry	92567		

Diagnosis/ICD-9: **V20.2**

I acknowledge receipt of medical services and authorize the release of any medical information necessary to process this claim for healthcare payment only. I do authorize payment to the provider.

Patient Signature _Sydney Nelson_

Total Estimated Charges: _____

Payment Amount: _____

Next Appointment: _____

Figure 3

Capital City Medical
Fee Schedule

New Patient OV			Punch Biopsy various codes	$80
Problem Focused 99201	$45		Nebulizer various codes	$45
Expanded Problem Focused 99202	$65		Cast Application various codes	$85
Detailed 99203	$85		Laryngoscopy 31505	$255
Comprehensive 99204	$105		Audiometry 92552	$85
Comprehensive/High Complex 99205	$115		Tympanometry 92567	$85
Well Exam infant (less than 1 year) 99381	$45		Ear Irrigation 69210	$25
Well Exam 1–4 yrs. 99382	$50		Diaphragm Fitting 57170	$30
Well Exam 5–11 yrs. 99383	$55		IV Therapy (up to one hour) 90760	$65
Well Exam 12–17 yrs. 99384	$65		Each additional hour 90761	$50
Well Exam 18–39 yrs. 99385	$85		Oximetry 94760	$10
Well Exam 40–64 yrs. 99386	$105		ECG 93000	$75
Established Patient OV			Holter Monitor various codes	$170
Post Op Follow Up Visit 99024	$0		Rhythm Strip 93040	$60
Minimum 99211	$35		Treadmill 93015	$375
Problem Focused 99212	$45		Cocci Skin Test 86490	$20
Expanded Problem Focused 99213	$55		X-ray, spine, chest, bone—any area various codes	$275
Detailed 99214	$65		Avulsion Nail 11730	$200
Comprehensive/High Complex 99215	$75		**Laboratory**	
Well exam infant (less than 1 year) 99391	$35		Amylase 82150	$40
Well Exam 1–4 yrs. 99392	$40		B12 82607	$30
Well Exam 5–11 yrs. 99393	$45		CBC & Diff 85025	$95
Well Exam 12–17 yrs. 99394	$55		Comp Metabolic Panel 80053	$75
Well Exam 18–39 yrs. 99395	$65		Chlamydia Screen 87110	$70
Well Exam 40–64 yrs. 99396	$75		Cholestrerol 82465	$75
Obstetrics			Digoxin 80162	$40
Total OB Care 59400	$1700		Electrolytes 80051	$70
Injections			Estrogen, Total 82672	$50
Administration 90772	$10		Ferritin 82728	$40
Allergy 95115	$35		Folate 82746	$30
DPT 90701	$50		GC Screen 87070	$60
Drug various codes	$35		Glucose 82947	$35
Influenza 90658	$25		Glycosylated HGB A1C 83036	$45
MMR 90707	$50		HCT 85014	$30
OPV 90712	$40		HDL 83718	$35
Pneumovax 90732	$35		HGB 85018	$30
TB Skin Test 86580	$15		Hep BSAG 83740	$40
TD 90718	$40		Hepatitis panel, acute 80074	$95
Tetanus Toxoid 90703	$40		HIV 86703	$100
Vaccine/Toxoid Administration for Younger			Iron & TIBC 83550	$45
Than 8 Years Old w/ counseling 90465	$10		Kidney Profile 80069	$95
Vaccine/Toxoid Administration for Adult 90471	$10		Lead 83665	$55
Arthrocentesis/Aspiration/Injection			Lipase 83690	$40
Small Joint 20600	$50		Lipid Panel 80061	$95
Interm Joint 20605	$60		Liver Profile 80076	$95
Major Joint 20610	$70		Mono Test 86308	$30
Trigger Point/Tendon Sheath Inj. 20550	$90		Pap Smear 88155	$90
Other Invasive/Noninvasive Procedures			Pap Collection/Supervision 88142	$95
Catheterization 51701	$55		Pregnancy Test 84703	$90
Circumcision 54150	$150		Obstetric Panel 80055	$85
Colposcopy 57452	$225		Pro Time 85610	$50
Colposcopy w/Biopsy 57454	$250		PSA 84153	$50
Cryosurgery Premalignant Lesion various codes	$160		RPR 86592	$55
Endometrial Biopsy 58100	$190		Sed. Rate 85651	$50
Excision Lesion Malignant various codes	$145		Stool Culture 87045	$80
Excision Lesion Benign various codes	$125		Stool O & P 87177	$105
Curettement Lesion			Strep Screen 87880	$35
Single 11055	$70		Theophylline 80198	$40
2–4 11056	$80		Thyroid Uptake 84479	$75
>4 11057	$90		TSH 84443	$50
Excision Skin Tags (1–15) 11200	$55		Urinalysis 81000	$35
Each Additional 10 11201	$30		Urine Culture 87088	$80
I & D Abscess Single/Simple 10060	$75		Drawing Fee 36415	$15
Multiple/Complex 10061	$95		Specimen Collection 99000	$10
I & D Pilonidal Cyst Simple 10080	$105			
I & D Pilonidal Cyst Complex 10081	$130			
Laceration Repair various codes	$60			

HEALTH INSURANCE CLAIM FORM

APPROVED BY NATIONAL UNIFORM CLAIM COMMITTEE 08/05

☐☐☐ PICA

1. MEDICARE MEDICAID TRICARE CHAMPVA GROUP FECA OTHER	1a. INSURED'S I.D. NUMBER (For Program in Item 1)

CHAMPUS HEALTH PLAN BLK LUNG

☐(Medicare #) ☐(Medicaid #) ☐(Sponsor's SSN) ☐(Member ID#) ☐(SSN or ID) ☐(SSN) ☐(ID)

2. PATIENT'S NAME (Last Name, First Name, Middle Initial)	3. PATIENT'S BIRTH DATE SEX	4. INSURED'S NAME (Last Name, First Name, Middle Initial)
	MM DD YY M☐ F☐	
5. PATIENT'S ADDRESS (No, Street)	6. PATIENT RELATIONSHIP TO INSURED	7. INSURED'S ADDRESS (No, Street)
	Self☐ Spouse☐ Child☐ Other☐	
CITY STATE	8. PATIENT STATUS	CITY STATE
	Single☐ Married☐ Other☐	
ZIP CODE TELEPHONE (Include Area Code) ( )	Full-Time Part-Time Employed☐ Student☐ Student☐	ZIP CODE TELEPHONE (Include Area Code) ( )
9. OTHER INSURED'S NAME (Last Name, First Name, Middle Initial)	10. IS PATIENT'S CONDITION RELATED TO:	11. INSURED'S POLICY GROUP OR FECA NUMBER
a. OTHER INSURED'S POLICY OR GROUP NUMBER	a. EMPLOYMENT? (Current or Previous) ☐YES ☐NO	a. INSURED'S DATE OF BIRTH SEX MM DD YY M☐ F☐
b. OTHER INSURED'S DATE OF BIRTH SEX MM DD YY M☐ F☐	b. AUTO ACCIDENT? PLACE (State) ☐YES ☐NO	b. EMPLOYER'S NAME OR SCHOOL NAME
c. EMPLOYER'S NAME OR SCHOOL NAME	c. OTHER ACCIDENT? ☐YES ☐NO	c. INSURANCE PLAN NAME OR PROGRAM NAME
d. INSURANCE PLAN NAME OR PROGRAM NAME	10d. RESERVED FOR LOCAL USE	d. IS THERE ANOTHER HEALTH BENEFIT PLAN? ☐YES ☐NO If yes, return to and complete item 9 a-d.

READ BACK OF FORM BEFORE COMPLETING & SIGNING THIS FORM.

12. PATIENT'S OR AUTHORIZED PERSON'S SIGNATURE I authorize the release of any medical or other information necessary to process this claim. I also request payment of government benefits either to myself or to the party who accepts assignment below.	13. INSURED'S OR AUTHORIZED PERSON'S SIGNATURE I authorize payment of medical benefits to the undersigned physician or supplier for services described below.
SIGNED _____ DATE _____	SIGNED _____

14. DATE OF CURRENT: ILLNESS (First symptom) OR MM DD YY INJURY (Accident) OR PREGNANCY (LMP)	15. IF PATIENT HAS HAD SAME OR SIMILAR ILLNESS, GIVE FIRST DATE MM DD YY	16. DATES PATIENT UNABLE TO WORK IN CURRENT OCCUPATION MM DD YY MM DD YY FROM TO
17. NAME OF REFERRING PHYSICIAN OR OTHER SOURCE	17a. 17b. NPI	18. HOSPITALIZATION DATES RELATED TO CURRENT SERVICES MM DD YY MM DD YY FROM TO
19. RESERVED FOR LOCAL USE		20. OUTSIDE LAB? $ CHARGES ☐YES ☐NO
21. DIAGNOSIS OR NATURE OF ILLNESS OR INJURY (Relate Items 1,2,3 or 4 to Item 24E by Line) 1. ⌊____.____ 3. ⌊____.____ 2. ⌊____.____ 4. ⌊____.____		22. MEDICAID RESUBMISSION CODE ORIGINAL REF. NO. 23. PRIOR AUTHORIZATION NUMBER

24. A. DATE(S) OF SERVICE From To MM DD YY MM DD YY	B. PLACE OF SERVICE	C. EMG	D. PROCEDURES, SERVICES, OR SUPPLIES (Explain Unusual Circumstances) CPT/HCPCS MODIFIER	E. DIAGNOSIS POINTER	F. $ CHARGES	G. DAYS OR UNITS	H. EPSDT Family Plan	I. ID. QUAL.	J. RENDERING PROVIDER ID. #
1								NPI	
2								NPI	
3								NPI	
4								NPI	
5								NPI	
6								NPI	

25. FEDERAL TAX I.D. NUMBER SSN EIN ☐☐	26. PATIENT'S ACCOUNT NO.	27. ACCEPT ASSIGNMENT? (For govt. claims, see back) ☐YES ☐NO	28. TOTAL CHARGE $	29. AMOUNT PAID $	30. BALANCE DUE $
31. SIGNATURE OF PHYSICIAN OR SUPPLIER INCLUDING DEGREES OR CREDENTIALS (I certify that the statements on the reverse apply to this bill and are made a part thereof.) SIGNED DATE	32. SERVICE FACILITY LOCATION INFORMATION a. NPI b.	33. BILLING PROVIDER INFO & PH. # ( ) a. NPI b.

NUCC Instruction Manual available at: www.nucc.org
WCMS-1500CS

APPROVED OMB 0938-0999 FORM CMS-1500 (08/05)

CARRIER

PATIENT AND INSURED INFORMATION

PHYSICIAN OR SUPPLIER INFORMATION

SECOND FOLD

FIRST FOLD WHCF-10-ENV / WHCF-10-ENV-SS

Figure 4

TEST 10: COMPLETE A MEDI-MEDI CLAIM

Directions: Using the source documents provided for patient Calvin Frew, and the Capital City Medical fee schedule (Figure 5), accurately complete a CMS-1500 claim form for this Medi-medi claim. Use the blank CMS-1500 claim form provided (Figure 6).

TEST 10

Capital City Medical—123 Unknown Boulevard, Capital City, NY 12345-2222 (555) 555-1234	Patient Information Form
	Tax ID: 75-0246810
Phil Wells, MD, Mannie Mends, MD, Bette R. Soone, MD	Group NPI: 1513171216

Patient Information:

Name: (Last, First) Frew, Calvin ☒ Male ☐ Female Birth Date: 12/29/1951

Address: 721 Braden Ln, Capital City, NY 12345 Phone: (555) 555-6227

Social Security Number: 303-03-1620 Full-Time Student: ☐ Yes ☒ No

Marital Status: ☐ Single ☐ Married ☒ Divorced ☐ Other

Employment:

Employer: Retired Phone: ( )

Address:

Condition Related to: ☐ Auto Accident ☐ Employment ☐ Other Accident

Date of Accident: State:

Emergency Contact: Phone: ( )

Primary Insurance: Medicare Phone: ( )

Address: P. O. Box 9834, Capital City, NY 12345

Insurance Policyholder's Name: Same ☐ M ☐ F DOB:

Address:

Phone: Relationship to Insured: ☒ Self ☐ Spouse ☐ Child ☐ Other

Employer: Phone: ( )

Employer's Address:

Policy/ID No: 521869954A Group No: Percent Covered: 80 % Copay Amt: $

Secondary Insurance: Medicaid Phone: ( )

Address: 4875 Capital Blvd, Capital City, NY 12345

Insurance Policyholder's Name: Same ☐ M ☐ F DOB:

Address:

Phone: Relationship to Insured: ☒ Self ☐ Spouse ☐ Child ☐ Other

Employer: Phone: ( )

Employer's Address:

Policy/ID No: 00665843324998 Group No: Percent Covered: % Copay Amt: $5.00

Reason for Visit: I woke up this morning with pain in my right thumb

Known Allergies:

Referred by:

TEST 10
SOAP

10/18/20XX
Assignment of Benefits: Y
Signature on File: Y
Referring Physician: N

S: Calvin Frew complains of pain in his right thumb since he woke up this morning. He can hardly move it.

O: Pt. denies any injury to his thumb. BP: 148/88. X-ray reveals dislocation. Put back in place without any complications.

A: 1. Right thumb dislocation—834.00

P: 1. Thumb placed back into joint successfully.

2. Keep appointment in 1 month for blood pressure checkup.

_____

Phil Wells, MD
Family Practice
NPI: 1234567890

TEST 10

Patient Name Calvin Frew

Capital City Medical
123 Unknown Boulevard, Capital City, NY 12345-2222

Date of Service
10-18-20XX

New Patient			Other Invasive/Noninvasive			Laboratory	
Problem Focused	99201		Arthrocentesis/Aspiration/Injection			Amylase	82150
Expanded Problem, Focused	99202		Small Joint	20600		B12	82607
Detailed	99203		Interm Joint	20605		CBC & Diff	85025
Comprehensive	99204		Major Joint	20610		Comp Metabolic Panel	80053
Comprehensive/High Complex	99205		**Other Invasive/Noninvasive**			Chlamydia Screen	87110
Well Exam Infant (up to 12 mos.)	99381		Audiometry	92552		Cholesterol	82465
Well Exam 1–4 yrs.	99382		Cast Application			Digoxin	80162
Well Exam 5–11 yrs.	99383		Location Long Short			Electrolytes	80051
Well Exam 12–17 yrs.	99384		Catheterization	51701		Ferritin	82728
Well Exam 18–39 yrs.	99385		Circumcision	54150		Folate	82746
Well Exam 40–64 yrs.	99386		Colposcopy	57452		GC Screen	87070
			Colposcopy w/Biopsy	57454		Glucose	82947
			Cryosurgery Premalignant Lesion			Glucose 1 HR	82950
			Location (s):			Glycosylated HGB A1C	83036
Established Patient			Cryosurgery Warts			HCT	85014
Post-Op Follow Up Visit	99024		Location (s):			HDL	83718
Minimum	99211		Curettement Lesion			Hep BSAG	87340
Problem Focused	99212		Single	11055		Hepatitis panel, acute	80074
Expanded Problem Focused	99213	X	2–4	11056		HGB	85018
Detailed	99214		>4	11057		HIV	86703
Comprehensive/High Complex	99215		Diaphragm Fitting	57170		Iron & TIBC	83550
Well Exam Infant (up to 12 mos.)	99391		Ear Irrigation	69210		Kidney Profile	80069
Well exam 1–4 yrs.	99392		ECG	93000		Lead	83655
Well Exam 5–11 yrs.	99393		Endometrial Biopsy	58100		Liver Profile	80076
Well Exam 12–17 yrs.	99394		Exc. Lesion Malignant			Mono Test	86308
Well Exam 18–39 yrs.	99395		Benign			Pap Smear	88155
Well Exam 40–64 yrs.	99396		Location			Pregnancy Test	84703
Obstetrics			Exc. Skin Tags (1–15)	11200		Obstetric Panel	80055
Total OB Care	59400		Each Additional 10	11201		Pro Time	85610
Injections			Fracture Treatment			PSA	84153
Administration Sub. / IM	90772		Loc			RPR	86592
Drug			w/Reduc	w/o Reduc		Sed. Rate	85651
Dosage			I & D Abscess Single/Simple	10060		Stool Culture	87045
Allergy	95115		Multiple or Comp	10061		Stool O & P	87177
Cocci Skin Test	86490		I & D Pilonidal Cyst Simple	10080		Strep Screen	87880
DPT	90701		Pilonidal Cyst Complex	10081		Theophylline	80198
Hemophilus	90646		IV Therapy—To One Hour	90760		Thyroid Uptake	84479
Influenza	90658		Each Additional Hour	90761		TSH	84443
MMR	90707		Laceration Repair			Urinalysis	81000
OPV	90712		Location Size Simp/Comp			Urine Culture	87088
Pneumovax	90732		Laryngoscopy	31505		Drawing Fee	36415
TB Skin Test	86580		Oximetry	94760		Specimen Collection	99000
TD	90718		Punch Biopsy			**Other:**	
Unlisted Immun	90749		Rhythm Strip	93040			
Tetanus Toxoid	90703		Treadmill	93015			
Vaccine/Toxoid Admin <8 Yr Old w/ Counseling	90465		Trigger Point or Tendon Sheath Inj.	20550			
Vaccine/Toxoid Administration for Adult	90471		Tympanometry	92567			

Diagnosis/ICD-9: **834.00**

I acknowledge receipt of medical services and authorize the release of any medical information necessary to process this claim for healthcare payment only. I do authorize payment to the provider.

Patient Signature _Calvin Frew_

Total Estimated Charges: _____

Payment Amount: _____

Next Appointment: _____

Figure 5

Capital City Medical
Fee Schedule

New Patient OV			Punch Biopsy various codes	$80
Problem Focused 99201	$45		Nebulizer various codes	$45
Expanded Problem Focused 99202	$65		Cast Application various codes	$85
Detailed 99203	$85		Laryngoscopy 31505	$255
Comprehensive 99204	$105		Audiometry 92552	$85
Comprehensive/High Complex 99205	$115		Tympanometry 92567	$85
Well Exam infant (less than 1 year) 99381	$45		Ear Irrigation 69210	$25
Well Exam 1–4 yrs. 99382	$50		Diaphragm Fitting 57170	$30
Well Exam 5–11 yrs. 99383	$55		IV Therapy (up to one hour) 90760	$65
Well Exam 12–17 yrs. 99384	$65		Each additional hour 90761	$50
Well Exam 18–39 yrs. 99385	$85		Oximetry 94760	$10
Well Exam 40–64 yrs. 99386	$105		ECG 93000	$75
Established Patient OV			Holter Monitor various codes	$170
Post Op Follow Up Visit 99024	$0		Rhythm Strip 93040	$60
Minimum 99211	$35		Treadmill 93015	$375
Problem Focused 99212	$45		Cocci Skin Test 86490	$20
Expanded Problem Focused 99213	$55		X-ray, spine, chest, bone—any area various codes	$275
Detailed 99214	$65		Avulsion Nail 11730	$200
Comprehensive/High Complex 99215	$75		**Laboratory**	
Well exam infant (less than 1 year) 99391	$35		Amylase 82150	$40
Well Exam 1–4 yrs. 99392	$40		B12 82607	$30
Well Exam 5–11 yrs. 99393	$45		CBC & Diff 85025	$95
Well Exam 12–17 yrs. 99394	$55		Comp Metabolic Panel 80053	$75
Well Exam 18–39 yrs. 99395	$65		Chlamydia Screen 87110	$70
Well Exam 40–64 yrs. 99396	$75		Cholestrerol 82465	$75
Obstetrics			Digoxin 80162	$40
Total OB Care 59400	$1700		Electrolytes 80051	$70
Injections			Estrogen, Total 82672	$50
Administration 90772	$10		Ferritin 82728	$40
Allergy 95115	$35		Folate 82746	$30
DPT 90701	$50		GC Screen 87070	$60
Drug various codes	$35		Glucose 82947	$35
Influenza 90658	$25		Glycosylated HGB A1C 83036	$45
MMR 90707	$50		HCT 85014	$30
OPV 90712	$40		HDL 83718	$35
Pneumovax 90732	$35		HGB 85018	$30
TB Skin Test 86580	$15		Hep BSAG 83740	$40
TD 90718	$40		Hepatitis panel, acute 80074	$95
Tetanus Toxoid 90703	$40		HIV 86703	$100
Vaccine/Toxoid Administration for Younger			Iron & TIBC 83550	$45
Than 8 Years Old w/ counseling 90465	$10		Kidney Profile 80069	$95
Vaccine/Toxoid Administration for Adult 90471	$10		Lead 83665	$55
Arthrocentesis/Aspiration/Injection			Lipase 83690	$40
Small Joint 20600	$50		Lipid Panel 80061	$95
Interm Joint 20605	$60		Liver Profile 80076	$95
Major Joint 20610	$70		Mono Test 86308	$30
Trigger Point/Tendon Sheath Inj. 20550	$90		Pap Smear 88155	$90
Other Invasive/Noninvasive Procedures			Pap Collection/Supervision 88142	$95
Catheterization 51701	$55		Pregnancy Test 84703	$90
Circumcision 54150	$150		Obstetric Panel 80055	$85
Colposcopy 57452	$225		Pro Time 85610	$50
Colposcopy w/Biopsy 57454	$250		PSA 84153	$50
Cryosurgery Premalignant Lesion various codes	$160		RPR 86592	$55
Endometrial Biopsy 58100	$190		Sed. Rate 85651	$50
Excision Lesion Malignant various codes	$145		Stool Culture 87045	$80
Excision Lesion Benign various codes	$125		Stool O & P 87177	$105
Curettement Lesion			Strep Screen 87880	$35
Single 11055	$70		Theophylline 80198	$40
2–4 11056	$80		Thyroid Uptake 84479	$75
>4 11057	$90		TSH 84443	$50
Excision Skin Tags (1–15) 11200	$55		Urinalysis 81000	$35
Each Additional 10 11201	$30		Urine Culture 87088	$80
I & D Abscess Single/Simple 10060	$75		Drawing Fee 36415	$15
Multiple/Complex 10061	$95		Specimen Collection 99000	$10
I & D Pilonidal Cyst Simple 10080	$105			
I & D Pilonidal Cyst Complex 10081	$130			
Laceration Repair various codes	$60			

HEALTH INSURANCE CLAIM FORM
APPROVED BY NATIONAL UNIFORM CLAIM COMMITTEE 08/05

			PICA							PICA	

1. MEDICARE	MEDICAID	TRICARE CHAMPUS	CHAMPVA	GROUP HEALTH PLAN	FECA BLK LUNG	OTHER	1a. INSURED'S I.D. NUMBER	(For Program in Item 1)
☐(Medicare #)	☐(Medicaid #)	☐(Sponsor's SSN)	☐(Member ID#)	☐(SSN or ID)	☐(SSN)	☐(ID)		

2. PATIENT'S NAME (Last Name, First Name, Middle Initial)

3. PATIENT'S BIRTH DATE   SEX
MM   DD   YY
M☐   F☐

4. INSURED'S NAME (Last Name, First Name, Middle Initial)

5. PATIENT'S ADDRESS (No., Street)

6. PATIENT RELATIONSHIP TO INSURED
Self☐   Spouse☐   Child☐   Other☐

7. INSURED'S ADDRESS (No, Street)

CITY   STATE

8. PATIENT STATUS
Single☐   Married☐   Other☐
Full-Time   Part-Time
Employed☐   Student☐   Student☐

CITY   STATE

ZIP CODE   TELEPHONE (Include Area Code)
(   )

ZIP CODE   TELEPHONE (Include Area Code)
(   )

9. OTHER INSURED'S NAME (Last Name, First Name, Middle Initial)

10. IS PATIENT'S CONDITION RELATED TO:

11. INSURED'S POLICY GROUP OR FECA NUMBER

a. OTHER INSURED'S POLICY OR GROUP NUMBER

a. EMPLOYMENT? (Current or Previous)
☐YES   ☐NO

a. INSURED'S DATE OF BIRTH   SEX
MM   DD   YY
M☐   F☐

b. OTHER INSURED'S DATE OF BIRTH   SEX
MM   DD   YY   M☐   F☐

b. AUTO ACCIDENT?   PLACE (State)
☐YES   ☐NO

b. EMPLOYER'S NAME OR SCHOOL NAME

c. EMPLOYER'S NAME OR SCHOOL NAME

c. OTHER ACCIDENT?
☐YES   ☐NO

c. INSURANCE PLAN NAME OR PROGRAM NAME

d. INSURANCE PLAN NAME OR PROGRAM NAME

10d. RESERVED FOR LOCAL USE

d. IS THERE ANOTHER HEALTH BENEFIT PLAN?
☐YES   ☐NO   If yes, return to and complete item 9 a-d.

READ BACK OF FORM BEFORE COMPLETING & SIGNING THIS FORM.

12. PATIENT'S OR AUTHORIZED PERSON'S SIGNATURE I authorize the release of any medical or other information necessary to process this claim. I also request payment of government benefits either to myself or to the party who accepts assignment below.

SIGNED _____   DATE _____

13. INSURED'S OR AUTHORIZED PERSON'S SIGNATURE I authorize payment of medical benefits to the undersigned physician or supplier for services described below.

SIGNED _____

14. DATE OF CURRENT: ◄ ILLNESS (First symptom) OR
MM   DD   YY   INJURY (Accident) OR
                      PREGNANCY (LMP)

15. IF PATIENT HAS HAD SAME OR SIMILAR ILLNESS,
GIVE FIRST DATE   MM   DD   YY

16. DATES PATIENT UNABLE TO WORK IN CURRENT OCCUPATION
MM   DD   YY   MM   DD   YY
FROM   TO

17. NAME OF REFERRING PHYSICIAN OR OTHER SOURCE

17a.
17b. NPI

18. HOSPITALIZATION DATES RELATED TO CURRENT SERVICES
MM   DD   YY   MM   DD   YY
FROM   TO

19. RESERVED FOR LOCAL USE

20. OUTSIDE LAB? $ CHARGES
☐YES   ☐NO

21. DIAGNOSIS OR NATURE OF ILLNESS OR INJURY (Relate Items 1,2,3 or 4 to Item 24E by Line)
1. _____ . _____   3. _____ . _____
2. _____ . _____   4. _____ . _____

22. MEDICAID RESUBMISSION
CODE   ORIGINAL REF. NO.

23. PRIOR AUTHORIZATION NUMBER

24. A. DATE(S) OF SERVICE						B. PLACE OF SERVICE	C. EMG	D. PROCEDURES, SERVICES, OR SUPPLIES (Explain Unusual Circumstances)		E. DIAGNOSIS POINTER	F. $ CHARGES	G. DAYS OR UNITS	H. EPSDT Family Plan	I. ID. QUAL.	J. RENDERING PROVIDER ID. #
From			To					CPT/HCPCS	MODIFIER						
MM	DD	YY	MM	DD	YY										
1														NPI	
2														NPI	
3														NPI	
4														NPI	
5														NPI	
6														NPI	

25. FEDERAL TAX I.D. NUMBER SSN EIN	26. PATIENT'S ACCOUNT NO.	27. ACCEPT ASSIGNMENT? (For govt. claims, see back)	28. TOTAL CHARGE	29. AMOUNT PAID	30. BALANCE DUE
☐☐		☐YES ☐NO	$	$	$

31. SIGNATURE OF PHYSICIAN OR SUPPLIER INCLUDING DEGREES OR CREDENTIALS
(I certify that the statements on the reverse apply to this bill and are made a part thereof.)

SIGNED _____   DATE _____

32. SERVICE FACILITY LOCATION INFORMATION

a. NPI   b.

33. BILLING PROVIDER INFO & PH. # (   )

a. NPI   b.

NUCC Instruction Manual available at: www.nucc.org
WCMS-1500CS

APPROVED OMB 0938-0999 FORM CMS-1500 (08/05)

Figure 6

TEST 11: COMPLETE A TRICARE CLAIM

Directions: Using the source documents provided for patient Gracie Lloyd and the Capital City Medical fee schedule (Figure 7), accurately complete a CMS-1500 claim form for TRICARE. Use the blank CMS-1500 claim form provided (Figure 8).

Complete the case on the basis of the following criteria:

- All patients have release of information and assignment of benefit signatures on file.

- All providers are participating and accept assignment.

- The group practice is the billing entity.

- The national transition to NPI numbers is complete, and legacy PINs of individual payers are no longer used.

- 2012 ICD-9-CM, ICD-10-CM/PCS, and CPT codes are used.

- Use eight-digit dates for birthdates. Use six-digit dates for all other dates.

- All street names should be entered with standard postal abbreviations, even if they are spelled out on the source documents.

- Enter ICD-9 and ICD-10 codes in the order in which they appear on the encounter form.

- When entering CPT codes, enter the E/M code first. Enter remaining codes in descending price order

TEST 11

Patient Information:

Name: (Last, First) Lloyd, Gracie   ❑ Male   ☒ Female   Birth Date: 11/03/1976

Address: 630 Jefferson Base, Capital City, NY 12345   Phone: (555) 555-3232

Social Security Number: 619-42-8736   Full-Time Student: ❑ Yes ❑ No

Marital Status: ❑ Single ☒ Married ❑ Divorced ❑ Other

Employment:

Employer: Jefferson Base   Phone: (555) 555-1600

Address: 600 Jefferson Base, Capital City, NY 12345

Condition Related to: ❑ Auto Accident ❑ Employment ❑ Other Accident

Date of Accident: _____ State: _____

Emergency Contact: _____ **Phone: ( )** _____

Primary Insurance: Medicare   Phone: ( ) _____

Address: 7594 Forces-Run Rd, Militaryville, NY 12345

Insurance Policyholder's Name: Same   ❑ M ❑ F DOB: _____

Address: _____

Phone: _____ Relationship to Insured: ☒ Self ❑ Spouse ❑ Child ❑ Other

Employer: _____ Phone: ( ) _____

Employer's Address: _____

Policy/ID No: 619428736   Group No: _____ Percent Covered: 80 % Copay Amt: $35.00

Secondary Insurance: _____ Phone: ( ) _____

Address: _____

Insurance Policyholder's Name: _____ ❑ M ❑ F DOB: _____

Address: _____

Phone: _____ Relationship to Insured: ❑ Self ❑ Spouse ❑ Child ❑ Other

Employer: _____ Phone: ( ) _____

Employer's Address: _____

Policy/ID No: _____ Group No: _____ Percent Covered: ___% Copay Amt: $_____

Reason for Visit: I think that I may be pregnant.

Known Allergies: _____

Referred by: _____

01/24/20XX
Assignment of Benefits: Y
Signature on File: Y
Referring Physician: N

S: Gracie Lloyd complains of missed menses ×2 weeks.
O: Pt. denies any N&V. Her last menstrual period was 12-10-20XX. She has one child, female, alive and well. She has no history of miscarriage or abortion.
A: 1. Absent menstruation—626.0 Pregnancy test V72.40
P: 1. Serum pregnancy today.
   2. Will call pt. with results.

_____
Phil Wells, MD
Family Practice
NPI: 1234567890

TEST 11

Capital City Medical
123 Unknown Boulevard, Capital City, NY 12345-2222

Date of Service
01-24-20XX

New Patient			Other Invasive/Noninvasive			Laboratory		
Problem Focused	99201		Arthrocentesis/Aspiration/Injection			Amylase	82150	
Expanded Problem, Focused	99202		Small Joint	20600		B12	82607	
Detailed	99203		Interm Joint	20605		CBC & Diff	85025	
Comprehensive	99204		Major Joint	20610		Comp Metabolic Panel	80053	
Comprehensive/High Complex	99205		**Other Invasive/Noninvasive**			Chlamydia Screen	87110	
Well Exam Infant (up to 12 mos.)	99381		Audiometry	92552		Cholesterol	82465	
Well Exam 1–4 yrs.	99382		Cast Application			Digoxin	80162	
Well Exam 5–11 yrs.	99383		Location Long Short			Electrolytes	80051	
Well Exam 12–17 yrs.	99384		Catheterization	51701		Ferritin	82728	
Well Exam 18–39 yrs.	99385		Circumcision	54150		Folate	82746	
Well Exam 40–64 yrs.	99386		Colposcopy	57452		GC Screen	87070	
			Colposcopy w/Biopsy	57454		Glucose	82947	
			Cryosurgery Premalignant Lesion			Glucose 1 HR	82950	
			Location (s):			Glycosylated HGB A1C	83036	
Established Patient			Cryosurgery Warts			HCT	85014	
Post-Op Follow Up Visit	99024		Location (s):			HDL	83718	
Minimum	99211		Curettement Lesion			Hep BSAG	87340	
Problem Focused	99212	X	Single	11055		Hepatitis panel, acute	80074	
Expanded Problem Focused	99213		2–4	11056		HGB	85018	
Detailed	99214		>4	11057		HIV	86703	
Comprehensive/High Complex	99215		Diaphragm Fitting	57170		Iron & TIBC	83550	
Well Exam Infant (up to 12 mos.)	99391		Ear Irrigation	69210		Kidney Profile	80069	
Well exam 1–4 yrs.	99392		ECG	93000		Lead	83655	
Well Exam 5–11 yrs.	99393		Endometrial Biopsy	58100		Liver Profile	80076	
Well Exam 12–17 yrs.	99394		Exc. Lesion Malignant			Mono Test	86308	
Well Exam 18–39 yrs.	99395		Benign			Pap Smear	88155	
Well Exam 40–64 yrs.	99396		Location			Pregnancy Test	84703	X
Obstetrics			Exc. Skin Tags (1–15)	11200		Obstetric Panel	80055	
Total OB Care	59400		Each Additional 10	11201		Pro Time	85610	
Injections			Fracture Treatment			PSA	84153	
Administration Sub. / IM	90772		Loc			RPR	86592	
Drug			w/Reduc w/o Reduc			Sed. Rate	85651	
Dosage			I & D Abscess Single/Simple	10060		Stool Culture	87045	
Allergy	95115		Multiple or Comp	10061		Stool O & P	87177	
Cocci Skin Test	86490		I & D Pilonidal Cyst Simple	10080		Strep Screen	87880	
DPT	90701		Pilonidal Cyst Complex	10081		Theophylline	80198	
Hemophilus	90646		IV Therapy—To One Hour	90760		Thyroid Uptake	84479	
Influenza	90658		Each Additional Hour	90761		TSH	84443	
MMR	90707		Laceration Repair			Urinalysis	81000	X
OPV	90712		Location Size Simp/Comp			Urine Culture	87088	
Pneumovax	90732		Laryngoscopy	31505		Drawing Fee	36415	
TB Skin Test	86580		Oximetry	94760		Specimen Collection	99000	
TD	90718		Punch Biopsy			**Other:**		
Unlisted Immun	90749		Rhythm Strip	93040				
Tetanus Toxoid	90703		Treadmill	93015				
Vaccine/Toxoid Admin <8 Yr Old w/ Counseling	90465		Trigger Point or Tendon Sheath Inj.	20550				
Vaccine/Toxoid Administration for Adult	90471		Tympanometry	92567				

Diagnosis/ICD-9: **626.0, V72.40**

I acknowledge receipt of medical services and authorize the release of any medical information necessary to process this claim for healthcare payment only. I do authorize payment to the provider.

Total Estimated Charges: _____

Payment Amount: _____

Patient Signature _Gracie Lloyd_

Next Appointment: _____

Figure 7

Capital City Medical
Fee Schedule

New Patient OV		Punch Biopsy various codes	$80
Problem Focused 99201	$45	Nebulizer various codes	$45
Expanded Problem Focused 99202	$65	Cast Application various codes	$85
Detailed 99203	$85	Laryngoscopy 31505	$255
Comprehensive 99204	$105	Audiometry 92552	$85
Comprehensive/High Complex 99205	$115	Tympanometry 92567	$85
Well Exam infant (less than 1 year) 99381	$45	Ear Irrigation 69210	$25
Well Exam 1–4 yrs. 99382	$50	Diaphragm Fitting 57170	$30
Well Exam 5–11 yrs. 99383	$55	IV Therapy (up to one hour) 90760	$65
Well Exam 12–17 yrs. 99384	$65	Each additional hour 90761	$50
Well Exam 18–39 yrs. 99385	$85	Oximetry 94760	$10
Well Exam 40–64 yrs. 99386	$105	ECG 93000	$75
Established Patient OV		Holter Monitor various codes	$170
Post Op Follow Up Visit 99024	$0	Rhythm Strip 93040	$60
Minimum 99211	$35	Treadmill 93015	$375
Problem Focused 99212	$45	Cocci Skin Test 86490	$20
Expanded Problem Focused 99213	$55	X-ray, spine, chest, bone—any area various codes	$275
Detailed 99214	$65	Avulsion Nail 11730	$200
Comprehensive/High Complex 99215	$75	**Laboratory**	
Well exam infant (less than 1 year) 99391	$35	Amylase 82150	$40
Well Exam 1–4 yrs. 99392	$40	B12 82607	$30
Well Exam 5–11 yrs. 99393	$45	CBC & Diff 85025	$95
Well Exam 12–17 yrs. 99394	$55	Comp Metabolic Panel 80053	$75
Well Exam 18–39 yrs. 99395	$65	Chlamydia Screen 87110	$70
Well Exam 40–64 yrs. 99396	$75	Cholestrerol 82465	$75
Obstetrics		Digoxin 80162	$40
Total OB Care 59400	$1700	Electrolytes 80051	$70
Injections		Estrogen, Total 82672	$50
Administration 90772	$10	Ferritin 82728	$40
Allergy 95115	$35	Folate 82746	$30
DPT 90701	$50	GC Screen 87070	$60
Drug various codes	$35	Glucose 82947	$35
Influenza 90658	$25	Glycosylated HGB A1C 83036	$45
MMR 90707	$50	HCT 85014	$30
OPV 90712	$40	HDL 83718	$35
Pneumovax 90732	$35	HGB 85018	$30
TB Skin Test 86580	$15	Hep BSAG 83740	$40
TD 90718	$40	Hepatitis panel, acute 80074	$95
Tetanus Toxoid 90703	$40	HIV 86703	$100
Vaccine/Toxoid Administration for Younger		Iron & TIBC 83550	$45
Than 8 Years Old w/ counseling 90465	$10	Kidney Profile 80069	$95
Vaccine/Toxoid Administration for Adult 90471	$10	Lead 83665	$55
Arthrocentesis/Aspiration/Injection		Lipase 83690	$40
Small Joint 20600	$50	Lipid Panel 80061	$95
Interm Joint 20605	$60	Liver Profile 80076	$95
Major Joint 20610	$70	Mono Test 86308	$30
Trigger Point/Tendon Sheath Inj. 20550	$90	Pap Smear 88155	$90
Other Invasive/Noninvasive Procedures		Pap Collection/Supervision 88142	$95
Catheterization 51701	$55	Pregnancy Test 84703	$90
Circumcision 54150	$150	Obstetric Panel 80055	$85
Colposcopy 57452	$225	Pro Time 85610	$50
Colposcopy w/Biopsy 57454	$250	PSA 84153	$50
Cryosurgery Premalignant Lesion various codes	$160	RPR 86592	$55
Endometrial Biopsy 58100	$190	Sed. Rate 85651	$50
Excision Lesion Malignant various codes	$145	Stool Culture 87045	$80
Excision Lesion Benign various codes	$125	Stool O & P 87177	$105
Curettement Lesion		Strep Screen 87880	$35
Single 11055	$70	Theophylline 80198	$40
2–4 11056	$80	Thyroid Uptake 84479	$75
>4 11057	$90	TSH 84443	$50
Excision Skin Tags (1–15) 11200	$55	Urinalysis 81000	$35
Each Additional 10 11201	$30	Urine Culture 87088	$80
I & D Abscess Single/Simple 10060	$75	Drawing Fee 36415	$15
Multiple/Complex 10061	$95	Specimen Collection 99000	$10
I & D Pilonidal Cyst Simple 10080	$105		
I & D Pilonidal Cyst Complex 10081	$130		
Laceration Repair various codes	$60		

(1500)

HEALTH INSURANCE CLAIM FORM

APPROVED BY NATIONAL UNIFORM CLAIM COMMITTEE 08/05

☐☐☐PICA   PICA☐☐☐

1. MEDICARE MEDICAID TRICARE CHAMPVA GROUP FECA OTHER	1a. INSURED'S I.D. NUMBER (For Program in Item 1)

1. MEDICARE   MEDICAID   TRICARE   CHAMPVA   GROUP HEALTH PLAN   FECA BLK LUNG   OTHER
CHAMPUS
☐ (Medicare #)   ☐ (Medicaid #)   ☐ (Sponsor's SSN)   ☐ (Member ID#)   ☐ (SSN or ID)   ☐ (SSN)   ☐ (ID)

1a. INSURED'S I.D. NUMBER (For Program in Item 1)

2. PATIENT'S NAME (Last Name, First Name, Middle Initial)

3. PATIENT'S BIRTH DATE   SEX
MM   DD   YY
M☐   F☐

4. INSURED'S NAME (Last Name, First Name, Middle Initial)

5. PATIENT'S ADDRESS (No., Street)

6. PATIENT RELATIONSHIP TO INSURED
Self☐   Spouse☐   Child☐   Other☐

7. INSURED'S ADDRESS (No, Street)

CITY   STATE

8. PATIENT STATUS
Single☐   Married☐   Other☐

CITY   STATE

ZIP CODE   TELEPHONE (Include Area Code)
(   )

Full-Time   Part-Time
Employed☐   Student☐   Student☐

ZIP CODE   TELEPHONE (Include Area Code)
(   )

9. OTHER INSURED'S NAME (Last Name, First Name, Middle Initial)

10. IS PATIENT'S CONDITION RELATED TO:

11. INSURED'S POLICY GROUP OR FECA NUMBER

a. OTHER INSURED'S POLICY OR GROUP NUMBER

a. EMPLOYMENT? (Current or Previous)
☐YES   ☐NO

a. INSURED'S DATE OF BIRTH   SEX
MM   DD   YY
M☐   F☐

b. OTHER INSURED'S DATE OF BIRTH   SEX
MM   DD   YY
M☐   F☐

b. AUTO ACCIDENT?   PLACE (State)
☐YES   ☐NO

b. EMPLOYER'S NAME OR SCHOOL NAME

c. EMPLOYER'S NAME OR SCHOOL NAME

c. OTHER ACCIDENT?
☐YES   ☐NO

c. INSURANCE PLAN NAME OR PROGRAM NAME

d. INSURANCE PLAN NAME OR PROGRAM NAME

10d. RESERVED FOR LOCAL USE

d. IS THERE ANOTHER HEALTH BENEFIT PLAN?
☐YES   ☐NO   If yes, return to and complete item 9 a-d.

READ BACK OF FORM BEFORE COMPLETING & SIGNING THIS FORM.

12. PATIENT'S OR AUTHORIZED PERSON'S SIGNATURE I authorize the release of any medical or other information necessary to process this claim. I also request payment of government benefits either to myself or to the party who accepts assignment below.

SIGNED _____   DATE_____

13. INSURED'S OR AUTHORIZED PERSON'S SIGNATURE I authorize payment of medical benefits to the undersigned physician or supplier for services described below.

SIGNED _____

14. DATE OF CURRENT: ILLNESS (First symptom) OR   INJURY (Accident) OR   PREGNANCY (LMP)
MM   DD   YY

15. IF PATIENT HAS HAD SAME OR SIMILAR ILLNESS, GIVE FIRST DATE   MM   DD   YY

16. DATES PATIENT UNABLE TO WORK IN CURRENT OCCUPATION
MM   DD   YY   MM   DD   YY
FROM   TO

17. NAME OF REFERRING PHYSICIAN OR OTHER SOURCE

17a.
17b.   NPI

18. HOSPITALIZATION DATES RELATED TO CURRENT SERVICES
MM   DD   YY   MM   DD   YY
FROM   TO

19. RESERVED FOR LOCAL USE

20. OUTSIDE LAB? $ CHARGES
☐YES   ☐NO

21. DIAGNOSIS OR NATURE OF ILLNESS OR INJURY (Relate Items 1,2,3 or 4 to Item 24E by Line)

1. |___.___| 3. |___.___|

2. |___.___| 4. |___.___|

22. MEDICAID RESUBMISSION
CODE   ORIGINAL REF. NO.

23. PRIOR AUTHORIZATION NUMBER

24. A. DATE(S) OF SERVICE			B. PLACE OF SERVICE	C. EMG	D. PROCEDURES, SERVICES, OR SUPPLIES (Explain Unusual Circumstances)		E. DIAGNOSIS POINTER	F. $ CHARGES	G. DAYS OR UNITS	H. EPSDT Family Plan	I. ID. QUAL.	J. RENDERING PROVIDER ID. #
From MM DD YY	To MM DD YY				CPT/HCPCS	MODIFIER						
1												NPI
2												NPI
3												NPI
4												NPI
5												NPI
6												NPI

25. FEDERAL TAX I.D. NUMBER SSN EIN ☐☐	26. PATIENT'S ACCOUNT NO.	27. ACCEPT ASSIGNMENT? (For govt. claims, see back) ☐YES ☐NO	28. TOTAL CHARGE $	29. AMOUNT PAID $	30. BALANCE DUE $

31. SIGNATURE OF PHYSICIAN OR SUPPLIER INCLUDING DEGREES OR CREDENTIALS (I certify that the statements on the reverse apply to this bill and are made a part thereof.)

SIGNED _____   DATE _____

32. SERVICE FACILITY LOCATION INFORMATION

a.   NPI   b.

33. BILLING PROVIDER INFO & PH. # (   )

a.   NPI   b.

NUCC Instruction Manual available at: www.nucc.org
WCMS-1500CS

APPROVED OMB 0938-0999 FORM CMS-1500 (08/05)

Figure 8

TEST 12: COMPLETE A
WORKERS' COMPENSATION CLAIM

Directions: Using the source documents provided for patient Devon Ulrich and the Capital City Medical fee schedule (Figure 9), accurately complete a CMS-1500 claim form for a Workers' Compensation claim. Use the blank CMS-1500 claim form provided (Figure 10).

Complete the case on the basis of the following criteria:

- All patients have release of information and assignment of benefit signatures on file, as a condition for Workers' Compensation. Items 12 and 13 should not be completed.

- By law, all providers are participating and accept assignment. Item 27 should not be marked.

- The group practice is the billing entity.

- The national transition to NPI numbers is complete, and legacy PINs of individual payers are no longer used. If legacy PINS are still being used by your state's Workers' Compensation program, your instructor may provide legacy PINs in addition to the NPI.

- 2012 ICD-9-CM, ICD-10-CM/PCS, and CPT codes are used.

- Use eight-digit dates for birthdates. Use six-digit dates for all other dates.

- All street names should be entered with standard postal abbreviations, even if they are spelled out on the source documents.

- Enter ICD-9 and ICD-10 codes in the order in which they appear on the encounter form.

- When entering CPT codes, enter the E/M code first. Enter remaining CPT codes in descending price order.

- Enter the Workers' Compensation assigned claim number in Item 1a. (Requirements will vary by state.)

TEST 12

Patient Information:

Name: (Last, First) Ulrich, Devon   ☒ Male   ☐ Female   Birth Date: 10/07/1971

Address: 42 Stone St, Township, NY 12345   Phone: (555) 555-7159

Social Security Number: 619-42-8736   Full-Time Student: ☐ Yes ☒ No

Marital Status: ☐ Single ☒ Married ☐ Divorced ☐ Other

Employment:

Employer: Curb Appeal Landscaping, Inc.   Phone: (555) 555-1291

Address: 600 Jefferson Base, Capital City NY 12345

Condition Related to: ☐ Auto Accident ☒ Employment ☐ Other Accident

Date of Accident: 09/06/20XX   State: NY

Emergency Contact: _____ Phone: ( ) _____

Primary Insurance: Capital Workers' Compensation Insurance Co.   Phone: ( ) _____

Address: 40, Hurt Rd, Capital City, NY 12345

Insurance Policyholder's Name: Curb Appeal Landscaping Inc.   ☐ M ☐ F DOB: _____

Address: _____

Phone: _____ Relationship to Insured: ☐ Self ☐ Spouse ☐ Child ☒ Other

Employer: Same as above   Phone: ( ) _____

Employer's Address: _____

Policy/ID No: WCDU1115   Group No: _____ Percent Covered: ___% Copay Amt: $_____

Secondary Insurance: _____   Phone: ( ) _____

Address: _____

Insurance Policyholder's Name: _____   ☐ M ☐ F DOB: _____

Address: _____

Phone: _____ Relationship to Insured: ☐ Self ☐ Spouse ☐ Child ☐ Other

Employer: _____   Phone: ( ) _____

Employer's Address: _____

Policy/ID No: _____   Group No: _____ Percent Covered: ___% Copay Amt: $_____

Reason for Visit: While working today I got excessively tired.

Known Allergies: _____

Referred by: _____

09/06/20XX
Assignment of Benefits: Y
Signature on File: Y
Referring Physician: N

S: New patient, Devon Ulrich, presents in the office today complaining of excessive tiredness. He was landscaping a client's yard today at work when he suddenly felt "weirdly exhausted."

O: HEENT: Normocephalic, atraumatic. Eyes clear. Nose clear. Throat: No masses. Chest clear. BP: 110/86, P: 74, R: 12, T: 97.6°. Abdomen is soft, nontender. No masses. Bowel sounds normal. Pt. shows signs of heat fatique. Lytes normal values.

A: 1. Heat exhaustion due to weather—992.5, E900.0.

P: 1. Plenty of rest.
2. Plenty of vitamin-rich liquids such as vitamin water.
3. Call office if no improvement or if dizziness, fainting, N&V occur.
4. Return in 3 days.
5. Off work until next appointment.
6. Please bill his workers' compensation. His info is as follows:
Capital Workers' Compensation Insurance Co.
40 Hurt Rd.
Capital City, NY 12345
Claim #WCDU1115
7. Phil Wells, MD state license #—MD-123456-L

_____

Phil Wells, MD
Family Practice
NPI: 1234567890

TEST 12

Patient Name Devon Ulrich

Capital City Medical
123 Unknown Boulevard, Capital City, NY 12345-2222

Date of Service
09-06-20XX

New Patient			Arthrocentesis/Aspiration/Injection		Laboratory		
Problem Focused	99201		Arthrocentesis/Aspiration/Injection		Amylase	82150	
Expanded Problem, Focused	99202		Small Joint	20600	B12	82607	
Detailed	99203		Interm Joint	20605	CBC & Diff	85025	
Comprehensive	99204	X	Major Joint	20610	Comp Metabolic Panel	80053	
Comprehensive/High Complex	99205		**Other Invasive/Noninvasive**		Chlamydia Screen	87110	
Well Exam Infant (up to 12 mos.)	99381		Audiometry	92552	Cholesterol	82465	
Well Exam 1–4 yrs.	99382		Cast Application		Digoxin	80162	
Well Exam 5–11 yrs.	99383		Location Long Short		Electrolytes	80051	X
Well Exam 12–17 yrs.	99384		Catheterization	51701	Ferritin	82728	
Well Exam 18–39 yrs.	99385		Circumcision	54150	Folate	82746	
Well Exam 40–64 yrs.	99386		Colposcopy	57452	GC Screen	87070	
			Colposcopy w/Biopsy	57454	Glucose	82947	
			Cryosurgery Premalignant Lesion		Glucose 1 HR	82950	
			Location (s):		Glycosylated HGB A1C	83036	
Established Patient			Cryosurgery Warts		HCT	85014	
Post-Op Follow Up Visit	99024		Location (s):		HDL	83718	
Minimum	99211		Curettement Lesion		Hep BSAG	87340	
Problem Focused	99212		Single	11055	Hepatitis panel, acute	80074	
Expanded Problem Focused	99213		2–4	11056	HGB	85018	
Detailed	99214		>4	11057	HIV	86703	
Comprehensive/High Complex	99215		Diaphragm Fitting	57170	Iron & TIBC	83550	
Well Exam Infant (up to 12 mos.)	99391		Ear Irrigation	69210	Kidney Profile	80069	
Well exam 1–4 yrs.	99392		ECG	93000	Lead	83655	
Well Exam 5–11 yrs.	99393		Endometrial Biopsy	58100	Liver Profile	80076	
Well Exam 12–17 yrs.	99394		Exc. Lesion Malignant		Mono Test	86308	
Well Exam 18–39 yrs.	99395		Benign		Pap Smear	88155	
Well Exam 40–64 yrs.	99396		Location		Pregnancy Test	84703	
Obstetrics			Exc. Skin Tags (1–15)	11200	Obstetric Panel	80055	
Total OB Care	59400		Each Additional 10	11201	Pro Time	85610	
Injections			Fracture Treatment		PSA	84153	
Administration Sub. / IM	90772		Loc		RPR	86592	
Drug			w/Reduc w/o Reduc		Sed. Rate	85651	
Dosage			I & D Abscess Single/Simple	10060	Stool Culture	87045	
Allergy	95115		Multiple or Comp	10061	Stool O & P	87177	
Cocci Skin Test	86490		I & D Pilonidal Cyst Simple	10080	Strep Screen	87880	
DPT	90701		Pilonidal Cyst Complex	10081	Theophylline	80198	
Hemophilus	90646		IV Therapy—To One Hour	90760	Thyroid Uptake	84479	
Influenza	90658		Each Additional Hour	90761	TSH	84443	
MMR	90707		Laceration Repair		Urinalysis	81000	
OPV	90712		Location Size Simp/Comp		Urine Culture	87088	
Pneumovax	90732		Laryngoscopy	31505	Drawing Fee	36415	X
TB Skin Test	86580		Oximetry	94760	Specimen Collection	99000	
TD	90718		Punch Biopsy		**Other:**		
Unlisted Immun	90749		Rhythm Strip	93040			
Tetanus Toxoid	90703		Treadmill	93015			
Vaccine/Toxoid Admin <8 Yr Old w/ Counseling	90465		Trigger Point or Tendon Sheath Inj.	20550			
Vaccine/Toxoid Administration for Adult	90471		Tympanometry	92567			

Diagnosis/ICD-9: **992.5, E900.0**

I acknowledge receipt of medical services and authorize the release of any medical information necessary to process this claim for healthcare payment only. I do authorize payment to the provider.

Total Estimated Charges: _____

Payment Amount: _____

Patient Signature _Devon Ulrich_____

Next Appointment: _____

Figure 9

Capital City Medical
Fee Schedule

New Patient OV			Punch Biopsy various codes	$80
Problem Focused 99201	$45		Nebulizer various codes	$45
Expanded Problem Focused 99202	$65		Cast Application various codes	$85
Detailed 99203	$85		Laryngoscopy 31505	$255
Comprehensive 99204	$105		Audiometry 92552	$85
Comprehensive/High Complex 99205	$115		Tympanometry 92567	$85
Well Exam infant (less than 1 year) 99381	$45		Ear Irrigation 69210	$25
Well Exam 1–4 yrs. 99382	$50		Diaphragm Fitting 57170	$30
Well Exam 5–11 yrs. 99383	$55		IV Therapy (up to one hour) 90760	$65
Well Exam 12–17 yrs. 99384	$65		Each additional hour 90761	$50
Well Exam 18–39 yrs. 99385	$85		Oximetry 94760	$10
Well Exam 40–64 yrs. 99386	$105		ECG 93000	$75
Established Patient OV			Holter Monitor various codes	$170
Post Op Follow Up Visit 99024	$0		Rhythm Strip 93040	$60
Minimum 99211	$35		Treadmill 93015	$375
Problem Focused 99212	$45		Cocci Skin Test 86490	$20
Expanded Problem Focused 99213	$55		X-ray, spine, chest, bone—any area various codes	$275
Detailed 99214	$65		Avulsion Nail 11730	$200
Comprehensive/High Complex 99215	$75		**Laboratory**	
Well exam infant (less than 1 year) 99391	$35		Amylase 82150	$40
Well Exam 1–4 yrs. 99392	$40		B12 82607	$30
Well Exam 5–11 yrs. 99393	$45		CBC & Diff 85025	$95
Well Exam 12–17 yrs. 99394	$55		Comp Metabolic Panel 80053	$75
Well Exam 18–39 yrs. 99395	$65		Chlamydia Screen 87110	$70
Well Exam 40–64 yrs. 99396	$75		Cholestrerol 82465	$75
Obstetrics			Digoxin 80162	$40
Total OB Care 59400	$1700		Electrolytes 80051	$70
Injections			Estrogen, Total 82672	$50
Administration 90772	$10		Ferritin 82728	$40
Allergy 95115	$35		Folate 82746	$30
DPT 90701	$50		GC Screen 87070	$60
Drug various codes	$35		Glucose 82947	$35
Influenza 90658	$25		Glycosylated HGB A1C 83036	$45
MMR 90707	$50		HCT 85014	$30
OPV 90712	$40		HDL 83718	$35
Pneumovax 90732	$35		HGB 85018	$30
TB Skin Test 86580	$15		Hep BSAG 83740	$40
TD 90718	$40		Hepatitis panel, acute 80074	$95
Tetanus Toxoid 90703	$40		HIV 86703	$100
Vaccine/Toxoid Administration for Younger			Iron & TIBC 83550	$45
Than 8 Years Old w/ counseling 90465	$10		Kidney Profile 80069	$95
Vaccine/Toxoid Administration for Adult 90471	$10		Lead 83665	$55
Arthrocentesis/Aspiration/Injection			Lipase 83690	$40
Small Joint 20600	$50		Lipid Panel 80061	$95
Interm Joint 20605	$60		Liver Profile 80076	$95
Major Joint 20610	$70		Mono Test 86308	$30
Trigger Point/Tendon Sheath Inj. 20550	$90		Pap Smear 88155	$90
Other Invasive/Noninvasive Procedures			Pap Collection/Supervision 88142	$95
Catheterization 51701	$55		Pregnancy Test 84703	$90
Circumcision 54150	$150		Obstetric Panel 80055	$85
Colposcopy 57452	$225		Pro Time 85610	$50
Colposcopy w/Biopsy 57454	$250		PSA 84153	$50
Cryosurgery Premalignant Lesion various codes	$160		RPR 86592	$55
Endometrial Biopsy 58100	$190		Sed. Rate 85651	$50
Excision Lesion Malignant various codes	$145		Stool Culture 87045	$80
Excision Lesion Benign various codes	$125		Stool O & P 87177	$105
Curettement Lesion			Strep Screen 87880	$35
Single 11055	$70		Theophylline 80198	$40
2–4 11056	$80		Thyroid Uptake 84479	$75
>4 11057	$90		TSH 84443	$50
Excision Skin Tags (1–15) 11200	$55		Urinalysis 81000	$35
Each Additional 10 11201	$30		Urine Culture 87088	$80
I & D Abscess Single/Simple 10060	$75		Drawing Fee 36415	$15
Multiple/Complex 10061	$95		Specimen Collection 99000	$10
I & D Pilonidal Cyst Simple 10080	$105			
I & D Pilonidal Cyst Complex 10081	$130			
Laceration Repair various codes	$60			

HEALTH INSURANCE CLAIM FORM
APPROVED BY NATIONAL UNIFORM CLAIM COMMITTEE 08/05

PICA

				PICA

1. MEDICARE ☐ (Medicare #) **MEDICAID** ☐ (Medicaid #) **TRICARE CHAMPUS** ☐ (Sponsor's SSN) **CHAMPVA** ☐ (Member ID#) **GROUP HEALTH PLAN** ☐ (SSN or ID) **FECA BLK LUNG** ☐ (SSN) **OTHER** ☐ (ID)

1a. INSURED'S I.D. NUMBER (For Program in Item 1)

2. PATIENT'S NAME (Last Name, First Name, Middle Initial)

3. PATIENT'S BIRTH DATE MM | DD | YY   **SEX** M ☐ F ☐

4. INSURED'S NAME (Last Name, First Name, Middle Initial)

5. PATIENT'S ADDRESS (No., Street)

6. PATIENT RELATIONSHIP TO INSURED Self ☐ Spouse ☐ Child ☐ Other ☐

7. INSURED'S ADDRESS (No, Street)

CITY | **STATE**

8. PATIENT STATUS Single ☐ Married ☐ Other ☐

CITY | **STATE**

ZIP CODE | **TELEPHONE** (Include Area Code) ( )

Employed ☐ Full-Time Student ☐ Part-Time Student ☐

ZIP CODE | **TELEPHONE** (Include Area Code) ( )

9. OTHER INSURED'S NAME (Last Name, First Name, Middle Initial)

10. IS PATIENT'S CONDITION RELATED TO:

11. INSURED'S POLICY GROUP OR FECA NUMBER

a. OTHER INSURED'S POLICY OR GROUP NUMBER

a. EMPLOYMENT? (Current or Previous) ☐ YES ☐ NO

a. INSURED'S DATE OF BIRTH MM | DD | YY   **SEX** M ☐ F ☐

b. OTHER INSURED'S DATE OF BIRTH MM | DD | YY   **SEX** M ☐ F ☐

b. AUTO ACCIDENT? ☐ YES ☐ NO   **PLACE** (State)

b. EMPLOYER'S NAME OR SCHOOL NAME

c. EMPLOYER'S NAME OR SCHOOL NAME

c. OTHER ACCIDENT? ☐ YES ☐ NO

c. INSURANCE PLAN NAME OR PROGRAM NAME

d. INSURANCE PLAN NAME OR PROGRAM NAME

10d. RESERVED FOR LOCAL USE

d. IS THERE ANOTHER HEALTH BENEFIT PLAN? ☐ YES ☐ NO   If yes, return to and complete item 9 a-d.

READ BACK OF FORM BEFORE COMPLETING & SIGNING THIS FORM.
12. PATIENT'S OR AUTHORIZED PERSON'S SIGNATURE I authorize the release of any medical or other information necessary to process this claim. I also request payment of government benefits either to myself or to the party who accepts assignment below.

SIGNED _____ DATE _____

13. INSURED'S OR AUTHORIZED PERSON'S SIGNATURE I authorize payment of medical benefits to the undersigned physician or supplier for services described below.

SIGNED _____

14. DATE OF CURRENT: MM | DD | YY   ILLNESS (First symptom) OR INJURY (Accident) OR PREGNANCY (LMP)

15. IF PATIENT HAS HAD SAME OR SIMILAR ILLNESS. GIVE FIRST DATE MM | DD | YY

16. DATES PATIENT UNABLE TO WORK IN CURRENT OCCUPATION FROM MM | DD | YY TO MM | DD | YY

17. NAME OF REFERRING PHYSICIAN OR OTHER SOURCE

17a.
17b. NPI

18. HOSPITALIZATION DATES RELATED TO CURRENT SERVICES FROM MM | DD | YY TO MM | DD | YY

19. RESERVED FOR LOCAL USE

20. OUTSIDE LAB? ☐ YES ☐ NO   **$ CHARGES**

21. DIAGNOSIS OR NATURE OF ILLNESS OR INJURY (Relate Items 1,2,3 or 4 to Item 24E by Line)

1. _____
2. _____
3. _____
4. _____

22. MEDICAID RESUBMISSION CODE | **ORIGINAL REF. NO.**

23. PRIOR AUTHORIZATION NUMBER

24. A. DATE(S) OF SERVICE From MM DD YY	To MM DD YY	B. PLACE OF SERVICE	C. EMG	D. PROCEDURES, SERVICES, OR SUPPLIES (Explain Unusual Circumstances) CPT/HCPCS	MODIFIER	E. DIAGNOSIS POINTER	F. $ CHARGES	G. DAYS OR UNITS	H. EPSDT Family Plan	I. ID. QUAL.	J. RENDERING PROVIDER ID. #
1										NPI	
2										NPI	
3										NPI	
4										NPI	
5										NPI	
6										NPI	

25. FEDERAL TAX I.D. NUMBER SSN ☐ EIN ☐

26. PATIENT'S ACCOUNT NO.

27. ACCEPT ASSIGNMENT? (For govt. claims, see back) ☐ YES ☐ NO

28. TOTAL CHARGE $

29. AMOUNT PAID $

30. BALANCE DUE $

31. SIGNATURE OF PHYSICIAN OR SUPPLIER INCLUDING DEGREES OR CREDENTIALS (I certify that the statements on the reverse apply to this bill and are made a part thereof.)

SIGNED _____ DATE _____

32. SERVICE FACILITY LOCATION INFORMATION

a. NPI | b.

33. BILLING PROVIDER INFO & PH. # ( )

a. NPI | b.

NUCC Instruction Manual available at: www.nucc.org
WCMS-1500CS

APPROVED OMB 0938-0999 FORM CMS-1500 (08/05)

CARRIER — *PATIENT AND INSURED INFORMATION* — *PHYSICIAN OR SUPPLIER INFORMATION*

SECOND FOLD — FIRST FOLD   WHCF-10-ENV / WHCF-10-ENV-SS

Figure 10

TEST 13: COMPLETE A CMS-1500 CLAIM FORM FOR COMMERCIAL INSURANCE

Directions: Using the source documents provided for patient Duncan Shelton and the Capital City Medical fee schedule (Figure 11), accurately complete a CMS-1500 claim form for commercial insurance carriers. Use the blank CMS-1500 claim form provided (Figure 12).

Complete the case on the basis of the following criteria:

- All patients have release of information and assignment of benefit signatures on file.

- All providers are participating and accept assignment, by contractual agreement. Item 27 is not marked.

- The group practice is the billing entity.

- The national transition to NPI numbers is complete, and legacy PINs of individual payers are no longer used. If legacy PINs are still being used by selected payers in your region, your instructor may provide legacy PINS in addition to the NPI.

- 2012 ICD-9-CM, ICD-12-CM/PCS, and CPT codes are used.

- Use eight-digit dates for birthdates. Use six-digit dates for all other dates.

- All street names should be entered with standard postal abbreviations, even if they are spelled out on the source documents.

- Enter ICD-9 and ICD-10 codes in the order in which they appear on the encounter form.

- When entering CPT codes, enter the E/M code first. Enter remaining codes in descending price order.

TEST 13

Patient Information:

Name: (Last, First) Shelton, Duncan   ☒ Male   ❑ Female   Birth Date: 02/11/1962

Address: 321 Skyline Dr, Capital City, NY 12345   Phone: (555) 555-8970

Social Security Number: 608-77-3458   Full-Time Student: ❑ Yes ☒ No

Marital Status: ❑ Single ☒ Married ❑ Divorced ❑ Other

Employment:

Employer: Capital City Hardware   Phone: (555) 555-6342

Address: 600 Jefferson Base, Capital City NY 12345

Condition Related to: ❑ Auto Accident ❑ Employment ❑ Other Accident

Date of Accident: _____ State: _____

Emergency Contact: _____ **Phone: ( )** _____

Primary Insurance: Blue Cross Blue Shield   Phone: ( ) _____

Address: 379 Blue Plaza, Capital City, NY 12345

Insurance Policyholder's Name: Shelton, Candy   ❑ M ☒ F DOB: 12/19/1964

Address: Same

Phone: _____ Relationship to Insured: ❑ Self ☒ Spouse ❑ Child ❑ Other

Employer: Channel 8 News   Phone: ( ) _____

Employer's Address: Channel 8 Center, News Drive, Capital City, NY 12345

Policy/ID No: YYJ34121269   Group No: 352257 Percent Covered: ____% Copay Amt: $ 20.00

Secondary Insurance: _____   Phone: ( ) _____

Address: _____

Insurance Policyholder's Name: _____   ❑ M ❑ F DOB: _____

Address: _____

Phone: _____ Relationship to Insured: ❑ Self ❑ Spouse ❑ Child ❑ Other

Employer: _____   Phone: ( ) _____

Employer's Address: _____

Policy/ID No: _____ Group No: _____ Percent Covered: ___% Copay Amt: $_____

Reason for Visit: I am here for a follow up on my test results for testicular pain

Known Allergies: _____

Referred by: _____

02/16/20XX
Assignment of Benefits: Y
Signature on File: Y
Referring Physician: N

S: Duncan Shelton is here to find out the results of his recent ultrasound of his testicles.

O: Pt. still complains of testicular pain ranging at 9. On exam, the testicles are still very swollen. He denies any new complaints. The ultrasound does reveal twisted veins in the testicles.

A: 1. Testicular torsion—608.20

P: 1. Pt. to see Mannie Mends, MD, for surgical consult ASAP.
2. Continue Percocet one p.o. q. 6h. p.r.n.

_____

Phil Wells, MD
Family Practice
NPI: 1234567890

TEST 13

Capital City Medical
123 Unknown Boulevard, Capital City, NY 12345-2222

Date of Service
02-16-20XX

New Patient			Other Invasive/Noninvasive			Laboratory	
Problem Focused	99201		Arthrocentesis/Aspiration/Injection			Amylase	82150
Expanded Problem, Focused	99202		Small Joint	20600		B12	82607
Detailed	99203		Interm Joint	20605		CBC & Diff	85025
Comprehensive	99204		Major Joint	20610		Comp Metabolic Panel	80053
Comprehensive/High Complex	99205		**Other Invasive/Noninvasive**			Chlamydia Screen	87110
Well Exam Infant (up to 12 mos.)	99381		Audiometry	92552		Cholesterol	82465
Well Exam 1–4 yrs.	99382		Cast Application			Digoxin	80162
Well Exam 5–11 yrs.	99383		Location ☒ Long Short			Electrolytes	80051
Well Exam 12–17 yrs.	99384		Catheterization	51701		Ferritin	82728
Well Exam 18–39 yrs.	99385		Circumcision	54150		Folate	82746
Well Exam 40–64 yrs.	99386		Colposcopy	57452		GC Screen	87070
			Colposcopy w/Biopsy	57454		Glucose	82947
			Cryosurgery Premalignant Lesion			Glucose 1 HR	82950
			Location (s):			Glycosylated HGB A1C	83036
Established Patient			Cryosurgery Warts			HCT	85014
Post-Op Follow Up Visit	99024		Location (s):			HDL	83718
Minimum	99211		Curettement Lesion			Hep BSAG	87340
Problem Focused	99212		Single	11055		Hepatitis panel, acute	80074
Expanded Problem Focused	99213	☒	2–4	11056		HGB	85018
Detailed	99214		>4	11057		HIV	86703
Comprehensive/High Complex	99215		Diaphragm Fitting	57170		Iron & TIBC	83550
Well Exam Infant (up to 12 mos.)	99391		Ear Irrigation	69210		Kidney Profile	80069
Well exam 1–4 yrs.	99392		ECG	93000		Lead	83655
Well Exam 5–11 yrs.	99393		Endometrial Biopsy	58100		Liver Profile	80076
Well Exam 12–17 yrs.	99394		Exc. Lesion Malignant			Mono Test	86308
Well Exam 18–39 yrs.	99395		Benign			Pap Smear	88155
Well Exam 40–64 yrs.	99396		Location			Pregnancy Test	84703
Obstetrics			Exc. Skin Taqs (1–15)	11200		Obstetric Panel	80055
Total OB Care	59400		Each Additional 10	11201		Pro Time	85610
Injections			Fracture Treatment			PSA	84153
Administration Sub. / IM	90772		Loc			RPR	86592
Drug			w/Reduc w/o Reduc			Sed. Rate	85651
Dosage			I & D Abscess Single/Simple	10060		Stool Culture	87045
Allergy	95115		Multiple or Comp	10061		Stool O & P	87177
Cocci Skin Test	86490		I & D Pilonidal Cyst Simple	10080		Strep Screen	87880
DPT	90701		Pilonidal Cyst Complex	10081		Theophylline	80198
Hemophilus	90646		IV Therapy—To One Hour	90760		Thyroid Uptake	84479
Influenza	90658		Each Additional Hour	90761		TSH	84443
MMR	90707		Laceration Repair			Urinalysis	81000
OPV	90712		Location Size Simp/Comp			Urine Culture	87088
Pneumovax	90732		Laryngoscopy	31505		Drawing Fee	36415
TB Skin Test	86580		Oximetry	94760		Specimen Collection	99000
TD	90718		Punch Biopsy			**Other:**	
Unlisted Immun	90749		Rhythm Strip	93040			
Tetanus Toxoid	90703		Treadmill	93015			
Vaccine/Toxoid Admin <8 Yr Old w/ Counseling	90465		Trigger Point or Tendon Sheath Inj.	20550			
Vaccine/Toxoid Administration for Adult	90471		Tympanometry	92567			

Diagnosis/ICD-9: **608.20**

I acknowledge receipt of medical services and authorize the release of any medical information necessary to process this claim for healthcare payment only. I do authorize payment to the provider.

Total Estimated Charges: _____

Payment Amount: _____

Patient Signature _Duncan Shelton_

Next Appointment: _____

Figure 11

Capital City Medical
Fee Schedule

New Patient OV		Punch Biopsy various codes	$80
Problem Focused 99201	$45	Nebulizer various codes	$45
Expanded Problem Focused 99202	$65	Cast Application various codes	$85
Detailed 99203	$85	Laryngoscopy 31505	$255
Comprehensive 99204	$105	Audiometry 92552	$85
Comprehensive/High Complex 99205	$115	Tympanometry 92567	$85
Well Exam infant (less than 1 year) 99381	$45	Ear Irrigation 69210	$25
Well Exam 1–4 yrs. 99382	$50	Diaphragm Fitting 57170	$30
Well Exam 5–11 yrs. 99383	$55	IV Therapy (up to one hour) 90760	$65
Well Exam 12–17 yrs. 99384	$65	Each additional hour 90761	$50
Well Exam 18–39 yrs. 99385	$85	Oximetry 94760	$10
Well Exam 40–64 yrs. 99386	$105	ECG 93000	$75
Established Patient OV		Holter Monitor various codes	$170
Post Op Follow Up Visit 99024	$0	Rhythm Strip 93040	$60
Minimum 99211	$35	Treadmill 93015	$375
Problem Focused 99212	$45	Cocci Skin Test 86490	$20
Expanded Problem Focused 99213	$55	X-ray, spine, chest, bone—any area various codes	$275
Detailed 99214	$65	Avulsion Nail 11730	$200
Comprehensive/High Complex 99215	$75	**Laboratory**	
Well exam infant (less than 1 year) 99391	$35	Amylase 82150	$40
Well Exam 1–4 yrs. 99392	$40	B12 82607	$30
Well Exam 5–11 yrs. 99393	$45	CBC & Diff 85025	$95
Well Exam 12–17 yrs. 99394	$55	Comp Metabolic Panel 80053	$75
Well Exam 18–39 yrs. 99395	$65	Chlamydia Screen 87110	$70
Well Exam 40–64 yrs. 99396	$75	Cholestrerol 82465	$75
Obstetrics		Digoxin 80162	$40
Total OB Care 59400	$1700	Electrolytes 80051	$70
Injections		Estrogen, Total 82672	$50
Administration 90772	$10	Ferritin 82728	$40
Allergy 95115	$35	Folate 82746	$30
DPT 90701	$50	GC Screen 87070	$60
Drug various codes	$35	Glucose 82947	$35
Influenza 90658	$25	Glycosylated HGB A1C 83036	$45
MMR 90707	$50	HCT 85014	$30
OPV 90712	$40	HDL 83718	$35
Pneumovax 90732	$35	HGB 85018	$30
TB Skin Test 86580	$15	Hep BSAG 83740	$40
TD 90718	$40	Hepatitis panel, acute 80074	$95
Tetanus Toxoid 90703	$40	HIV 86703	$100
Vaccine/Toxoid Administration for Younger		Iron & TIBC 83550	$45
Than 8 Years Old w/ counseling 90465	$10	Kidney Profile 80069	$95
Vaccine/Toxoid Administration for Adult 90471	$10	Lead 83665	$55
Arthrocentesis/Aspiration/Injection		Lipase 83690	$40
Small Joint 20600	$50	Lipid Panel 80061	$95
Interm Joint 20605	$60	Liver Profile 80076	$95
Major Joint 20610	$70	Mono Test 86308	$30
Trigger Point/Tendon Sheath Inj. 20550	$90	Pap Smear 88155	$90
Other Invasive/Noninvasive Procedures		Pap Collection/Supervision 88142	$95
Catheterization 51701	$55	Pregnancy Test 84703	$90
Circumcision 54150	$150	Obstetric Panel 80055	$85
Colposcopy 57452	$225	Pro Time 85610	$50
Colposcopy w/Biopsy 57454	$250	PSA 84153	$50
Cryosurgery Premalignant Lesion various codes	$160	RPR 86592	$55
Endometrial Biopsy 58100	$190	Sed. Rate 85651	$50
Excision Lesion Malignant various codes	$145	Stool Culture 87045	$80
Excision Lesion Benign various codes	$125	Stool O & P 87177	$105
Curettement Lesion		Strep Screen 87880	$35
Single 11055	$70	Theophylline 80198	$40
2–4 11056	$80	Thyroid Uptake 84479	$75
>4 11057	$90	TSH 84443	$50
Excision Skin Tags (1–15) 11200	$55	Urinalysis 81000	$35
Each Additional 10 11201	$30	Urine Culture 87088	$80
I & D Abscess Single/Simple 10060	$75	Drawing Fee 36415	$15
Multiple/Complex 10061	$95	Specimen Collection 99000	$10
I & D Pilonidal Cyst Simple 10080	$105		
I & D Pilonidal Cyst Complex 10081	$130		
Laceration Repair various codes	$60		

1500

HEALTH INSURANCE CLAIM FORM
APPROVED BY NATIONAL UNIFORM CLAIM COMMITTEE 08/05

☐☐☐ PICA

PICA ☐☐☐

| 1. MEDICARE | MEDICAID | TRICARE CHAMPUS | CHAMPVA | GROUP HEALTH PLAN | FECA BLK LUNG | OTHER | 1a. INSURED'S I.D. NUMBER | (For Program in Item 1) |
| ☐ (Medicare #) | ☐ (Medicaid #) | ☐ (Sponsor's SSN) | ☐ (Member ID#) | ☐ (SSN or ID) | ☐ (SSN) | ☐ (ID) | | |

2. PATIENT'S NAME (Last Name, First Name, Middle Initial)

3. PATIENT'S BIRTH DATE MM ┊ DD ┊ YY   SEX   M☐ F☐

4. INSURED'S NAME (Last Name, First Name, Middle Initial)

5. PATIENT'S ADDRESS (No., Street)

6. PATIENT RELATIONSHIP TO INSURED
Self☐ Spouse☐ Child☐ Other☐

7. INSURED'S ADDRESS (No., Street)

CITY   STATE

8. PATIENT STATUS
Single☐ Married☐ Other☐

Employed☐ Full-Time Student☐ Part-Time Student☐

CITY   STATE

ZIP CODE   TELEPHONE (Include Area Code) ( )

ZIP CODE   TELEPHONE (Include Area Code) ( )

9. OTHER INSURED'S NAME (Last Name, First Name, Middle Initial)

10. IS PATIENT'S CONDITION RELATED TO:

11. INSURED'S POLICY GROUP OR FECA NUMBER

a. OTHER INSURED'S POLICY OR GROUP NUMBER

a. EMPLOYMENT? (Current or Previous)
☐ YES ☐ NO

a. INSURED'S DATE OF BIRTH MM ┊ DD ┊ YY   SEX   M☐ F☐

b. OTHER INSURED'S DATE OF BIRTH MM ┊ DD ┊ YY   SEX   M☐ F☐

b. AUTO ACCIDENT?   PLACE (State)
☐ YES ☐ NO

b. EMPLOYER'S NAME OR SCHOOL NAME

c. EMPLOYER'S NAME OR SCHOOL NAME

c. OTHER ACCIDENT?
☐ YES ☐ NO

c. INSURANCE PLAN NAME OR PROGRAM NAME

d. INSURANCE PLAN NAME OR PROGRAM NAME

10d. RESERVED FOR LOCAL USE

d. IS THERE ANOTHER HEALTH BENEFIT PLAN?
☐ YES ☐ NO   If yes, return to and complete item 9 a-d.

READ BACK OF FORM BEFORE COMPLETING & SIGNING THIS FORM.
12. PATIENT'S OR AUTHORIZED PERSON'S SIGNATURE I authorize the release of any medical or other information necessary to process this claim. I also request payment of government benefits either to myself or to the party who accepts assignment below.

SIGNED _____ DATE _____

13. INSURED'S OR AUTHORIZED PERSON'S SIGNATURE I authorize payment of medical benefits to the undersigned physician or supplier for services described below.

SIGNED _____

14. DATE OF CURRENT: MM ┊ DD ┊ YY   ◄ ILLNESS (First symptom) OR INJURY (Accident) OR PREGNANCY (LMP)

15. IF PATIENT HAS HAD SAME OR SIMILAR ILLNESS, GIVE FIRST DATE MM ┊ DD ┊ YY

16. DATES PATIENT UNABLE TO WORK IN CURRENT OCCUPATION
FROM MM ┊ DD ┊ YY   TO MM ┊ DD ┊ YY

17. NAME OF REFERRING PHYSICIAN OR OTHER SOURCE

17a.
17b. NPI

18. HOSPITALIZATION DATES RELATED TO CURRENT SERVICES
FROM MM ┊ DD ┊ YY   TO MM ┊ DD ┊ YY

19. RESERVED FOR LOCAL USE

20. OUTSIDE LAB? $ CHARGES
☐ YES ☐ NO

21. DIAGNOSIS OR NATURE OF ILLNESS OR INJURY (Relate Items 1,2,3 or 4 to Item 24E by Line)

1. ┃___.___   3. ┃___.___
2. ┃___.___   4. ┃___.___

22. MEDICAID RESUBMISSION
CODE   ORIGINAL REF. NO.

23. PRIOR AUTHORIZATION NUMBER

24. A. DATE(S) OF SERVICE From To MM DD YY MM DD YY	B. PLACE OF SERVICE	C. EMG	D. PROCEDURES, SERVICES, OR SUPPLIES (Explain Unusual Circumstances) CPT/HCPCS MODIFIER	E. DIAGNOSIS POINTER	F. $ CHARGES	G. DAYS OR UNITS	H. EPSDT Family Plan	I. ID. QUAL.	J. RENDERING PROVIDER ID. #
1									NPI
2									NPI
3									NPI
4									NPI
5									NPI
6									NPI

25. FEDERAL TAX I.D. NUMBER   SSN EIN ☐☐

26. PATIENT'S ACCOUNT NO.

27. ACCEPT ASSIGNMENT? (For govt. claims, see back)
☐ YES ☐ NO

28. TOTAL CHARGE $

29. AMOUNT PAID $

30. BALANCE DUE $

31. SIGNATURE OF PHYSICIAN OR SUPPLIER INCLUDING DEGREES OR CREDENTIALS (I certify that the statements on the reverse apply to this bill and are made a part thereof.)

SIGNED _____ DATE _____

32. SERVICE FACILITY LOCATION INFORMATION

a. NPI   b.

33. BILLING PROVIDER INFO & PH. # ( )

a. NPI   b.

NUCC Instruction Manual available at: www.nucc.org
WCMS-1500CS

APPROVED OMB 0938-0999 FORM CMS-1500 (08/05)

Text along left margin: SECOND FOLD   WHCF-10-ENV / WHCF-10-ENV-SS   FIRST FOLD

Text along right margin: CARRIER   PATIENT AND INSURED INFORMATION   PHYSICIAN OR SUPPLIER INFORMATION

Figure 12

Directions: Using the source documents provided for patient Clair Carter, accurately complete a UB-04 claim form. Use the blank UB-04 form provided (Figure 13).

TEST 14

Capital City General Hospital
1000 Cherry Street
Capital City, NY 12345-2222
(555) 555-1000

Patient Information:	Clair Carter
	1409 Gunner Road, Capital City, NY 12345
	555-555-1791
DOB:	10-19-1974
Sex:	Female
SSN:	222-88-2010
Status:	Single **Student:** No
Employer:	Plastics Unlimited
	5792 Kiln Way, Capital City, NY 12345
	555-555-5792
Responsible Party:	Clair Carter
Insurance Information:	Aetna
	1625 Healthcare Bldg., Capital City, NY 12345
ID #:	423381 **Group #:** 7619
Insured's Name:	Same **Relationship to Patient:** Self
Insured's DOB:	**Insured's Sex:** F
Insured's Address:	
Insured's Employer:	
Authorization:	68235498432 **Approved # of Days:** 4
Attending Physician:	Phil Wells, MD
Federal Tax ID #:	75-0246810
Group NPI:	1234567890

Reason for visit: Heroin overdose.

TEST 14

HPI: This is a Caucasian female admitted through the emergency department on May 13, 20XX, at 1:30 a.m. for a heroin overdose. Pt. was found unresponsive in her apartment by boyfriend. Pt. has been abusing heroin for about 2 months, per the boyfriend. There is evidence of track marks on both upper and lower extremities. The freshest mark is on the right lower extremity. Pt. has no evidence of organ failure at this time. Pt. was discharged to rehab clinic on May 17, 20XX, at 11:00 a.m.

Patient Control #:	900521	**Type of Admission:**	1
MR #:	1846533422	**Source of Admission:**	7
Hospital NPI:	1212121212	**Discharge Status:**	05
Hospital Tax ID:	75-7575757	**Type of Bill Code:**	111

Fees:

Revenue Codes	Units	Total Charges	Dates of Service
110 Room/Board/Semi	4	$ 400.00/day	05/13/20XX–05/17/20XX
250 Pharmacy	5	$1250.00	05/13/20XX–05/17/20XX
260 IV Therapy	4	$1000.00	05/13/20XX–05/16/20XX
270 Med/Surg Supplies	4	$ 400.00	05/13/20XX–05/16/20XX
300 Laboratory	3	$ 300.00	05/14/20XX–05/17/20XX
001 TOTAL		$3450.00	

Principal DX:	965.01, E850.0, 304.00, 780.09
Admitting DX:	965.01, E850.0
Principal Procedure Code:	99.29

| 5 FED. TAX NO. | 6 STATEMENT COVERS PERIOD FROM THROUGH | 7 |

| 8 PATIENT NAME | a | | 9 PATIENT ADDRESS | a | | | | c | d | | e |
| b | | | b | | | | | | | | |

| 10 BIRTHDATE | 11 SEX | 12 DATE | ADMISSION 13 HR | 14 TYPE | 15 SRC | 16 DHR | 17 STAT | 18 | 19 | 20 | 21 | CONDITION CODES 22 23 24 25 26 27 28 | 29 ACDT STATE | 30 |

31 OCCURRENCE CODE DATE	32 OCCURRENCE CODE DATE	33 OCCURRENCE CODE DATE	34 OCCURRENCE CODE DATE	35 OCCURRENCE SPAN CODE FROM THROUGH	36 OCCURRENCE SPAN CODE FROM THROUGH	37
a						
b						

38		39 VALUE CODES CODE AMOUNT	40 VALUE CODES CODE AMOUNT	41 VALUE CODES CODE AMOUNT
	a			
	b			
	c			
	d			

42 REV.CD.	43 DESCRIPTION	44 HCPCS/RATE/HPPS CODE	45 SERV. DATE	46 SERV. UNITS	47 TOTAL CHARGES	48 NON-COVERED CHARGES	49
1							1
2							2
3							3
4							4
5							5
6							6
7							7
8							8
9							9
10							10
11							11
12							12
13							13
14							14
15							15
16							16
17							17
18							18
19							19
20							20
21							21
22							22
23	PAGE ____ OF ____	CREATION DATE		TOTALS ➤			23

50 PAYER NAME	51 HEALTH PLAN ID	52 REL. INFO	53 ASG. BEN.	54 PRIOR PAYMENTS	55 EST. AMOUNT DUE	56 NPI	
A							57 OTHER PRV ID	A
B								B
C								C

58 INSURED'S NAME	59 P. REL	60 INSURED'S UNIQUE ID	61 GROUP NAME	62 INSURANCE GROUP NO.
A				
B				
C				

63 TREATMENT AUTHORIZATION CODES	64 DOCUMENT CONTROL NUMBER	65 EMPLOYER NAME
A		
B		
C		

66 DX	67	A	B	C	D	E	F	G	H	68
		I	J	K	L	M	N	O	P	Q	
69 ADMIT DX	70 PATIENT REASON DX a b c	71 PPS CODE	72 ECI a b c	73

74 PRINCIPAL PROCEDURE CODE DATE	a. OTHER PROCEDURE CODE DATE	b. OTHER PROCEDURE CODE DATE	75	76 ATTENDING NPI QUAL
				LAST FIRST
c. OTHER PROCEDURE CODE DATE	d. OTHER PROCEDURE CODE DATE	e. OTHER PROCEDURE CODE DATE		77 OPERATING NPI QUAL
				LAST FIRST

80 REMARKS	81CC a		78 OTHER NPI QUAL
	b		LAST FIRST
	c		79 OTHER NPI QUAL
	d		LAST FIRST

UB-04 CMS-1450 NLCF-UB04-1   APPROVED OMB NO. 0938-0997 OCR/Original   **NUBC** National Uniform Billing Committee   THE CERTIFICATIONS ON THE REVERSE APPLY TO THIS BILL AND ARE MADE A PART HEREOF.

Figure 13

NOTES

NOTES

NOTES

NOTES

NOTES

NOTES

NOTES

NOTES

NOTES

NOTES

Notes